PSORIASIS
A Closer Look

PSORIASIS
A Closer Look

2nd Edition

Editor
Jayakar Thomas
MD DD MNAMS FRCP FRCPCH IFAAD PhD DSc
Professor and Head
Department of Dermatology
Chettinad Hospital and Research Institute
Chennai, Tamil Nadu, India

Co-Editor
Parimalam Kumar
MD DD MNAMS FRCP IFAAD
Professor and Head
Department of Dermatology
Madras Medical College and Hospital
Chennai, Tamil Nadu, India

Foreword
UR Dhanalakshmi

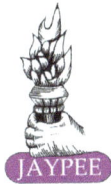

JAYPEE

JAYPEE BROTHERS MEDICAL PUBLISHERS

The Health Sciences Publisher

New Delhi | London

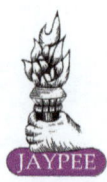 **Jaypee Brothers Medical Publishers (P) Ltd**

Headquarters
EMCA House
23/23-B, Ansari Road, Daryaganj
New Delhi 110 002, India
Landline: +91-11-23272143, +91-11-23272703
+91-11-23282021, +91-11-23245672
E-mail: jaypee@jaypeebrothers.com

Corporate Office
Jaypee Brothers Medical Publishers (P) Ltd.
4838/24, Ansari Road, Daryaganj
New Delhi 110 002, India
Phone: +91-11-43574357
Fax: +91-11-43574314
E-mail: jaypee@jaypeebrothers.com

Overseas Office
JP Medical Ltd.
83, Victoria Street, London
SW1H 0HW (UK)
Phone: +44-20 3170 8910
Fax: +44(0)20 3008 6180
E-mail: info@jpmedpub.com

Website: www.jaypeebrothers.com
Website: www.jaypeedigital.com

© 2023, Jaypee Brothers Medical Publishers

The views and opinions expressed in this book are solely those of the original contributor(s)/author(s) and do not necessarily represent those of editor(s) or publisher of the book.

All rights reserved by the author. No part of this publication may be reproduced, stored or transmitted in any form or by any means, electronic, mechanical, photocopying, recording or otherwise, without the prior permission in writing of the publishers.

All brand names and product names used in this book are trade names, service marks, trademarks or registered trademarks of their respective owners. The publisher is not associated with any product or vendor mentioned in this book.

Medical knowledge and practice change constantly. This book is designed to provide accurate, authoritative information about the subject matter in question. However, readers are advised to check the most current information available on procedures included and check information from the manufacturer of each product to be administered, to verify the recommended dose, formula, method and duration of administration, adverse effects and contraindications. It is the responsibility of the practitioner to take all appropriate safety precautions. Neither the publisher nor the author(s)/editor(s) assume any liability for any injury and/or damage to persons or property arising from or related to use of material in this book.

This book is sold on the understanding that the publisher is not engaged in providing professional medical services. If such advice or services are required, the services of a competent medical professional should be sought.

Every effort has been made where necessary to contact holders of copyright to obtain permission to reproduce copyright material. If any have been inadvertently overlooked, the publisher will be pleased to make the necessary arrangements at the first opportunity.

Inquiries for bulk sales may be solicited at: jaypee@jaypeebrothers.com

Psoriasis: A Closer Look / Jayakar Thomas

First Edition: 2014

Second Edition: **2023**

ISBN: 978-93-5465-980-5

DEDICATED TO

The many dermatologists who provide care to the patients with psoriasis,

Our committed teachers of Dermatology,

The patients who were willing to permit us to take their photographs, and

Most of all to our beloved family for their care, love, and affection without which this humble piece of work would not have been a reality.

Jayakar Thomas
Editor

Parimalam Kumar
Co-Editor

Foreword

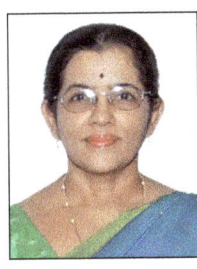

Professor UR Dhanalakshmi MB DD MD DNB
Former Professor and Head
Department of Dermatology
Madras Medical College
Chennai, Tamil Nadu, India

It is a privilege to write the "Foreword" for the book *Psoriasis—A Closer Look (Second Edition)*, edited by Professor Jayakar Thomas. I have listened to numerous orations and talks delivered by him as well as gone through a lot of his books, chapters in books and articles.

In medicine, it is important to diagnose and treat common conditions more effectively rather than concentrating on rare disorders since the bulk of our patients fall into the former category.

Psoriasis is among the common conditions encountered in clinical practice and it is also one of the most psychologically crippling disorders. The social and psychological aspects are very important notably because they continue from childhood to adulthood.

Psoriasis—A Closer Look (Second Edition) covers every aspect of this disease and should be read by every dermatologist since the bulk of patients coming to a dermatologist have this problem. The images and legends are especially informative and help in easy understanding.

I congratulate the co-editor Professor Parimalam Kumar for working alongside Professor Jayakar Thomas in compiling this book. I also convey my best wishes to all the contributors to this book and hope that they come up with similar work in the future.

Preface to the Second Edition

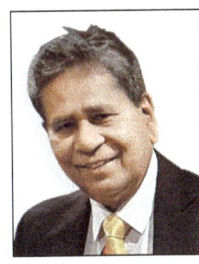

Jayakar Thomas
Editor

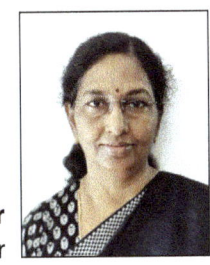

Parimalam Kumar
Co-Editor

"Knowledge, if not shared is of no use at all"

The engine of change driving innovation in diseases of the skin is nowhere near slowing down. Physicians and dermatologists should look forward to near-term breakthroughs that could change the way they diagnose and manage these challenging situations: hence the need for this *"Psoriasis—A Closer Look (Second Edition)"*.

We have tried our best to address the following: *Disease Modification in Psoriasis: How Do We Define It and What Evidence Do We Have so Far?*

This book, *Psoriasis—A Closer Look (Second Edition)*, is designed as an academic project with the target readers as both postgraduate students and practicing dermatologists. All chapters encompass glimpses of existing knowledge in the light of recent advances in the segment of "Psoriasis", complications, and the comorbidities. The treatment challenges, both oral and systemic, have been addressed in this edition. Yet another unique addition is the chapter on "Dermoscopy".

We hope this book is a helpful tool—not only for the student who needs an expert source of basic knowledge, but also for the pressured practitioner who needs a clear, concise, and balanced distillation of the best information on which to base daily clinical decisions.

At times, the science presented might seem overwhelming. But, one can start reading from any chapter, based on one's interests, tastes, and preferences.

Preface to the First Edition

Knowledge, if not shared is of no use at all.

Over the years, psoriasis has emerged as a common disease of the skin, affecting millions the world over. Yet, the paucity of sufficient printed learning and teaching material on the disease exists palpably. *Psoriasis A Closer Look* is intended to serve three sections of dermatologists—postgraduate students, postgraduate teachers and practicing dermatologists.

We have included knowingly same basics along with robust information on psoriasis. It is hoped that the publication of this book will enhance the spread of ideas that are currently trickling through the scientific literature.

We wish you happy and fruitful reading!

Jayakar Thomas
Parimalam Kumar
Sindhu Ragavi Balaji

Contents

Chapter 1:	Introduction	1
Chapter 2:	Epidemiology	2
Chapter 3:	Etiopathogenesis and Immunology	5
Chapter 4:	Clinical Aspects	12
Chapter 5:	Pediatric Psoriasis	40
Chapter 6:	Psoriasis and Pregnancy	64
Chapter 7:	Psoriasis in HIV	69
Chapter 8:	Psoriasis as a Systemic Disease	73
Chapter 9:	Investigations	83
Chapter 10:	Treatment	86
Chapter 11:	Complications and "The Psoriatic March"	113
Chapter 12:	Psychological Aspects, Course and Prognosis, Follow-up, and Rehabilitation	117
Chapter 13:	Dermoscopy in Psoriasis	120
Index		141

Introduction

Psoriasis is a T-cell mediated chronic inflammatory disorder of the skin seen in about 3.5% of the population.[1] One-third of psoriasis cases in a dermatology center are seen in pediatric age-group.[2] Psoriasis is a lifelong inflammatory disorder of the skin that can vary widely in its presentation but is characterized by the common features of erythema, skin thickening and scaling. The diagnosis is usually made on clinical grounds by any well-trained clinician. Despite considerable research into its etiology, there are still no definitive genetic or biochemical markers for psoriasis, and it continues to be diagnosed primarily based on skin manifestations. Its impact on a patient depends not only on the percentage of body surface area of the lesions, but also on their location. Involvement of the hands, feet, scalp and genital areas can have a disproportionate effect on quality of life and disability. Additionally, in a significant subset of psoriasis patients, the disease process involves progressive damage to the articular joints. Moreover, clinical studies have increasingly revealed associations of psoriasis and its treatments with many systemic diseases. Although establishing causality in these associations remains problematic, these associations have immediate diagnostic and therapeutic implications.

Timely diagnosis and appropriate management cannot only arrest progression, but also minimize the psychosocial burden imposed by this illness. Thereby disfiguring states and its evolution into a metabolic syndrome requiring extensive treatment can well be averted. This book will cover almost all aspects of pediatric psoriasis including the rare clinical form like congenital erythrodermic psoriasis and present the latest update, especially on the etiopathogenesis and treatment options. An evidence-based approach has been given while discussing these issues. There is increasing awareness the world over that psoriasis is more than "skin deep" and is now emerging as a systemic disease. It is attempted to emphasize the role of inflammation as a major factor, leading to multiple organ dysfunction. Similarly, the concept "psoriatic march" is also thrashed out though it is not yet formally proven. Finally the reader will accept that a holistic approach, including education, aggressive treatment wherever necessary along with psychological support in the form of empathy rather than sympathy, is all that is needed for care of psoriatic patients. The main aim of treatment should be to reduce the burden of the disease over time by controlling symptoms, helping the patient to cope with the chronic nature of the disease, limiting psychological and relational consequences, and preventing systemic complications and comorbidity.

REFERENCES

1. Kurd SK, Gelfand JM. The prevalence of previously diagnosed and undiagnosed psoriasis in US adults: results from NHANES 2003-2004. J Am Acad Dermatol. 2009;60(2):218-24.
2. Raychaudhuri SP, Gross J. A comparative study of pediatric onset psoriasis with adult onset psoriasis. Pediatr Dermatol. 2000;17(3):174-8.

Epidemiology

There is considerable racial variation in the prevalence of psoriasis from country to country which may be attributable to many factors like climate, genetic susceptibility and lifestyle.

Psoriasis occurs worldwide and has no gender preference; however, its prevalence varies considerably. However, according to Basko-Plluska JL and Petronic-Rosic V, the prevalence of psoriasis has not changed with time; according to epidemiological studies, in contrast to other autoimmune diseases whose prevalence rates have increased.[1] In the United States (US), psoriasis affects approximately 2% of the population, although rates as high as 4.6% have been reported.[2,3] Bell et al. showed an age- and sex-adjusted annual incidence of 60.4 in 100,000 for Rochester, MN, between the period of 1980 and 1983.[4] More recently, Huerta et al. reported an incidence rate of 14 per 10,000 person-years.[5] The difference in reported incidence rate can be attributed to the different case definitions used in these studies. Psoriasis is extremely rare to absent in certain ethnic groups such as Africans, African-Americans, Japanese, Alaskans, Australians and Norwegian Lapps.[3,6,7]

According to Kurd SK, Gelfand JM, psoriasis is seen in about 3.5% of the population.[8] One-third of psoriasis cases in a dermatology center are seen in pediatric age-group.[9] In India, the prevalence of psoriasis varies from 0.44 to 2.8%; it is twice more common in males compared to females, and most of the patients are in their third or fourth decade at the time of presentation.[10]

Psoriasis has a bimodal distribution of age of onset. Those individuals with early onset appear, in general, to have more severe disease and are much more likely to have an affected first-degree relative with psoriasis. One-third of adults with psoriasis report onset in childhood. Ethnic variation is not clear, with some studies quoting incidence highest in Caucasians, black then Asian populations.[11] It is alarming to note that 40,000 children under 10 years of age were afflicted by psoriasis.[12] The distribution of psoriasis is almost equal in boys and girls. However, female preponderance has been observed by some authors. The occurrence of psoriatic diaper rash in younger children and its inclusion increases incidence of psoriasis in children under 2 years of age.[11] The exact age distribution is not clear, though literature states that nearly 30% of patients with psoriasis develop the disease before the age of 18 years.[13] It is of interest to note that in the age group <20 years, the frequency of psoriasis was 20% higher in girls than in boys, in contrast to adults.[14] Compared with 37% in adult-onset patients, 49% of pediatric-onset patients had first-degree family members affected with psoriasis. Some studies have reported familial incidence in childhood cases of psoriasis as high as 89%.[15]

According to Basko-Plluska JL and Petronic-Rosic V, psoriasis can first appear at any age; however, a bimodal distribution of the age of onset is characteristic. The majority of cases, approximately 75%, presents before the age of 40 years, with a peak at 20–30 years old. The remaining cases present after the age of 40 years. Patients with early disease onset tend to have a positive family history of psoriasis, frequent association with histocompatibility antigen [human leukocyte antigen (HLA)]-Cw6, and more severe disease. Those with onset after the age of 40 years usually have a negative family history and a normal frequency of the Cw6 allele.[1]

Involvement of joints with psoriatic arthritis is less prevalent in younger patients; however, it does occur in childhood disease and should be considered in the differential of pediatric arthritis.[16] The heritability of psoriasis is as high as 91%, which is supported by many studies, documenting a concordance in incidence of as high as 73% and 20% in monozygotic and dizygotic twins, respectively.[17]

Involvement of multiple genes makes the genetic basis of psoriasis complex, and hence, it is difficult to draw a conclusion about the correct heritability of the disease. The heritability of psoriasis has been estimated to be 60–90%, based on twin studies. Thus making psoriasis a highly heritable disease, the heritability seems to be highest of all multifactorial genetic diseases.[18,19] Concordance rates as high as 70% have been reported among monozygotic twins, versus 12–30% in dizygotic twins.[20] According to family studies, it was shown that if both parents have psoriasis, the offsprings have a 50% chance of developing the disease. The risk decreases to 16%, if only one parent has psoriasis. The siblings of a psoriatic child with unaffected parents have an 8% risk of developing the disease. Males have a higher risk of transmitting psoriasis to offspring than females, which is likely due to genomic imprinting.[21] HLA studies have shown that psoriasis is associated with several

HLA antigens, most frequently HLA-Cw6, which confers a relative risk of 10 for developing the disease in the Caucasian population. However, only approximately 10% of individuals who express the HLA-Cw6 allele go on to develop psoriasis.[22] In addition, HLA-Cw6 influences the age of onset of the disease. HLA-Cw6 is expressed in about 85–90% of patients with early-onset psoriasis, but in only 15% of patients with late-onset disease.[23]

Human leukocyte antigens-B13, HLA-B17, HLA-B37 and HLA-Bw16 have also been associated with plaque psoriasis. HLA-B27 is expressed with an increased frequency in pustular psoriasis and acrodermatitis continua of Hallopeau. A significant association between guttate psoriasis and erythrodermic psoriasis with HLA-B13 and HLA-B17 expression has been reported.

Protein tyrosine phosphatase N22 (PTPN22) and its association to psoriasis have been extensively analyzed. There seems to be a positive association between psoriasis and the PTPN22, the significance of which is yet to be proved beyond doubt.[24]

Many analytic epidemiologic studies have identified multiple risk factors like smoking, obesity, alcohol consumption, diet, infections, medications, and stressful life events to play an important role in the disease manifestation.

European studies have also confirmed that current smoking and obesity are independent risk factors for developing psoriasis.[25] One of the largest studies estimated that 30% of new psoriasis cases were due to being overweight (body mass index > 25).[26] A higher prevalence of psoriasis has been demonstrated in current smokers than never- or ex-smokers.[27] Many studies suggest that alcohol plays an important role in the exacerbation of psoriasis. It was noted that heavy drinkers have a tendency to develop more extensive and inflamed skin lesions.[28-30]

Infections are known factors to be associated with psoriasis. Acute bacterial and viral infections have been associated with the onset or exacerbation of psoriasis.[31] Streptococcal infections are often triggers of guttate psoriasis, especially in children and young adults.[32] There are reports to show the association of HIV infection and psoriasis. Medications, including beta-blockers, lithium, antimalarials, tetracycline antibiotics, nonsteroidal anti-inflammatory drugs (NSAIDs), and steroid withdrawal have been associated with the onset or exacerbation of psoriasis, mostly based in case reports.[33] Antimalarial drugs may exacerbate preexisting psoriasis in up to 40% of patients by inhibiting the enzyme transglutaminase and causing epidermal proliferation.[34] The role of psychological stress has long been attributed in the exacerbation of psoriasis. Acute psychosocial stress was shown to induce altered hypothalamic–pituitary–adrenal (HPA) responses in patients with psoriasis—particularly in those who experienced a flare of disease with stress.[35]

REFERENCES

1. Basko-Plluska JL, Petronic-Rosic V. Psoriasis: epidemiology, natural history, and differential diagnosis. Psoriasis: Targets and Therapy. 2012;2:67-76.
2. Naldi L. Epidemiology of psoriasis. Curr Drug Targets Inflamm Allergy. 2004;3(2):121-8.
3. Raychaudhuri SP, Farber EM. The prevalence of psoriasis in the world. J Eur Acad Dermatol Venereol. 2001;15(1):16-7.
4. Bell LM, Sedlack R, Beard CM, et al. Incidence of psoriasis in Rochester, Minn, 1980-1983. Arch Dermatol. 1991;127(8):1184-7.
5. Huerta C, Rivero E, Rodriguez LA. Incidence and risk factors for psoriasis in the general population. Arch Dermatol. 2007;143(12):1559-65.
6. Christophers E. Psoriasis—epidemiology and clinical spectrum. Clin Exp Dermatol. 2001;26(4):314-20.
7. Gelfand JM, Stern RS, Nijsten T, et al. The prevalence of psoriasis in African Americans: results from a population-based study. J Am Acad Dermatol. 2005;52(1):23-6.
8. Kurd SK, Gelfand JM. The prevalence of previously diagnosed and undiagnosed psoriasis in US adults: results from NHANES 2003-2004. J Am Acad Dermatol. 2009;60(2):218-24.
9. Raychaudhuri SP, Gross J. A comparative study of pediatric onset psoriasis with adult onset psoriasis. Pediatr Dermatol. 2000;17(3):174-8.
10. Dogra S, Yadav S. Psoriasis in India: prevalence and pattern. Indian J Dermatol Venereol Leprol. 2013;76(6):595-601.
11. Sharma V, Orchards D. Paediatric psoriasis. Paediatr Child Health. 2011;21(3):126-31.
12. Sticherling M, Augusti M, Boehncke W, et al. Therapy of psoriasis in childhood and adolescence: a German expert consensus. J Dtsch Dermatol Ges. 2011;9(10):815-23.
13. Augustin M, Glaeske G, Radtke MA, et al. Epidemiology and comorbidity of psoriasis in children. Br J Dermatol. 2010;162(3):633-6.
14. Swanbeck G, Inerot A, Martinsson T, et al. Age at onset and different types of psoriasis. Br J Dermatol. 1995;133(5):768-73.
15. Farber EM, Mullen RH, Jacobs AH, et al. Infantile psoriasis: a follow-up study. Pediatr Dermatol. 1986;3(3):237-43.
16. Kumar B, Jain R, Sandhu K, et al. Epidemiology of childhood psoriasis: a study of 419 patients from northern India. Int J Dermatol. 2004;43(9):654-8.
17. Farber EM, Nall ML, Watson W. Natural history of psoriasis in 61 twin pairs. Arch Dermatol. 1974;109(2):207-11.
18. Elder J, Nair R, Guo S, et al. The genetics of psoriasis. Arch Dermatol. 1994;130(2):216-24.
19. Elder JT, Nair RP, Henseler T, et al. The genetics of psoriasis 2001: the odyssey continues. Arch Dermatol. 2001;137(11):1447-54.
20. Valdimarsson H. The genetic basis of psoriasis. Clin Dermatol. 2007;25(6):563-7.
21. Rahman PE. Genetic epidemiology of psoriasis and psoriatic arthritis. Ann Rheum Dis. 2005;64(Suppl 2): ii37-9.
22. Trembath R, Clough RL, Rosbotham JL, et al. Identification of a major susceptibility locus on chromosome 6p and evidence for further disease loci revealed by a two stage genome-wide search in psoriasis. Hum Mol Genet. 1997;6(5):813-20.

23. Richardson SK, Gelfand J. Update on the natural history and systemic treatment of psoriasis. Adv Dermatol. 2008;24:171-96.
24. Chen YF, Chang J. PTPN2 C1858T and the risk of psoriasis: a meta-analysis. Mol Bio Rep. 2012;39(8):7861-70.
25. Naldi L, Chatenoud L, Linder D, et al. Cigarette smoking, body mass index, and stressful life events as risk factors for psoriasis: results from an Italian case-control study. J Invest Dermatol. 2005;125(1):61-7.
26. Setty AR, Curhan G, Choi HK. Obesity, wait circumference, weight change, and the risk of psoriasis in women: Nurses' Health Study II. Arch Intern Med. 2007;167(15):1670-5.
27. Schäfer T. Epidemiology of psoriasis: review and the German perspective. Dermatology. 2006;212(4):327-37.
28. Poikolainen K, Reunala T, Karvonen J, et al. Alcohol intake: a risk factor for psoriasis in young and middle aged men? BMJ. 1990;300(6727):780-3.
29. Naldi L, Peli L, Parazzini F. Association of early-stage psoriasis with smoking and male alcohol consumption: evidence from an Italian case-control study. Arch Dermatol. 1999;135(12):1479-84.
30. Higgins EM, du Vivier AW. Alcohol and the skin. Alcohol Alcohol. 1992;27(6):595-602.
31. Naldi L, Peli L, Parazzini F, et al. Family history of psoriasis, stressful life event, and recent infectious diseases are risk factors for a first episode of acute guttate psoriasis: results of a case-control study. J Am Acad Dermatol. 2001;44(3):433-8.
32. Zhao G, Feng X, Na A, et al. Acute guttate psoriasis patients have positive *Streptococcus hemolyticus* throat cultures and elevated antistreptococcal M6 protein titers. J Dermatol. 2005;32(2):91-6.
33. Tsankov N, Irena A, Kasandjieva J. Drug-induced psoriasis: recognition and management. Am J Clin Dermatol. 2000;1(3):159-65.
34. Fry L, Baker BS. Triggering psoriasis: the role of infections and medications. Clin Dermatol. 2007;25(6):606-15.
35. Richards HL, Ray DW, Kirby B, et al. Response of the hypothalamic-pituitary-adrenal axis to psychosocial stress in patients with psoriasis. Br J Dermatol. 2005;153(6):1114-20.

Etiopathogenesis and Immunology

ETIOLOGICAL AND PRECIPITATING FACTORS

Psoriasis is a systemic, immune-mediated disorder, characterized by inflammatory skin and joint manifestations. The exact etiopathogenesis of psoriasis has not been completely elucidated.

This chapter briefly discusses about the various etiological and precipitating factors **(Box 1)** and a succinct discussion on the pathogenesis of psoriasis.

Genetic Factors

Major gene for psoriasis susceptibility is thought mainly to be located on chromosome 6, the site of human leukocyte antigens (HLA) class I (associated with early-onset disease) and II (late-onset disease) which are thought to produce differing subtypes of the disease. Individuals with the Cw0602 allele are four times more likely to develop guttate psoriasis. A series of genes have been isolated in which mutations have been associated with psoriatic disease, including interleukin (IL)12-B9 (1p31.3), IL-13 (5q31.1), IL-23R (1p31.3), HLA-BW6, psoriasis susceptibility locus 6 (PSORS6), signal transducer and activator of transcription 2 gene (*STAT2*)/IL-23A (12q13.2), tumor necrosis factor alpha-induced protein 3 gene (*TNF-α-IP3*) (6q23.3) and TNFAIP3-interacting protein 1 gene (*TNIP1*) (5q33.1). These genes play a role in helper T type 2 (Th2) cell and Th17 cell activity which have been noted in psoriatic lesions.[1,2] Several attempts have been made to detect psoriasis susceptibility loci by linkage studies. Up to now, at least nine loci are known (PSORS1-9).[3] There is a strong association exists in early-onset psoriasis for the HLA-Cw6 allele.[4] Concordance of psoriasis is much higher in monozygotic than heterozygotic twins. The deletion of two late cornified envelope genes (LCE3C and LCE3B) is a common genetic factor for susceptibility to psoriasis in different populations.[5]

In the susceptible genetic background, precipitating factors are more important in pediatric than in adult-onset psoriasis. They largely include trauma, infections, drugs, sunlight, metabolic causes, alcohol, smoking, stress, and obesity. Streptococcal pharyngitis or perianal streptococcal dermatitis typically provokes guttate psoriasis. Infection with human immunodeficiency virus (HIV) can induce or exacerbate psoriasis.

Trauma

A wide range of injurious local stimuli, in any form including physical, chemical, electrical, surgical, infective and inflammatory insults, has been recognized to elicit psoriatic lesions, which is clinically observed as Koebner's phenomenon.

Infection

In children, streptococcal throat infection is strongly associated with guttate psoriasis. There is also evidence that streptococcal infection may be important in chronic plaque psoriasis. It is interesting to note that episodes of guttate psoriasis are much more common in individuals

---

BOX 1: Etiological and precipitating factors.

- Genetic
- Trauma
- Infection
- Drugs
- Sunlight
- Metabolic factors
- Pregnancy
- Alcohol and smoking
- Stress
- Obesity

> **BOX 2: Drugs exacerbating psoriasis.**
>
> - Antimalarials
> - Beta blockers
> - Bupropion
> - Calcium-channel blockers
> - Captopril
> - Fluoxetine
> - Glyburide
> - Granulocyte colony-stimulating factor
> - Interferons (IFNs)
> - Interleukins (ILs)
> - Lipid-lowering drugs
> - Lithium
> - Penicillin
> - Terbinafine

with a family history of plaque psoriasis. The association between HIV infection and psoriatic arthropathy is not yet fully explained. However, the role of T cell seems to be an important factor.

Drugs

Drugs play an important role in the onset or exacerbation of psoriasis: Lithium salts, antimalarials, beta-adrenergic blocking agents, nonsteroidal anti-inflammatory drugs, angiotensin-converting enzyme inhibitors and the withdrawal of corticosteroids.

The list of drugs exacerbating psoriasis is given in **Box 2**.

Sunlight

Though sunlight is beneficial to psoriasis, in some sunlight can exacerbate psoriasis. Females are more prone for photoexaggeration of psoriasis. It is also found that photoexaggerated psoriasis is associated with HLA-CW6 and early-onset disease.

Metabolic Factors

Hypocalcemia is known to precipitate psoriasis. It can worsen pustular psoriasis.

Pregnancy

Pregnancy has dual effect on psoriasis. As most of them feel better, the disease can worsen in some. Impetigo herpetiformis is a form of pustular psoriasis, which occurs only during pregnancy, and recur with every pregnancy.

Alcohol and Smoking

Alcohol though is not known to induce psoriasis, it is well documented to exacerbate preexisting disease in many. Excess drinking can also be a consequence of the disease that leads to treatment resistance and reduced therapeutic compliance. Abstinence has been reported to induce remission.

Smoking seems to be associated with development of palmoplantar pustular psoriasis.

Stress

It is suggested that psoriasis is a stress-related disease, and can be exacerbated by perceived stress. Increased concentrations of neurotransmitters in psoriatic plaques support this view.

Obesity

Obesity is considered as a risk factor for psoriasis, and can increase the severity of psoriasis.[6,7] Children with obesity and overweight get more adipose tissue. Onset or worsening of psoriasis with weight gain and/or improvement with weight loss is observed. The adipose tissue is a vigorous endocrine organ capable of secreting multiple proinflammatory adipocytokines such as IL-6, IL-1, TNF-α-11 and adiponectin which play an important role in the pathogenesis of psoriasis.

Expression of the disease much depends on the capacity of the epidermis to express the same. This is a complex process, linked to interaction of cells of the epidermis, dermis, immune system and humoral elements. The inherent phenotype has a capacity of the keratinocyte for hyperproliferation and altered differentiation, both of which are genetically controlled. A genetic aberration can therefore trigger the cascade of inflammatory events in the evolution of the disease.

PATHOLOGY

From a histological point of view, psoriasis is a dynamic dermatosis that changes during the evolution of an individual lesion. Lesions are usually diagnostic only in early stages or near the margin of advancing plaques. Hyperkeratosis, parakeratosis, Munro microabscesses, spongiform pustule of Kogoj, diminished or absent granular layer, regular acanthosis, papillomatosis, tortuosity and dilatation of papillary capillaries, and chronic inflammation in the upper dermis are the common features seen in psoriasis. However, Munro microabscesses and Kogoj's micropustules are diagnostic clues of psoriasis, but they are not always present in all cases at all stages. All other features can be found in various types of eczemas and other dermatoses.[8] Depending on type, site and stage of the disease, histological features tend to differ **(Figs. 1 to 11)**.

CHAPTER 3 Etiopathogenesis and Immunology

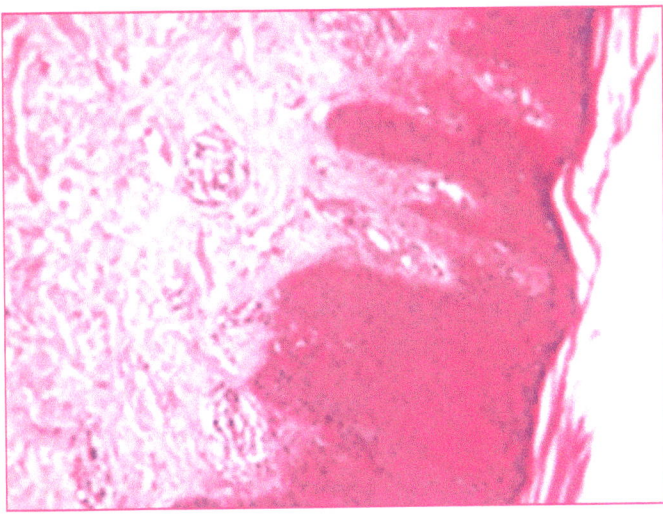

Fig. 1: Classical picture showing hyperkeratosis, parakeratosis, thin granular layer and regular acanthosis.

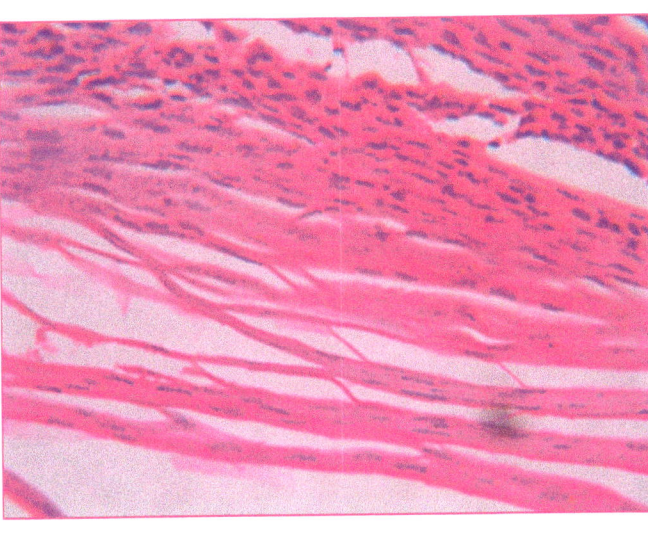

Fig. 4: High-power view showing hyperkeratosis and parakeratosis of a plaque on the sole.

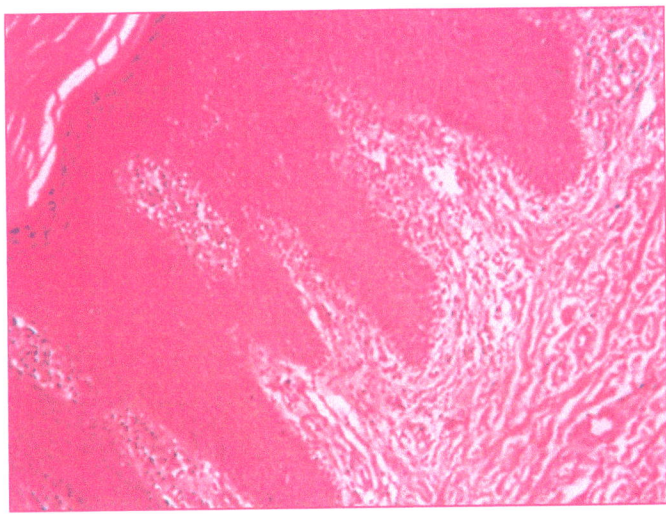

Fig. 2: Early papule showing papillae with squirting neutrophils.

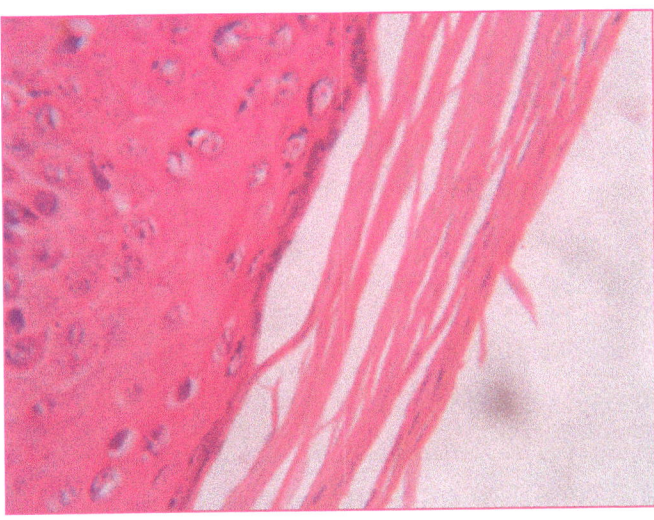

Fig. 5: High-power view showing hyperkeratosis and parakeratosis with the attenuated granular layer.

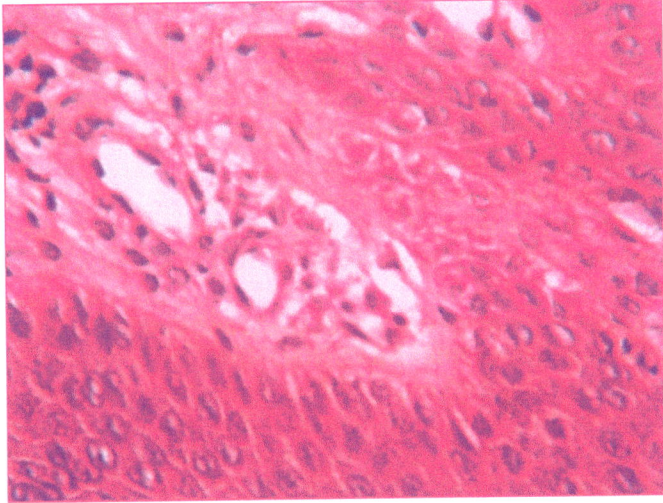

Fig. 3: Dilated tortuous capillary under high power.

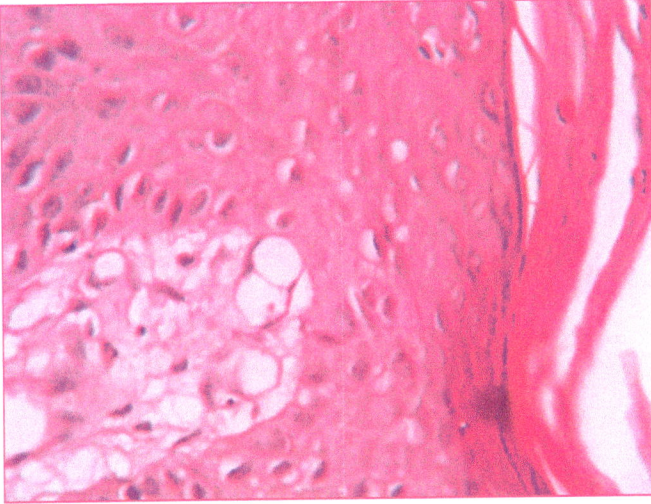

Fig. 6: High-power view of formation of Munro's microabscess.

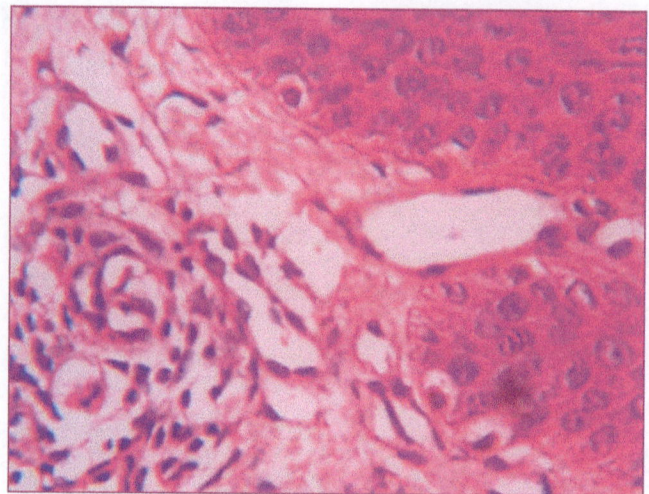

Fig. 7: High-power view of spongiform pustule.

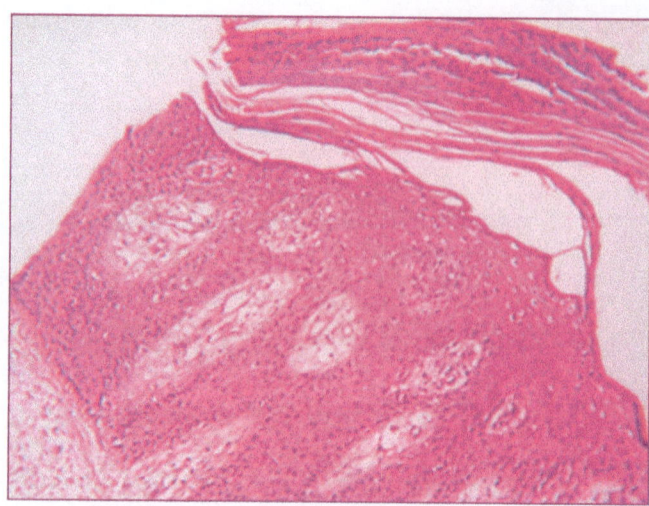

Fig. 10: Psoriasis of the sole with gross hyperkeratosis and psoriasis form acanthosis.

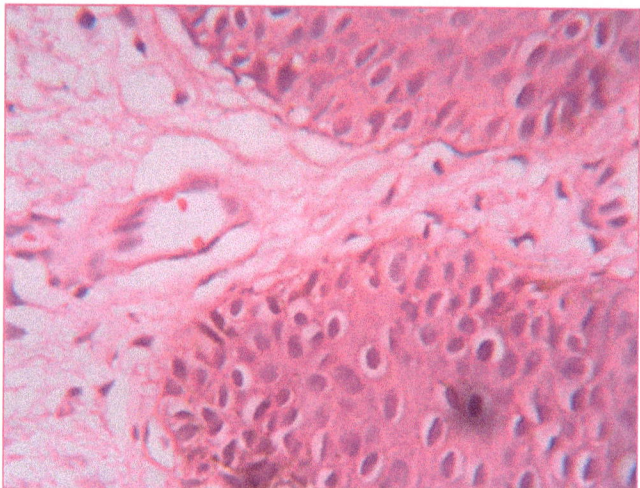

Fig. 8: High-power view of the dilated papillary capillary.

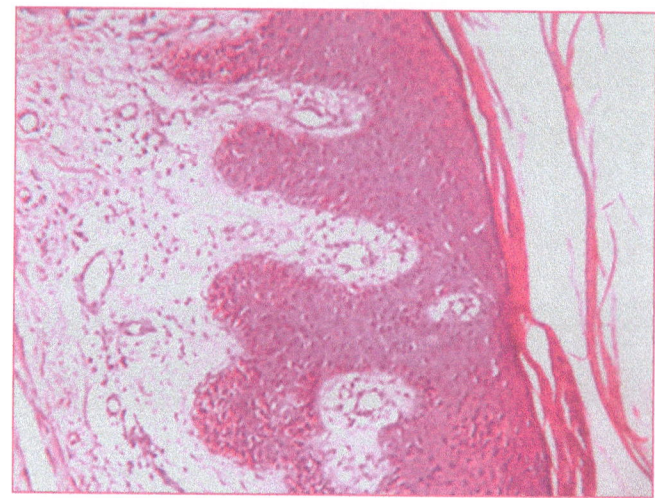

Fig. 11: Reduction in epidermal thickening and formation of granular layer after treatment.

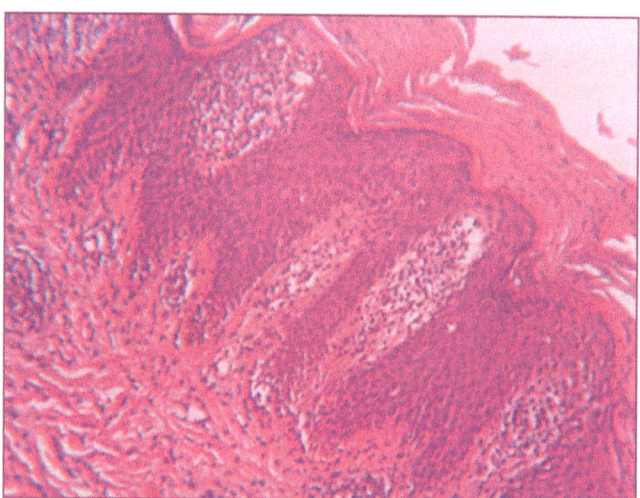

Fig. 9: Psoriasis of the palm showing massive hyperkeratosis, parakeratosis, suprapapillary thinning of epidermis, regular acanthosis, dilated papillary capillary with neutrophils.

The histology in erythrodermic psoriasis will not show all the classical findings in all cases. In infants, the most consistent feature of congenital erythrodermic psoriasis are regular acanthosis and dilatation of papillary capillaries with neutrophilic squirting into the epidermis.[9] The mean accuracy of the histopathological diagnoses was <55%, even in adult erythroderma.[10]

Histological confirmation of psoriasis is not always mandatory as most of the cases are clinically diagnosed even as children. However, early skin biopsy is helpful in the diagnosis of neonatal and infantile erythroderma where the etiology of erythroderma can be made and timely diagnosis will help manage the child better. Histology does help in adults to rule out other causes of erythroderma. It also helps differentiate atopic dermatitis (AD) from psoriasis in both children and adults. However there are instances where both diseases can coexist[9] **(Fig. 12)**.

Though recruitment of T cells into the skin and their effector responses are the key features in the pathogenesis of

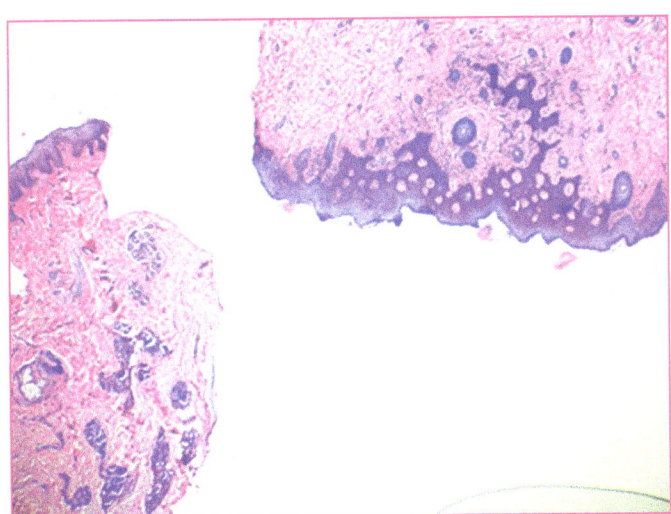

Fig. 12: Child with erythroderma showing features of both psoriasis (chest) and eczema (leg) at the same time.

AD and psoriasis, the clinical presentation depends on the localization of the subset of immune cells into inflamed skin which further mediate their clinical difference. According to some, the inflammatory infiltrate appears to be the central reason for the entire pathogenesis of psoriasis. Abnormal regulation of T cells coupled with interaction between keratinocytes and complex cytokine network is involved in the pathogenesis of the disease. There is dilatation and elongation of vertical dermal capillary loops in lesional skin and a fourfold increase in endothelium of superficial but not deep microvasculature, indicating that these changes are confined to the upper plexus. There is localization of endothelial proliferation and microvascular expansion in active plaque psoriasis. Theses vascular changes may point toward the importance of angiogenesis, in the pathogenesis of psoriasis. Marked proliferation of cutaneous nerves and increased levels of neuropeptides have been detected in lesional psoriatic skin, potentially contributing to the development of psoriasis.[10]

IMMUNOPATHOGENESIS

Psoriasis is now recognized as the most prevalent autoimmune disease caused by inappropriate activation of the cellular immune system. The disease is defined by a series of linked cellular changes in the skin: Hyperplasia of epidermal keratinocytes, vascular hyperplasia and ectasia, and infiltration of T lymphocytes, neutrophils and other types of leukocyte in affected skin. Rapid progress has been made toward dissecting cellular and molecular pathways of inflammation that contribute to disease pathogenesis that encompasses, genetic basis; cellular basis and epidermal proliferation; angiogenesis and vascular changes; immunologic basis and immunologic events including an immunogenetic spin off which determines the clinical manifestation.

Psoriasis and associated psoriatic arthritis (PsA) are complex genetic diseases with environmental and genetic components.

One of the most compelling susceptibility factors for psoriasis is the presence of HLA-Cwa 0602. Other susceptibility loci for psoriasis reside on chromosomes 1q21, 3q21, 4q, 7p, 8, 11, 16q, 17q and 20p. It is postulated that alternative pathways of leukocyte activation would converge to activate type 1 inflammatory genes which, in turn, regulate end-stage inflammation in skin and the appearance of the psoriasis phenotype.[11]

The immunologic evolution of psoriasis can be studied in three phases: (1) The sensitization phase, (2) The silent phase and (3) The effector phase.[12]

In the first phase, specific effector Th17 and Th1 cells evolve from naïve T cells under the influence of dendritic cells (DCs) in secondary lymphatic organs such as the lymph nodes or tonsils. This sensitization phase is followed by the second phase, which remains silent for a variable period of time, without any clinical manifestation. As long as the sensitization phase is not associated with an infection, it is clinically unnoticeable and not characterized by any skin alterations; followed by a silent phase of variable duration. In the presence of precipitating or triggering factor like infection or trauma, the third phase namely the effector phase begins with the skin infiltration of various immune cells monocytes/macrophages, various subpopulations of DCs, various subpopulations of T cells and neutrophilic granulocytes.

It has been demonstrated that epidermal keratinocytes are the primary source of angiogenic activity. The expression of P- and E-selectin in dermal blood vessels makes it easier for the infiltration. Immigration of these immune cells activate local tissue macrophages, DCs and mast cells which liberate their products. Aberrant production of IL-8 and thrombospondin-1 by psoriatic keratinocytes mediates angiogenesis.

As this phase continues, the biology of the keratinocytes changes resulting in a massively increased proliferation of these cells and their altered terminal differentiation. While most studies suggest a primary role for the immune system in psoriasis pathogenesis (see below), it has been argued that vascular change precedes the immune response. Investigations of the "active" edge of plaque psoriasis showed vascular proliferation to precede changes in epidermal keratin. In the absence of adequate control of inflammation, in the form of treatment, skin lesions persist leading to other consequences.

The sequence of the immunologic events that are theorized to occur in psoriasis would be:[13]

- Antigenic stimuli contribute to the activation of plasmacytoid DCs and other innate immune cells in the skin
- Proinflammatory cytokines produced by innate immune cells, including interferon alpha (IFN-α), stimulate the activation of myeloid DCs in the skin

- Myeloid DCs produce cytokines such as IL-23 and IL-12 that stimulate the attraction, activation and differentiation of T cells
- Recruited T cells produce cytokines that stimulate keratinocytes to proliferate and produce proinflammatory antimicrobial peptides and cytokines
- Cytokines produced by immune cells and keratinocytes perpetuate the inflammatory process via participation in positive feedback loops.

The formation of the pustules in impetigo herpetiformis, could be related to imbalance of the skin elastase and its inhibitors as a result of low levels of skin-derived antileukoproteinase (SKALP).

Keratinocytes of patients with AD and psoriasis show an intrinsically abnormal and different chemokine production profile and favor the recruitment of distinct leukocyte subsets into the skin. However, in spite of their differences, both AD and psoriasis share epidermal hyperplasia, aberrant immunity and skin barrier anomalies. Genetic studies of both psoriasis and AD suggest that defects affecting cells of the skin need to be as seriously considered as defects in adaptive immunity. The epidermal differentiation complex has been implicated in both AD and psoriasis. It transcribes within terminally differentiating keratinocytes, and contains many genes that may modify immune processes in the epithelium. The colocalization of AD to psoriasis loci indicates that AD is influenced by genes that modulate dermal responses independently from atopic mechanisms. What spins off the immune system and decides on the pathogenesis, clinical presentation in a genetically prone individual needs further elucidation.[14]

BIOMARKERS

Ever since research has tried to pin down the exact cause for psoriasis, the need for a marker to predict the chances of the disease in any individual and also the chances of comorbidities in an affected individual has been the target. Various genetic, cellular and biochemical markers are discovered in association with psoriasis. It is also scientifically proved that few of these are shared between other associated conditions as well.

Genetic Markers

The HLA region (specifically the version of the *HLA-C* gene called HLA-Cwa 0602) was the first genetic marker to be associated with psoriasis.[15] Linkage analysis studies have identified nine chromosomal loci associated with psoriasis named PSORS1 to PSORS9, the major psoriasis genetic determinant being PSORS1, located within the major histocompatibility complex (MHC) on chromosome 6p which probably accounts for 35–50% of the heritability of the disease. Psoriasis has a strong genetic component; a child with two affected parents has a 50% chance of developing it; siblings have a three- to sixfold risk. But the genes responsible for psoriasis have not yet been completely understood.

There is an association between psoriasis and various HLA markers: HLA-B13, B16, B17, B37, Cw6 and DR7 are associated with skin disease; HLA-B27, B38, B39, DR4 and DR7 are associated with skin plus joint disease; the relative risk is 9–15 times normal for HLA-Cw6. There is linkage disequilibrium for HLAs Cw6, B13 and Bw57 as well as an early onset in type I psoriasis, frequently showing positive family history. Whereas type II psoriasis manifesting at a later age, is more frequently associated with Cw2 and B27 than normal.

Cellular Markers

Keratins can be used as biomarkers of psoriasis severity. Immunostaining with antikeratins K16, K6, K1 and K10 antibodies reflects abnormal hyperproliferation and differentiation of keratinocytes, whereas K1 and K10, representing markers of terminal differentiation of keratinocytes are downregulated in psoriatic skin lesions. Keratins (K16 and K17) have been identified as markers of keratinocyte hyperproliferation in psoriasis in vivo and in vitro. At least six markers of abnormal keratinocyte differentiation have been found and all have implications in the pathogenesis of the disease. These include aberrations of keratinocyte transglutaminase type I (TGase K), SKALP, migration inhibitory factor-related protein-8 (MRP-8), involucrin, filaggrin and keratin expression.[16]

Serum and Inflammatory Biomarkers

Higher levels of C-reactive protein have been demonstrated in patients with psoriasis compared with controls with a significant correlation to disease severity. Vascular endothelial growth factor (VEGF) levels were found to be increased and to correlate with disease severity. Indeed, circulating levels of VEGF were higher during active psoriasis and in the presence of psoriatic arthritis, and were lowered during disease remission. Adiponectin, leptin, ghrelin, resistin, inflammatory cytokines [ILs 6, 8, 17, 18, 23, 1 beta (β); TNFs, plasminogen activator inhibitor 1], uric acid, C-reactive protein and lipid abnormalities. Many other molecules have been proposed as biomarkers of cutaneous psoriasis, including metalloproteinase-1 (a marker of tissue damage), transforming growth factor-β1 and tissue inhibitor of metalloproteinase-1. Expression of Toll-like receptor 4 (TLR4) has been found in guttate psoriasis, spectrum that is known to be precipitated by bacterial infection.

Comorbidity

From the genetic point of view, patients with the cutaneous form of psoriasis and those with psoriatic arthritis share the majority of the predisposing gene variants, in particular an association with HLA-Cw6. Other class I antigens are also associated with psoriatic arthritis, including HLA-B13,

HLA-B57, HLA-B39 and HLA-Cw7. From linkage analysis studies, only one locus, i.e., PSORAS1 (PSORS8), seems to be specifically associated with psoriatic arthritis. Basal IL-1β, IL-6 and IL-22 levels in synovial fluid were correlated with C-reactive protein levels and these cytokines were significantly reduced after this therapy. Other markers that have been detected in the circulation of patients with psoriatic arthritis reflect cartilage destruction and bone remodeling. These include metalloproteinase-3, osteoprotegerin, and the ratio between C-propeptide of type II collagen and collagen fragment neoepitopes (CPII: C2C). The serum level of the receptor activator of nuclear factor kappa-B ligand (RANKL) reflects the extent of bone erosion, and has been proposed as a predictive marker of progressive joint damage. Circulating osteoclast precursors in patients with psoriatic arthritis have also been proposed as cellular biomarkers of disease severity because of their correlation with bone erosion. Leptin and resistin could be investigated further as candidate biomarkers for prediction of development of insulin resistance and atherosclerosis in patients with psoriatic disease.

Biomarkers not only provide insights into the mechanisms involved in the pathogenesis of the disease, but also help to some extent in the distinction between the different clinical variants of the disease, assessment of disease activity and severity and prediction of the outcome of a therapeutic intervention. Biomarkers could also allow the selection of patient-tailored therapy to maximize the beneficial effect. A field of great importance is the use of biomarkers for prediction of development of comorbidities such as arthritis, cardiovascular disease and metabolic syndrome.[17]

REFERENCES

1. Lowes MA, Kikuchi T, Fuentes-Duculan J, et al. Psoriasis vulgaris lesions contain discrete populations of Th1 and Th17 T cells. J Invest Dermatol. 2008;128(5):1207-11.
2. Hüffmeier U, Lascorz J, Becker T, et al. Characterization of psoriasis susceptibility locus 6 (PSORS6) in patients with early onset psoriasis and evidence for interaction with PSORS1. J Med Genet. 2009;46(11):736-44.
3. Schäfer T. Epidemiology of psoriasis. Review and the German perspective. Dermatology. 2006;212(4):327-37.
4. Henseler T. The genetics of psoriasis. J Am Acad Dermatol. 1997;37(2):S1-11.
5. Riveira-Munoz E, He SM, Escaramís G, et al. Meta-analysis confirms the LCE3C_LCE3B deletion as a risk factor for psoriasis in several ethnic groups and finds interaction with HLA-Cw6. J Invest Dermatol. 2011;131(5):1105-9.
6. Takahashi H, Tsuji H, Takahashi I, et al. Plasma adiponectin and leptin levels in Japanese patients with psoriasis. Br J Dermatol. 2008;159(5):1207-8.
7. Takahashi H, Tsuji H, Takahashi I, et al. Prevalence of obesity/adiposity in Japanese psoriasis patients: adiposity is correlated with the severity of psoriasis. J Dermatol Sci. 2009;54(1):61-3.
8. Mobini N, Toussaint S, Kamino H. Papulosquamous disorders. In: Elder DE, Elenitsas R, Johnson BL, Murphy GF, Xu X (Eds). Lever's Histopathology of the Skin, 10th edition. New York, USA: Lippincott Williams & Wilkins Company; 2008. pp. 169-203.
9. Parimalam K, Thomas J, Dineshkumar D. Histology of infantile erythrodermic psoriasis—a study of eight cases. E-Journal of the Indian Society of Teledermatology. 2012;6(1):28-33.
10. Chiricozzi A, Chimenti S. Effective Topical Agents and Emerging Perspectives in the Treatment of Psoriasis. Expert Rev Dermatol. 2012;7:283-93.
11. Krueger JG, Bowcock A. Psoriasis pathophysiology: current concepts of pathogenesis. Ann Rheum Dis. 2005;64(Suppl 2):ii30-6.
12. Sabat R, Philipp S, Höflich C, et al. Immunopathogenesis of psoriasis. Exp Dermatol. 2007;16(10):779-98.
13. Nestle FO, Kaplan DH, Barker J. Psoriasis. N Eng J Med. 2009;361(5):496-509.
14. Parimalam K, Thomas J. Congenital erythrodermic psoriasis with atopic dermatitis: an example of immunogenetic spinoff. Indian J Pathol Microbiol. 2013;56(1):72-3.
15. Walter H, Brachtel R, Eckes L, et al. Psoriasis vulgaris and genetic markers. Hum Genet. 1977;37(2):169-81.
16. Molteni S, Reali E. Biomarkers in the pathogenesis, diagnosis, and treatment of psoriasis. Psoriasis: Targets and Therapy. 2012;2:55-66.
17. Gerkowicz A, Pietrzak A, Szepietowski JC, et al. Biochemical markers of psoriasis as a metabolic disease. Folia Histochem Cytobiol. 2012;50(2):155-70.

Clinical Aspects

INTRODUCTION

Over 125 million people worldwide, approximately 2 to 3% of the total population, have psoriasis. Studies show that between 10 and 30% of people with psoriasis also develop psoriatic arthritis (PsA). Psoriasis in children is not uncommon. About one out of three people with psoriasis report having a relative with psoriasis. If one parent has psoriasis, a child has about a 10% chance of having psoriasis. If both parents have psoriasis, a child has approximately a 50% chance of developing the disease. A positive family history, precipitating trigger factors and age of onset can all, to some extent, predict the prognosis of the disease in children. A positive family history has been reported in 23.4 to 71% of children with psoriasis.[1,2] Identical twins have more chances of manifesting psoriasis than fraternal twins.[3]

This portion of the topic will be dealt under the following headings:
- History and evaluation
- Clinical variants
- Associations.

HISTORY AND EVALUATION

It is an art to elicit history and evaluate a patient with any disease, more so with a disease like psoriasis, which is now a systemic disorder with psychological implications and lot of associated comorbidities. Thorough knowledge will help elicit proper history which will help appropriate treatment. Spending time with the patient while eliciting history is of utmost importance to develop a good patient doctor report, which has got long way to go in effective control of the disease. Winning the patient's confidence is the first step in getting good patient compliance.

The following aspects should be necessarily concentrated upon while evaluating the patient:
- Age of onset
- Triggering and exacerbating factors
- Signals of psoriasis
- Grading
- Associations.

Age of Onset

Variations exist between studies regarding the age of onset of psoriasis. The first manifestation of psoriasis may occur at any age from birth to old age, females tending to present the disease earlier than males. The mean age of onset for the first presentation of psoriasis can range from 15 years to 20 years of age, with a second peak occurring at 55 years to 60 years.[4] Peak age of onset in childhood psoriasis is between 8 years and 12 years.[5] Family history of psoriasis predicts early disease.[6] The disease duration may vary from a few weeks to a whole lifetime. The course is unpredictable and the variations are numerous. Psoriasis type I and type II are distinguished by a bimodal age at onset **(Figs. 1 and 2)**.

Type I begins on or before the age of 40 years; type II begins after the age of 40 years. Type I disease accounts for >75% of the cases.

Triggering and Exacerbating Factors

Precipitating factors are more important in pediatric than in adult-onset psoriasis. They largely include trauma,

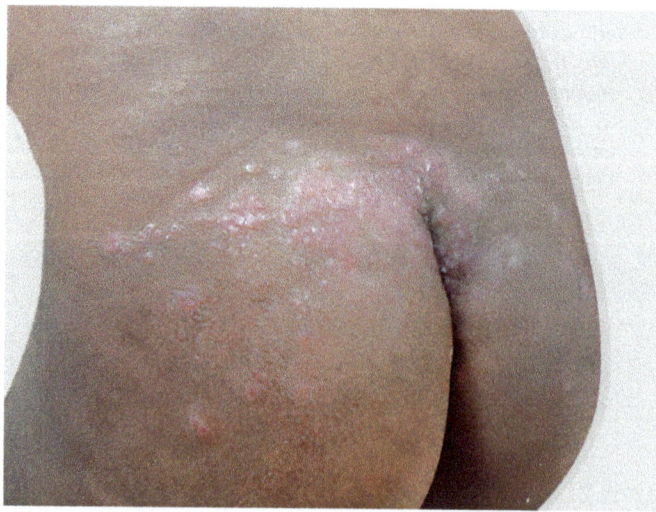

Fig. 1: Type I psoriasis with onset in childhood.

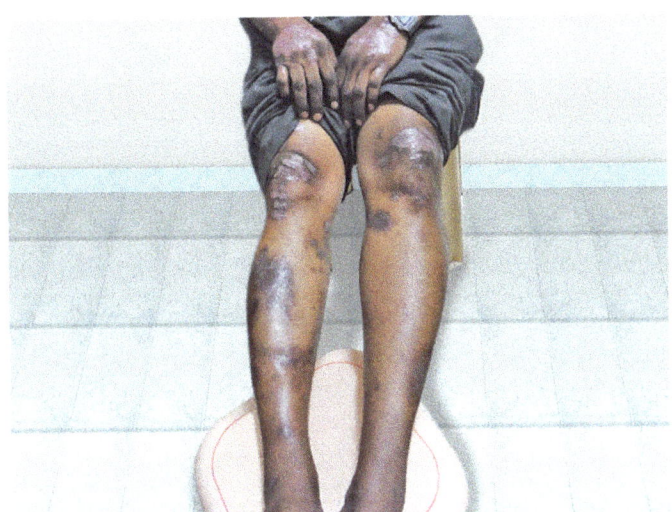

Fig. 2: Type II psoriasis having onset during adult lifes.

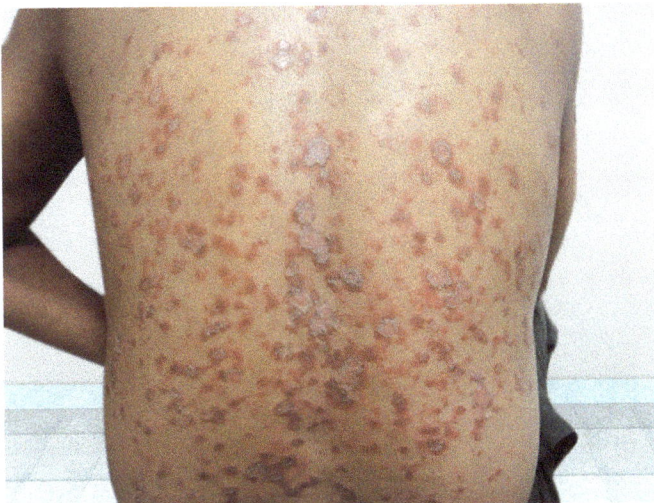

Fig. 4: Same man as in **Figure 3** showing exacerbation with beta blocker.

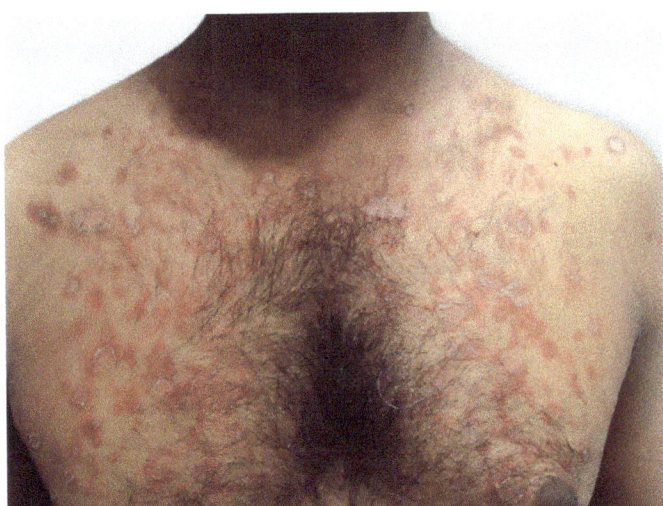

Fig. 3: Man who's psoriasis got exacerbated with beta blocker.

infections, drugs and stress. The appearance of psoriatic lesions in uninvolved skin at sites of former trauma is known as isomorphic response or Koebner phenomenon. Any form of trauma including physical, chemical, thermal, surgical, or inflammatory trauma can result in exacerbation of psoriasis. Streptococcal pharyngitis or perianal streptococcal dermatitis typically provokes guttate psoriasis and childhood pustular psoriasis can be elicited by the streptococcal antigen.[7,8] Infection with human immunodeficiency virus can induce or exacerbate psoriasis.[9] Whereas the use of β-blocking agents and lithium is a well-known trigger of psoriasis in adult patients **(Figs. 3 and 4)**, antimalarials and withdrawal of oral or topical corticosteroids play a more important role in rebound or induction of childhood psoriasis.[10-12] In addition, several studies emphasize the influence of psychological and psychosomatic factors like stress or lack of social support in the course of psoriasis.[13] Inflammatory focus was the most frequent trigger factor observed by Barisic-Drusko and Rucevic.[14] One must understand that gradation exists among psoriatic patients and in the same individual over time, ranging from apparently healthy to minor signs to overt clinical manifestations.

Even before development of classical papule or plaque of psoriasis, patient may present with any one of the following subtle symptoms which should not be brushed aside:

- Worsening of a pre-existing erythematous plaque
- Sudden onset of pustules
- Recent infection, especially streptococcal sore throat or tonsillitis
- Pain in an asymptomatic plaque in the vicinity of affected joint
- Pruritus (sometimes in guttate psoriasis)
- Dystrophic nails
- Long-term rash with recent presentation of joint pain
- Joint pain without any visible skin findings

The so called minor signs, usually considered as "stigmata" of psoriasis, are easily missed out and the diagnosis is delayed if not looked for **(Figs. 5 to 14)**.[15]

Signals of Psoriasis (Box 1)

The most common skin manifestations are scaling erythematous macules, papules and plaques. Typically, the macules are seen first and these progresses to maculopapules and ultimately well-demarcated, noncoherent, silvery plaques overlying a glossy homogeneous erythema. The area of skin involvement varies with the form of psoriasis. The clinical types of psoriasis are more or less the same as in adults and children with some variation in the incidence of different types.

Plaque type psoriasis, scalp psoriasis, guttate psoriasis, nail psoriasis, flexural psoriasis, napkin psoriasis, unstable psoriasis, pustular psoriasis are the types of psoriasis commonly encountered in children. Congenital psoriasis,

CHAPTER 4 Clinical Aspects

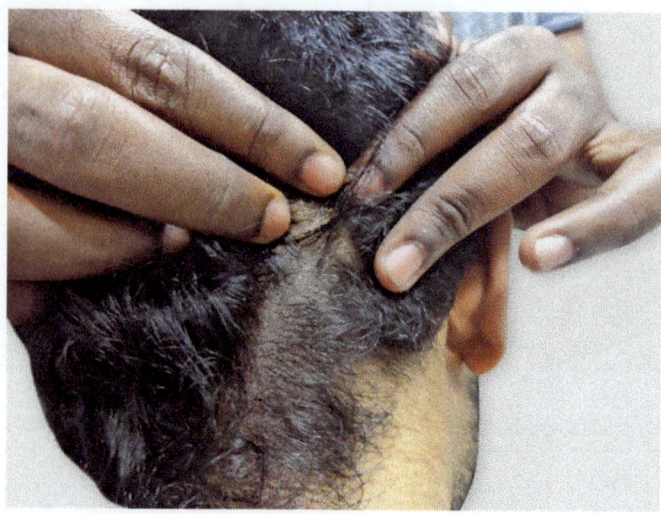

Fig. 5: Severe seborrheic dermatitis in a college student, an indicator of psoriasis.

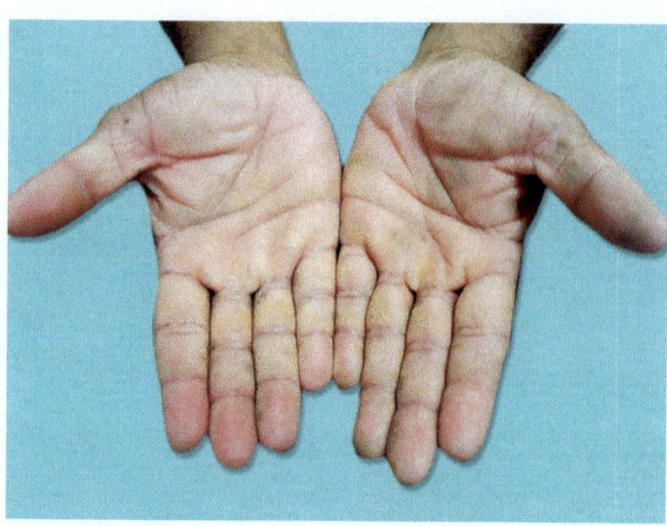

Fig. 8: Keratolysis punctata like lesions on the palms—an early sign of psoriasis.

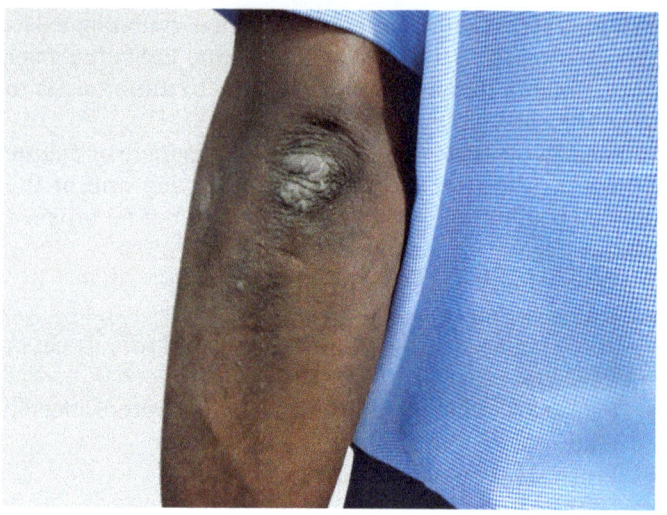

Fig. 6: Hyperkeratotic non-scaly plaque on the elbow of a man—a signal of psoriasis.

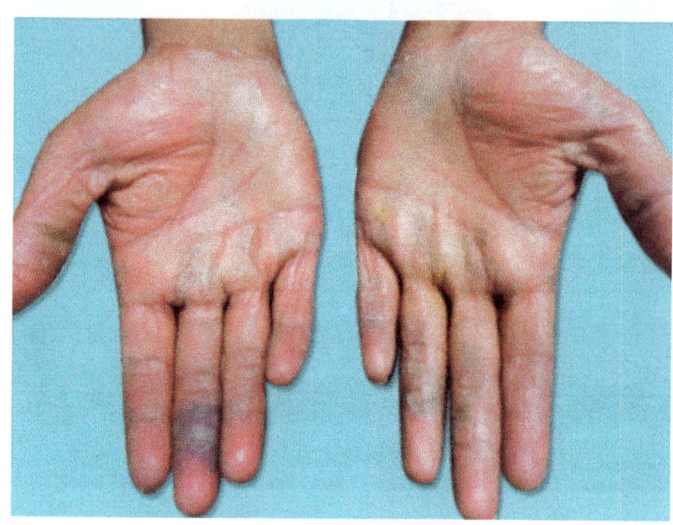

Fig. 9: Eczematous patch on the palms of a young man signaling psoriasis. He also had severe dandruff.

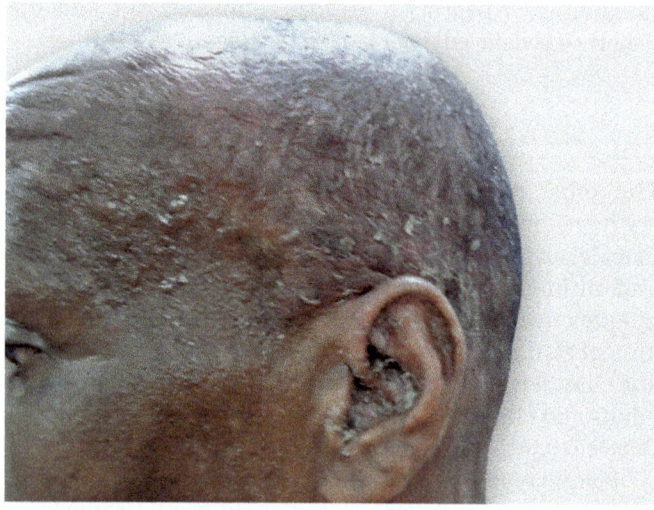

Fig. 7: Psoriasis can be missed in patients presenting with recalcitrant otitis externa.

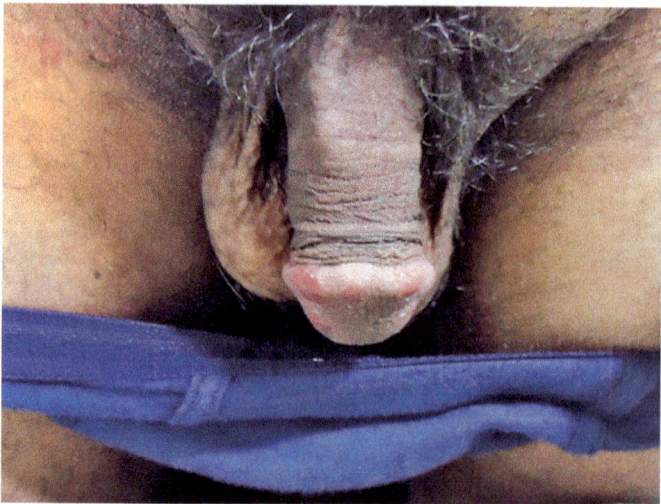

Fig. 10: Sharply marginated erythema of the penile skin should arouse suspicion of psoriasis.

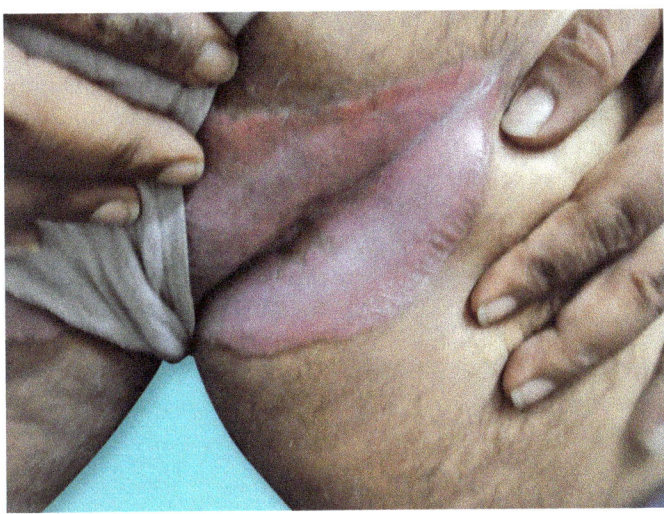

Fig. 11: Intertrigo with sharply marginated erythema may be a sign of psoriasis.

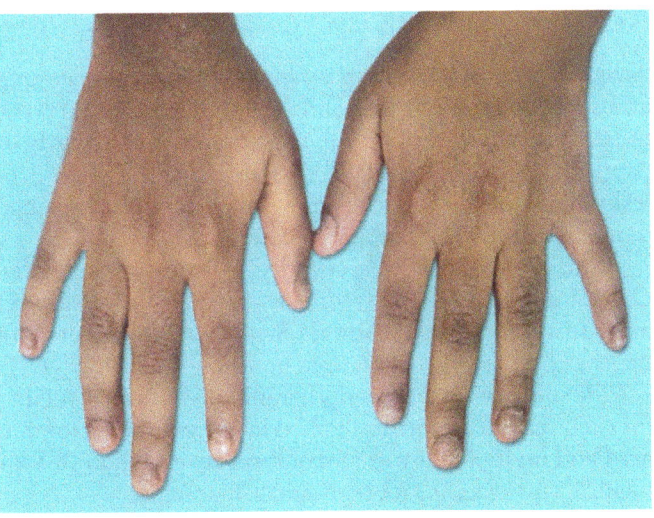

Fig. 13: Nail pitting is a sign of psoriasis.

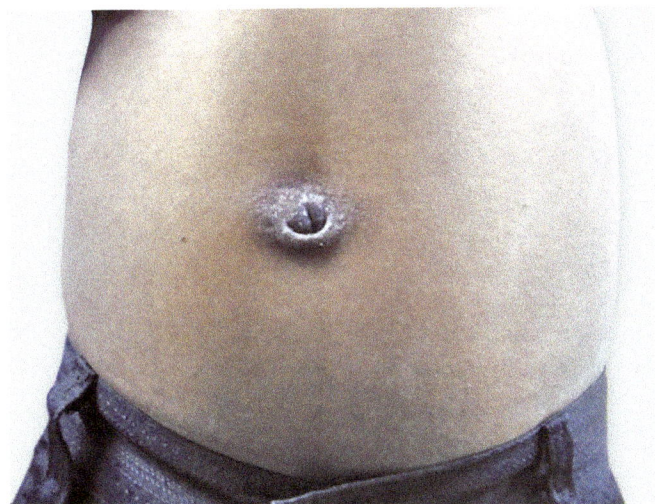

Fig. 12: Periumbilical erythema and scaling may be a sign of flexural psoriasis which can be easily missed in colored skin.

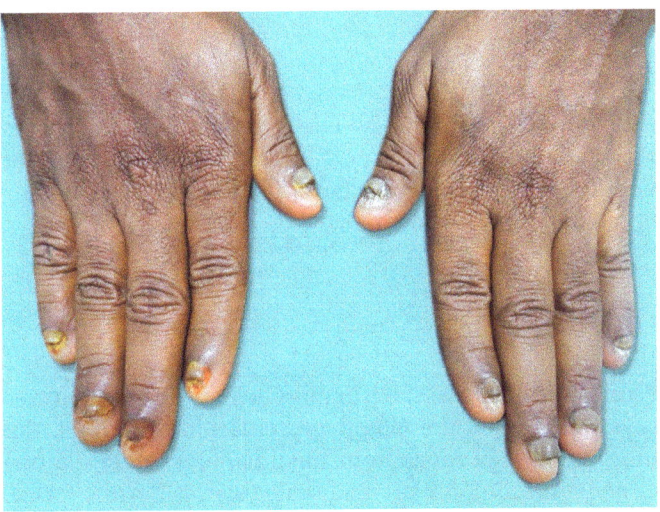

Fig. 14: Subungual hyperkeratosis with onycholysis indicating psoriasis.

> **BOX 1: Signals of psoriasis.**
>
> - Severe dandruff
> - Hyperkeratotic non-scaly plaques on extensor surfaces
> - Recalcitrant scaly otitis externa
> - Keratolysis-like lesions of the palms and soles
> - Eczematous patches on palms and soles
> - Sharply marginated areas of erythema over the penile skin
> - Intertrigo with sharp margination of erythema
> - Nail pittings
> - Subungual hyperkeratosis and onycholysis
> - Sterile multiple paronychia

congenital psoriatic erythroderma and infantile psoriasis are rare forms of psoriasis seen in the first year of life. Erythrodermic psoriasis and PsA are less frequent when compared to adulthood psoriasis. Mucosal involvement has been rare in Indian children.[16] Psoriasis can now be considered as a disease manifesting from "womb to tomb".

The disease in children is more pruritic and the lesions are relatively thinner, softer and less scaly. The classical erythematous scaly papule or plaque will mostly give a clue for diagnosis.

The following features are pertinent and helpful in the clinical diagnosis of psoriasis:[17]

- The isomorphic response or Koebner phenomenon, which is occurrence of lesions in areas of trauma
- The Auspitz sign—pinpoint bleeding at the base of scale that has been removed
- Presence of nail pitting, which can aid in diagnosis of the disease
- Altered pigmentation with lesional clearance.

The first two findings are useful to assess the disease activity.

Grading

Severity grading for psoriasis is usually based on surface area and severity. Psoriasis Area and Severity Index (PASI) is the most widely used tool for the measurement of severity of psoriasis. PASI combines the assessment of the severity of lesions and the area affected into a single score in the range 0 (no disease) to 72 (maximal disease).

Within each area, the severity is estimated by three clinical signs: erythema (redness), induration (thickness) and desquamation (scaling). Severity parameters are measured on a scale of 0–4, from none to maximum.

The sum of all three severity parameters is then calculated for each section of skin, multiplied by the area score for that area and multiplied by weight of respective section (0.1 for head, 0.2 for arms, 0.3 for body and 0.4 for legs).

A simpler way to assess the severity would be mild, moderate and severe which are represented as <3, 3 to 10% and >10% body surface area (BSA), respectively.[18]

Associations

A detailed history must be elicited to find all the known associations of psoriasis. It is important to elicit relevant findings about the other systems whenever systemic therapy or phototherapy is contemplated.

CLINICAL VARIANTS

Psoriasis is highly variable in morphology, distribution and severity. Despite the classic presentation described, the morphology can range from small papules (guttate form) to generalized erythema and scale (erythrodermic form). In addition, there can be involvement of one or more of the following: skin, nail, mucosa, and joint. The disease can be asymptomatic, localized, or widespread and disabling. Further, psoriasis may have a variable course presenting as chronic, stable plaques, or may present acutely with a rapid progression and widespread involvement. Psoriasis may be symptomatic with patients complaining of intense pruritus or burning. The different spectrum of psoriasis is outlined in **Box 2**.

Type of Disease

Plaque Type Psoriasis

Psoriasis vulgaris or plaque-type psoriasis is by far the commonest clinical type of psoriasis both in children and adults accounting to as high as 80%. Classical plaque is characterized by erythema and silvery white scales; the scale may be scraped away to reveal inflamed skin beneath showing multiple pinpoint bleeding spots, the Auspitz sign. However, in dark skinned patients, erythema and scaling are not so obvious. The common sites involved include scalp, post auricular area, elbows, knees, umbilical region and buttocks. The lesions may initially begin as erythematous macules (flat and < 1 cm) or papules, extend peripherally and coalesce to form plaques of one to several centimeters in diameter **(Figs. 15 to 20)**.

A white blanching ring, known as Woronoff's ring, may be observed in the skin surrounding a psoriatic plaque.

Scale is typically present in psoriasis that is characteristically silvery white and can vary in thickness.

> **BOX 2: Clinical spectrum of psoriasis based on.**
>
> - *Type of disease*:
>   - Plaque
>   - Guttate
>   - Linear
>   - Pustular
>   - Erythrodermic
>   - Unstable
> - *Site of involvement*:
>   - Scalp
>   - Flexural
>   - Palmoplantar
>   - Mucosal
>   - Ocular
>   - Nail
>   - Arthropathic
> - *Disease manifestation*:
>   - Latent
>   - Mild
>   - Moderate
>   - Moderate-to-severe
>   - Severe
>   - Gaurded prognosis

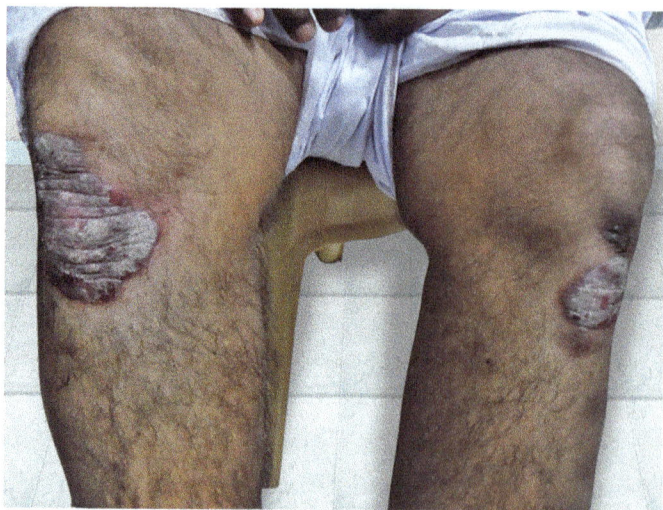

Fig. 15: Plaque psoriasis showing Auspitz sign.

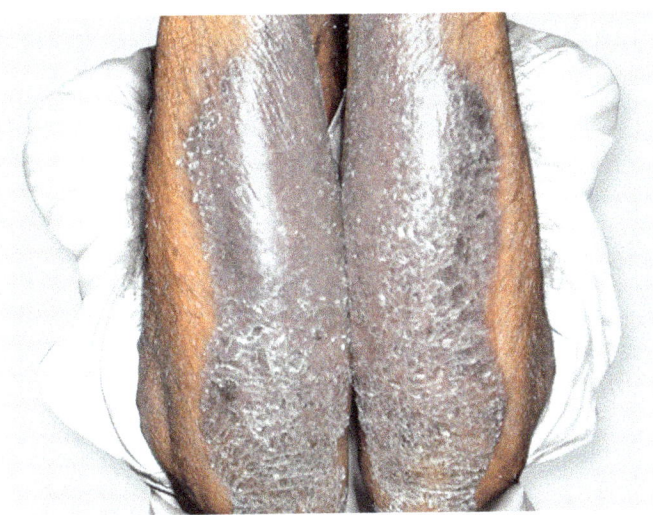

Fig. 16: Persistence of plaque psoriasis due to constant friction acting as Koebnerization.

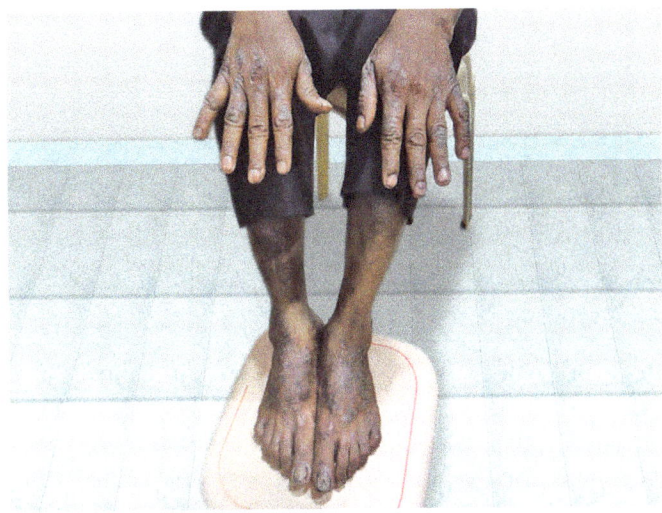

Fig. 19: Plaque type psoriasis of the hands and feet.

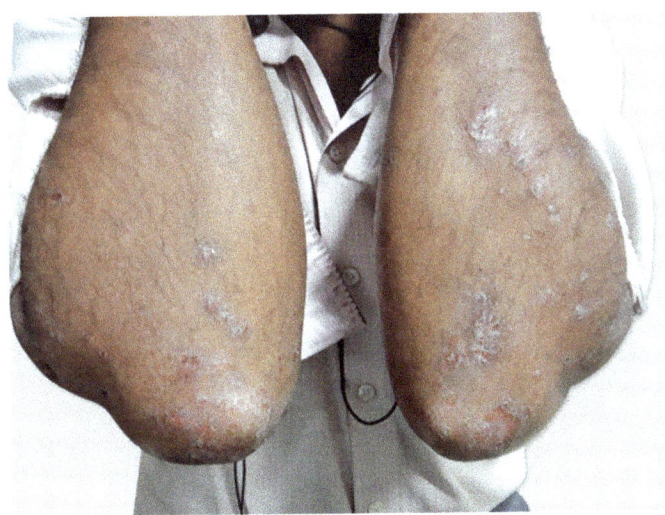

Fig. 17: Plaque type psoriasis affecting the extensor surface.

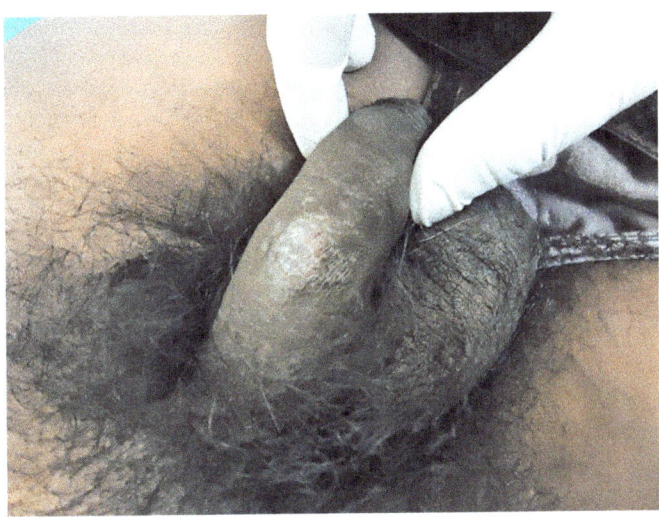

Fig. 20: Rare site for a plaque type psoriasis.

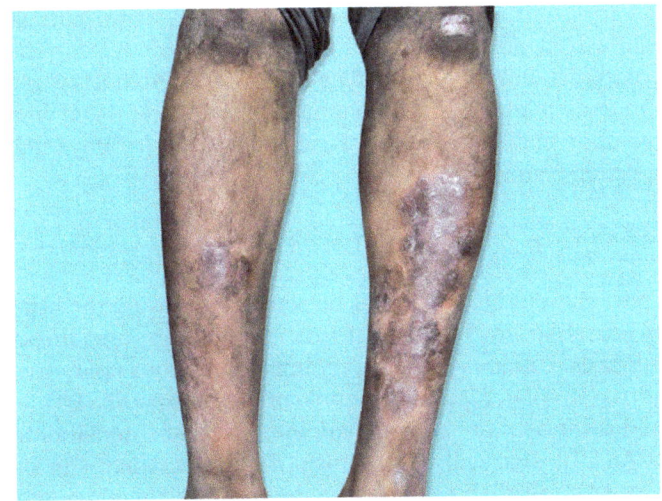

Fig. 18: Psoriasis vulgaris affecting the shin.

Removal of scale may reveal tiny bleeding points (Auspitz sign). The amount of scaling varies among patients and even at different sites on a given patient. In acute inflammatory or exanthematic psoriasis, scaling can be minimal and erythema may be the predominant clinical sign.[19] Scalp is the most common initial site affected. Facial involvement in children is a frequent observation in majority of the reports which varies from 18 to 46%.[20]

Presence of Koebners' response (development of isomorphic skin lesion along the line of trauma) is an indicator of disease activity. Eczema can sometimes closely mimic psoriasis when the scales are loose. However, demonstration of Auspitz sign will help diagnosing psoriasis though Auspitz sign is not pathognomonic. It is always advisable to examine the hidden features of psoriasis as they are sometimes the true signals. Bowen's disease and cutaneous T-cell lymphoma should be ruled out by

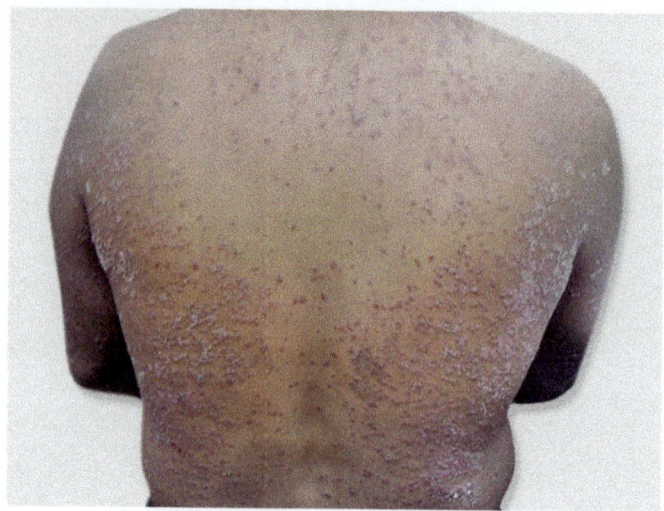

Fig. 21: Guttate psoriasis in an adult.

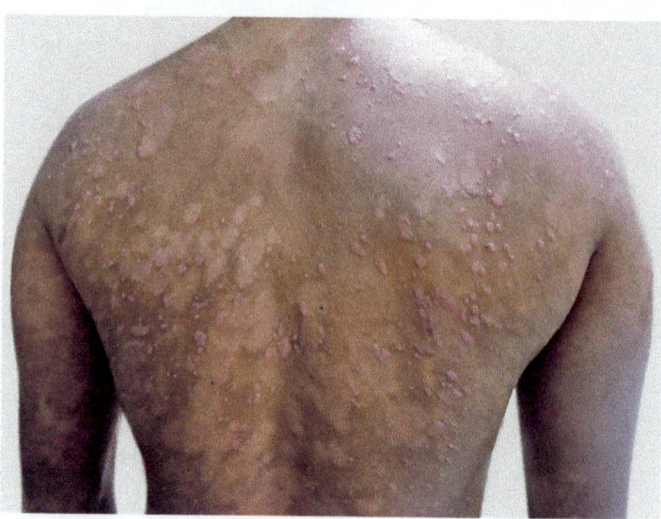

Fig. 23: Guttate lesions in adult evolving to psoriasis vulgaris.

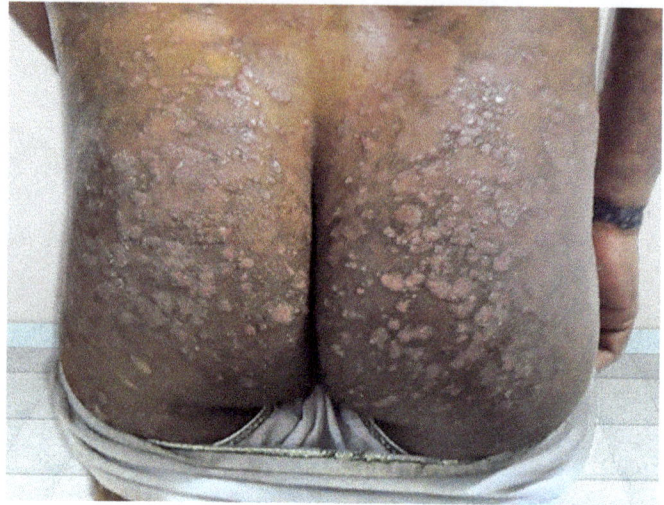

Fig. 22: Guttate lesions in adult evolving to psoriasis vulgaris.

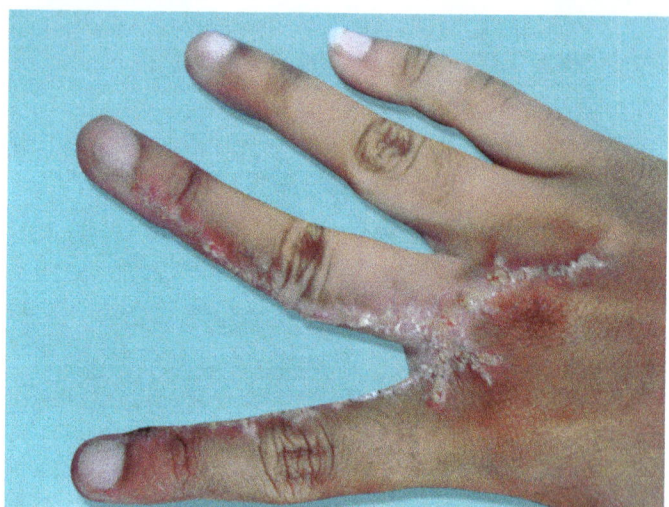

Fig. 24: Linear psoriasis in an adult.

pathological study in a chronic plaque of psoriasis that does not respond to treatment.

Guttate Psoriasis

Guttate (*gutta* meaning a droplet) psoriasis presents as small salmon-pink papules, 1-10 mm in diameter, predominately on the trunk **(Figs. 21 to 23)**.

These are usually distributed in a centripetal fashion although guttate lesions can also involve the head and limbs. The lesions may be scaly. It frequently appears suddenly, 2-3 weeks after an upper respiratory infection (URI) with group A beta-hemolytic streptococci which can be the presenting episode of psoriasis in children, or occasionally adults. Guttate psoriasis has been reported to follow Kawasaki disease.[21] The number of lesions may range from 5 or 10 to over 100. Guttate psoriasis accounts for 2% of the total cases of psoriasis. In children, an acute episode of guttate psoriasis is usually self-limiting; in adults, guttate flares may complicate chronic plaque disease. Although few studies have assessed the long term prognosis of children with acute guttate psoriasis, nearly one-third of patients with guttate psoriasis eventually develop plaque type of psoriasis. Pityriasis rosea and early papule of lichen planus can be differentiated with evolution of the disease, apart from the intense itching noted in lichen planus.

Linear Psoriasis

Erythematous scaly papules or plaques following the lines of Blaschko are features of this rare, variant and linear psoriasis. Unlike, inflammatory linear verrucous epidermal nevus (ILVEN), there is no or only mild pruritus **(Fig. 24)**.

Presence of Koebner's phenomenon and demonstration of Auspitz sign will help clinical diagnosis which can be further confirmed with biopsy, the histology of which will show psoriasiform features. Family history for psoriasis is often positive in patients with Blaschko's linear psoriasis.[22]

There is lower expression of keratin 10 in psoriasis as compared to normal levels in ILVEN. Whereas lower levels of cell surface expression markers of T-cell subsets, such as CD8, CD45RO, CD2, CD94 and CD161, are features of ILVEN.[23]

Pustular Psoriasis

Pustular psoriasis presents as sterile pustules appearing locally or diffusely over the body **(Figs. 25 to 34)**.

Pustular psoriasis may cycle through erythema, pustules and then scaling. Pustular psoriasis can develop *de novo* or in a patient with psoriasis vulgaris. For clinical approach, pustular psoriasis can be classified as localized or generalized **(Box 3)**. Localized pustular psoriasis predominantly involves the hands and feet, whereas generalized pustular psoriasis (GPP) affects the entire body surface when it presents as erythroderma which can lead to multi-organ failure.

Palmoplantar pustulosis: The relationship of palmoplantar pustulosis (PPP) to psoriasis vulgaris is controversial.[24,25] Smoking has been shown as a probable provocative factor.[26] PPP was previously considered to be a localized form of pustular psoriasis but about 10–20% of patients with PPP have psoriasis elsewhere. It is now known that they are distinct conditions with different genetic backgrounds. Palmoplantar pustulosis is much more common in. It is thought that activated nicotine receptors in the sweat glands cause an inflammatory process.[27]

Acrodermatitis continua of hallopeau: Often starts at the tip of the digit, the skin becoming red and scaly and pustules develop, subsequently nail bed may be involved leading to nail dystrophy and even onycholysis. Vesiculo pustules are followed by a fringe of undermined epidermis with a red glazed skin.

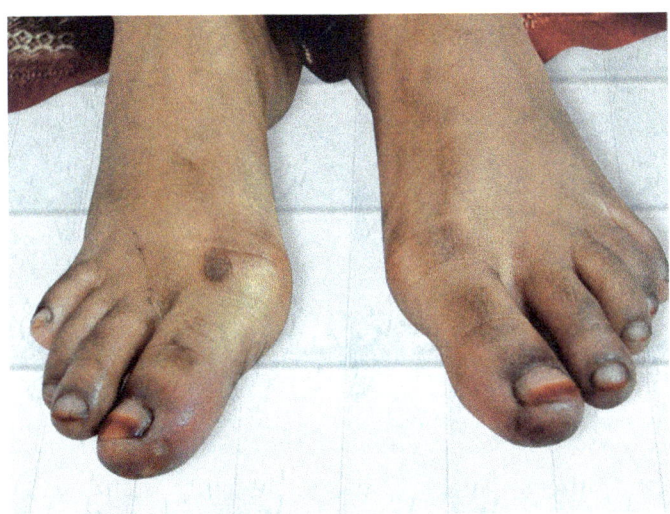

Fig. 25: Localized pustular psoriasis of the feet.

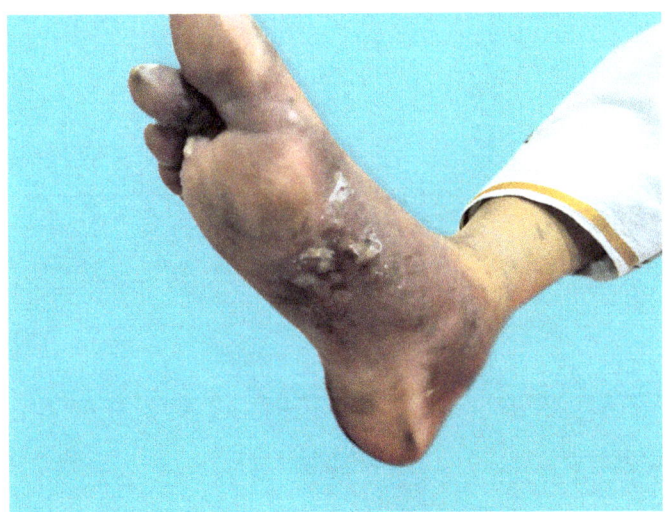

Fig. 27: Localized pustular psoriasis of the sole.

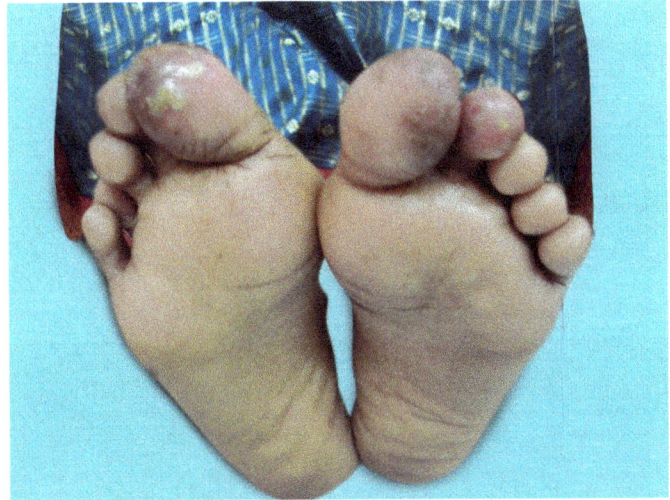

Fig. 26: Note pustules with erythema and scaling early stage of acrodermatitis continua.

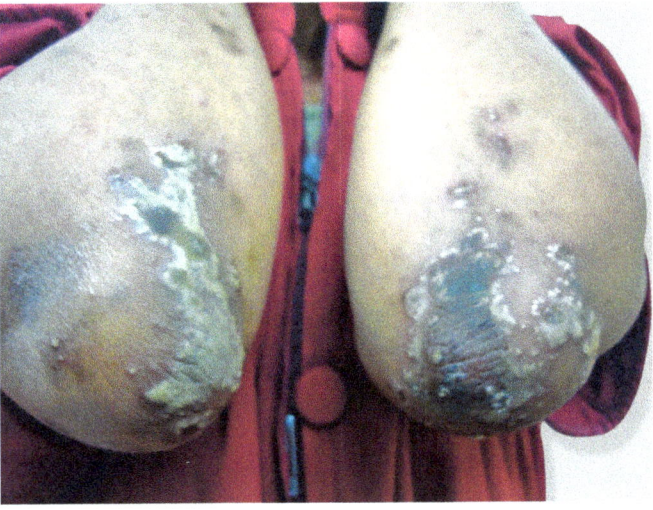

Fig. 28: Localized form of pustular psoriasis in an adolescent boy who was having plaque type psoriasis.

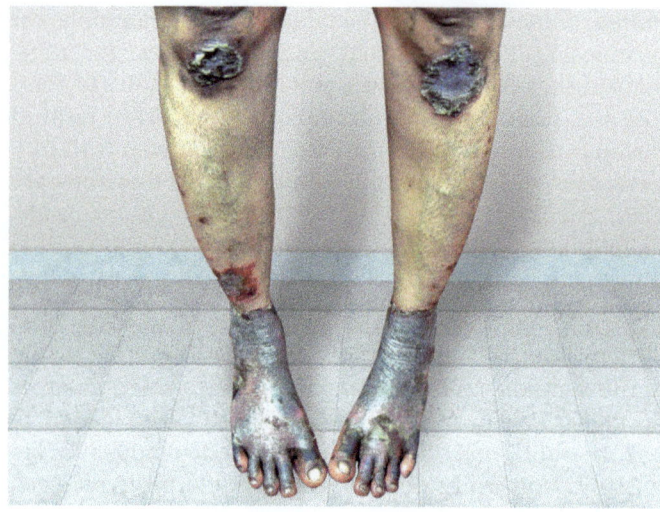

Fig. 29: Localized form of generalized pustular psoriasis resolving after therapy and resuming the original plaque morphology.

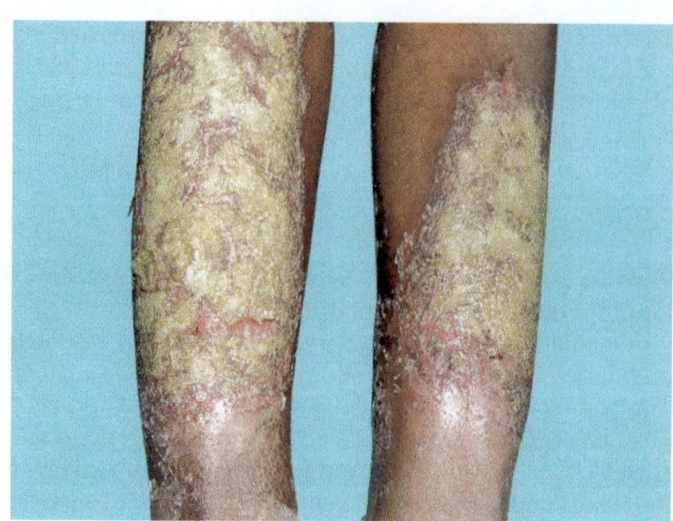

Fig. 32: Lake of pus in acute generalized pustular psoriasis.

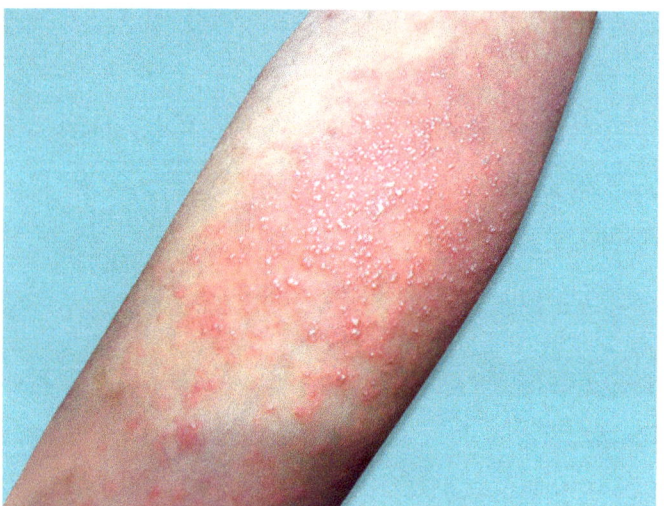

Fig. 30: Pin point pustules in early pustular psoriasis.

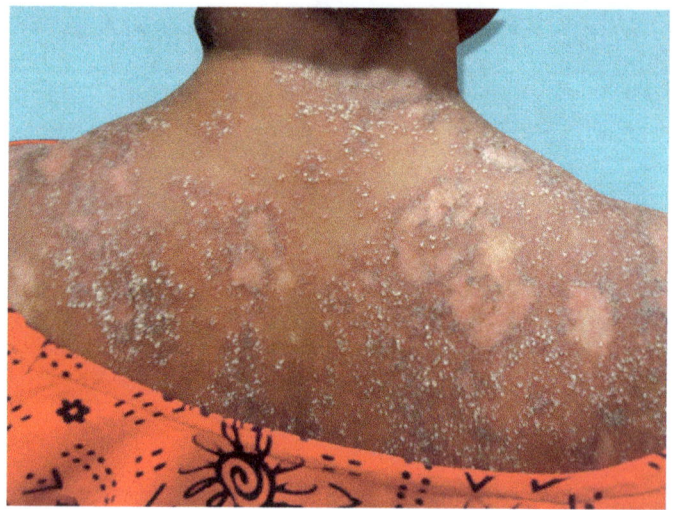

Fig. 33: Acute generalized pustular psoriasis of von Zumbusch.

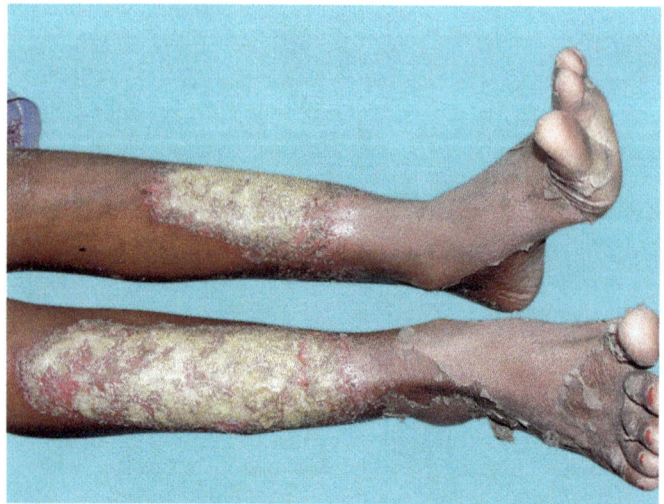

Fig. 31: Superficial pustules after sudden withdrawal of systemic steroids.

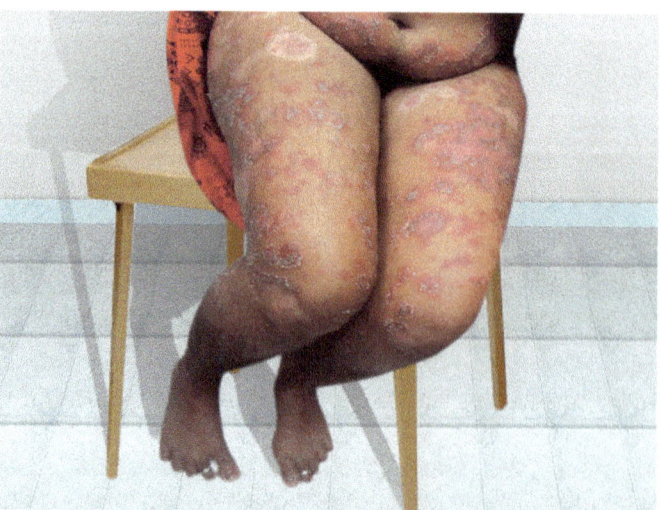

Fig. 34: Acute generalized pustular psoriasis of von Zumbusch.

BOX 3: Types of pustular psoriasis.

- *Localized pustular psoriasis*:
  - Palmoplantar pustulosis
  - Acrodermatitis continua
- *Generalized pustular psoriasis (GPP)*:
  - Acute
  - Of pregnancy
  - Infantile and juvenile
  - Circinate, annular, linear
  - Localized form of GPP

BOX 4: Drugs precipitating generalized pustular psoriasis.

- Salicylates
- Iodide
- Lithium
- Phenylbutazone
- Oxyphenbutazone
- Progesterone
- Terbinafine
- Amfebutamone
- Withdrawal of cyclosporine

Bony changes can occur leading to osteolysis of the tuft of the distal phalanx. The free end of the digit may become wasted and tapered with disturbance in the vasculature. Acrodermatitis continua, though is a disease of children, in affected adults may evolve into GPP. The tongue may become involved with fissuring or the annulus migrans of pustular psoriasis. Tinea manuum is usually asymmetric in distribution and demonstration of the fungal element will help in establishing the diagnosis which is sometimes challenging. Contact dermatitis can be confirmed with a patch test.

Parakeratosis pustulosa in children can mimic acrodermatitis continua. However, the occurrence of pustules is rare. There is predominant scaling along with nail dystrophy.[28] Histological examination will confirm psoriasis which will show neutrophilic micro abscess.

Generalized pustular psoriasis: Amongst the many predisposing factors, steroid withdrawal seems to be the most common. There are many drugs that can precipitate GPP **(Box 4)**.

Acute generalized pustular psoriasis (von Zumbusch): Two main groups have been distinguished. In the first, typical psoriasis of early onset develops into pustular psoriasis after some years, often after a triggering factor. In the second, late onset psoriasis undergoes spontaneous progression to the generalized pustular form.[29] The onset may be preceded by sensation of burning followed by dryness of the skin.

An abrupt onset of high fever and severe malaise precedes development of generalized eruption of pinpoint pustules. Sheets of erythema and pustulation spread to involve previously unaffected skin, the flexures and genital regions being particularly involved. Different configurations like, isolated pustules, lakes of pus, circinate lesions, plaques of erythema with pustular collarets or a generalized erythroderma can be seen. Waves of pustulation may succeed each other and the pustules dry.

The nails become thickened or separated by subungual lakes of pus. The buccal mucosa and tongue may be involved, 'geographic' tongue and fissured tongue are the common oral manifestations.[30] Remission occurs within days or weeks. Exhaustion, toxicity or infection are the common cause of death in untreated cases. Remission is followed by erythroderma or return to the original state. Relapses are common.

Pustular psoriasis in infants and children: Childhood pustular psoriasis is a rare disease which usually appears at 2-10 years of age, constituting <1% of childhood psoriasis.[31,32] A review of 1,262 cases of childhood psoriasis found a 0.6% rate of pustular variants. Four clinical patterns of pustular psoriasis have been described in children: namely, GPP or von Zumbusch, annular pustular psoriasis (APP), exanthematic pustular psoriasis and localized pustular psoriasis. Annular form seems to be the commonest presentation. They are not necessarily mutually exclusive and mixed variants are also possible.[33] In children, the clinical pattern of GPP (an acute, episodic and potentially life-threatening form of psoriasis) classically presents as widespread sheets of sterile pustules on bright erythematous skin that resolves within 3–4 days, with recurrent waves of inflammation. The acute pustulation is typically associated with fever and toxic changes.[34,35] Compared with the adult forms, the first manifestation of GPP in children is usually more severe, presenting with high fever accompanied by generalized pustules. Few of these cases eventually develop psoriasis vulgaris.[36] The younger the age of onset, the more severe the patient's condition can be.

Circinate, annular and linear forms of pustular psoriasis: Circinate type of pustular psoriasis appears as discrete areas of erythema which become raised and edematous. Pustules appear at the edges of the round lesions, creating rings, spread centrifugally and may mimic erythema annulare centrifugum. The pustules dry out and leave a trail of scale as the lesion grows. Annular and other patterned lesions may be seen in acute GPP, but are more characteristic of the subacute or chronic forms of widespread pustular psoriasis. It may occur alone or as a phase in the evolution of GPP. Linear forms of pustular psoriasis are occasionally observed within the context of more generalized pustulosis.

Localized form of GPP: These must be distinguished from PPP or acropustulosis. The term "psoriasis with pustules" is perhaps more appropriate. One or more plaques of psoriasis vulgaris may develop pustules, especially after excessively irritant topical therapy.

Erythrodermic Psoriasis

Erythrodermic psoriasis presents as generalized erythema, pain, itching and fine scaling; various pustular forms also exist. It typically encompasses nearly the entire BSA (**Figs. 35 to 45**).

It may be accompanied by fever, chills, hypothermia and dehydration, secondary to the large BSA involvement. Patients with severe pustular or erythrodermic psoriasis may require hospital admission for metabolic and pain management. Older patients with erythrodermic psoriasis may experience cardiac instability and hypotension due to massive vascular shunting in the skin.

Pedal edema, especially around the ankles, may also develop along with infection. Disruption in the thermoregulatory mechanism leads to shivering episodes. Infection, pneumonia and congestive heart failure brought on by erythrodermic psoriasis can be life threatening.

Erythrodermic psoriasis is a particularly inflammatory form of psoriasis that often affects most of the body surface. It generally appears on people who have unstable plaque psoriasis where lesions are not clearly defined. It is characterized by periodicity and widespread and fiery redness of the skin. Histopathological confirmation to establish the cause of erythroderma as psoriasis is not always possible during the acute stages. When the patient presents with erythroderma for the first time without a definite history of psoriasis, one has to wait for the acute phase to settle to establish the diagnosis. Systemic steroids should be used with extreme caution in such case.

Erythrodermic psoriasis in children: Erythrodermic psoriasis is a rare clinical presentation in childhood psoriasis. It may arise from any type, commonly from the plaque type. It may arise from any type of psoriasis. Drugs, environmental, psychological and metabolic factors can trigger the onset

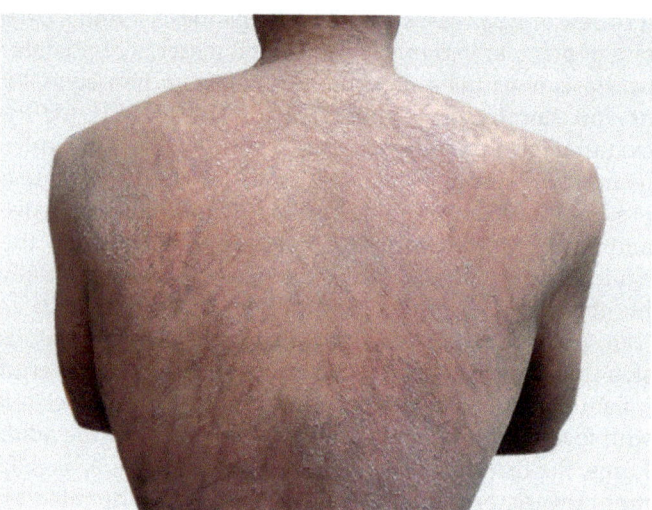

Fig. 35: Erythrodermic psoriasis in a college student.

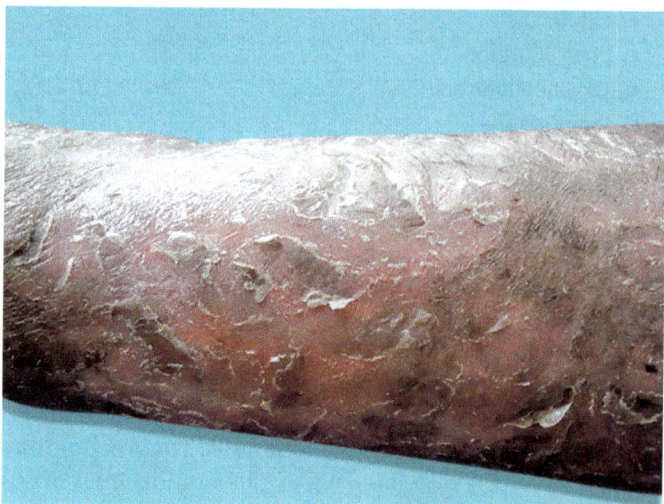

Fig. 37: Closer view of scaling and erythema of erythrodermic psoriasis.

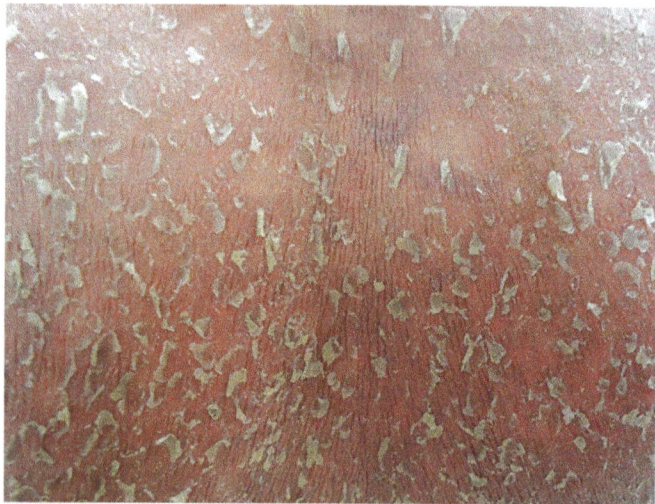

Fig. 36: Note crimson red erythema of psoriatic erythroderma.

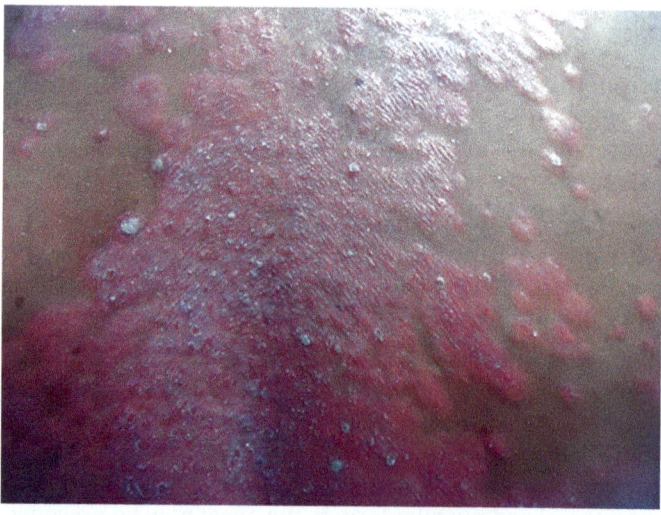

Fig. 38: Plaque psoriasis evolving into erythroderma.

CHAPTER 4 Clinical Aspects

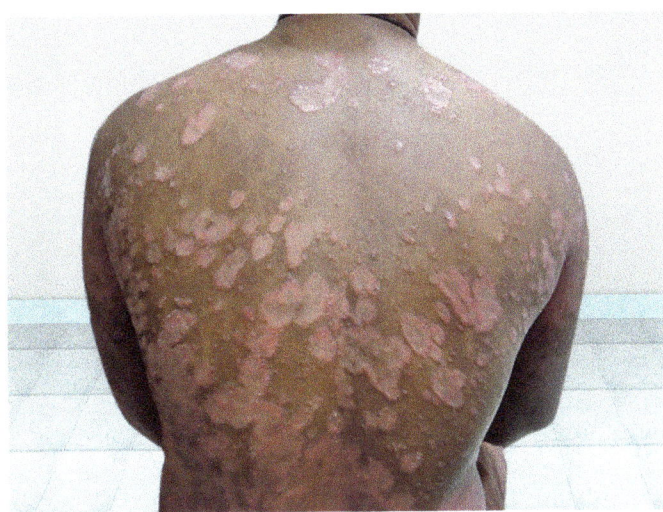

Fig. 39: Psoriasis starting as guttate lesion progressing to plaque type and rapidly evolving to erythroderma—an unstable form of psoriasis.

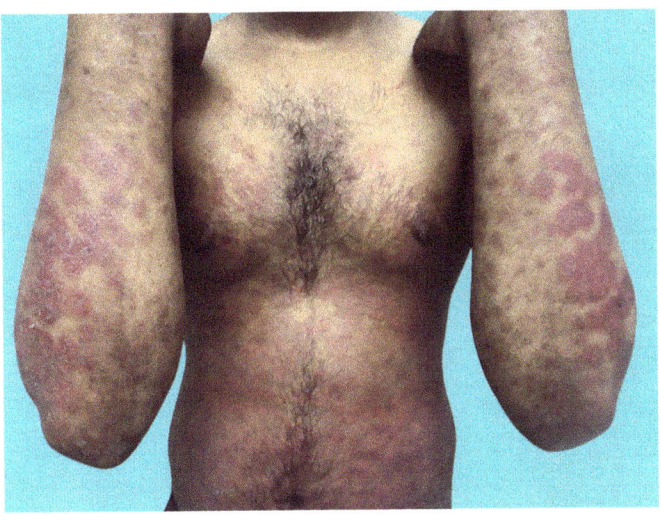

Fig. 42: Large easily removable scales with intense erythema in erythrodermic psoriasis.

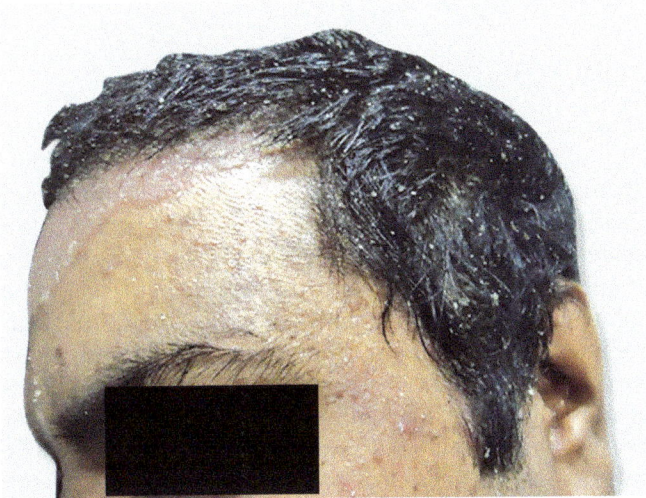

Fig. 40: Note involvement of scalp in erythrodermic psoriasis.

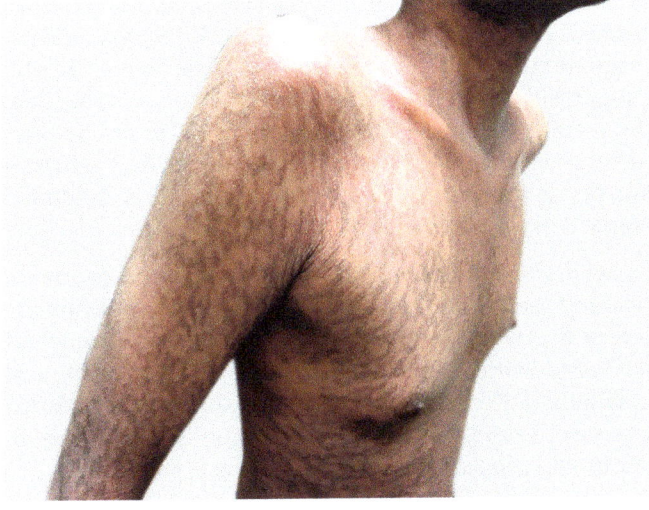

Fig. 43: Erythrodermic psoriasis recalcitrant to treatment.

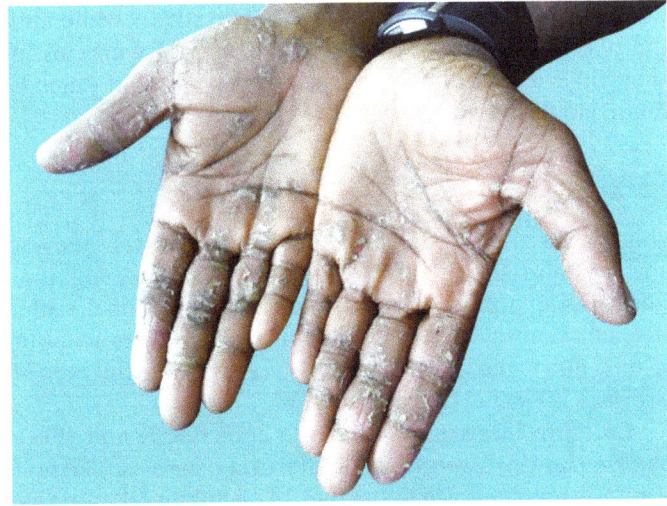

Fig. 41: Involvement of palm in erythrodermic psoriasis.

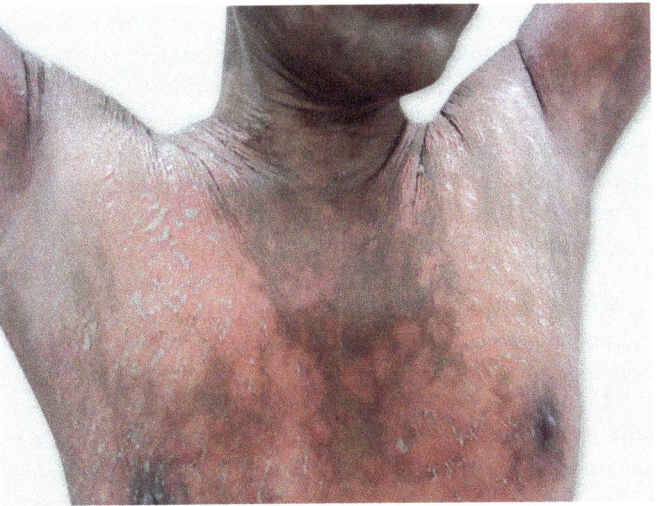

Fig. 44: Psoriatic erythroderma with relative sparing of the face and sun exposed skin.

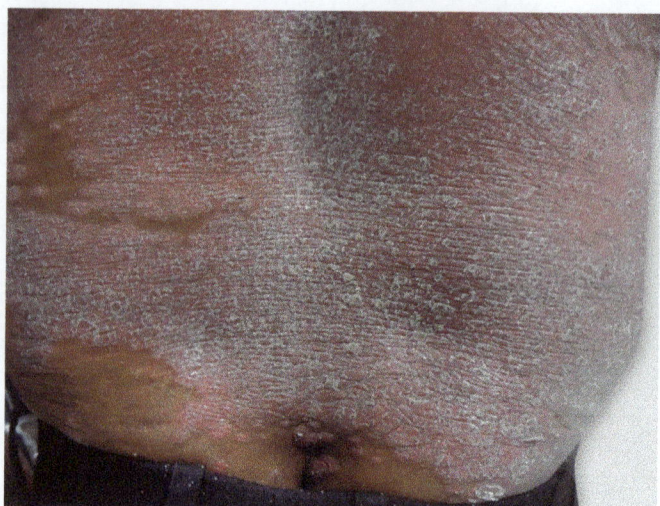

Fig. 45: Erythrodermic psoriasis with guarded prognosis.

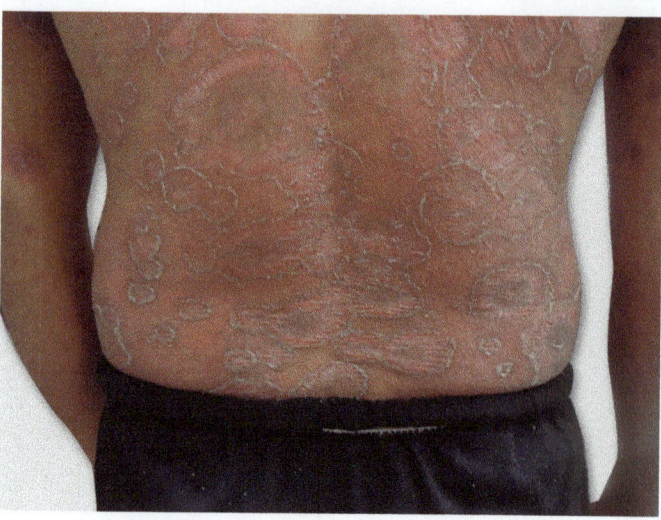

Fig. 46: Unstable psoriasis; note the fiery red erythema.

of erythrodermic form of the disease. This spectrum of psoriasis is characterized by generalized erythema, edema, desquamation and systemic compromise. The child will present with fever, dehydration, malaise and malnutrition. The overall presentation can range from mild to severe form. The erythrodermic form occurs in about 1.4% of psoriasis cases in children and adolescents. Overall, <3% of childhood psoriasis manifests with erythrodermat.

Congenital erythrodermic psoriasis: Congenital psoriasis, meaning psoriasis present at birth or appearing during the neonatal period is exceptional. Congenital occurrence of psoriasis, defined as the development of any of its clinical variants at birth or during very first days of life, is considered very rare. Clinicopathologic correlation is mandatory in confirming congenital erythroderma due to psoriasis.

Unstable Psoriasis

Unstable psoriasis is a dermatological emergency. People with stable chronic plaque psoriasis may suddenly progress to unstable psoriasis. It also involves forms like the erythrodermic form and the pustular form that can rapidly progress and cause dangerous or even fatal medical complications, even death. The erythema and scaling of the skin are often accompanied by severe itching and pain. Erythrodermic psoriasis is a particularly inflammatory form of psoriasis that often affects most of the body surface. When it appears on people who have unstable plaque psoriasis, where lesions are not clearly defined, it is characterized by periodicity and widespread and fiery redness of the skin **(Fig. 46)**.

Such erythrodermic psoriasis "throws off" the body chemistry causing protein and fluid loss that can lead to severe illness. Common triggers include infections, drugs, alcohol and abrupt cessation of steroids. The course of disease is unpredictable and the condition is a medical emergency and will require inpatient multidisciplinary care.

Site of Involvement

Scalp Psoriasis

Scalp psoriasis affects approximately 50% of patients. Scalp is the commonest site involved both in children and adults. Itching and hair loss are common symptoms though not a feature seen in all. Scalp can be involved either as an isolated site of affection or as part of plaque type psoriasis, pustular psoriasis and erythrodermic psoriasis. The scaling and erythema typically transgress the frontal hair line feature that helps in differentiating from seborrheic dermatitis. Circumscribed scaly plaques are sometimes the only presentation. Plaque of pityriasis amiantacea over the scalp is characterized by the presence of asbestos-like scales. Localized hair loss can be seen in children with pityriasis amiantacea. There can be diffuse hair loss in those with erythrodermic psoriasis. It presents as erythematous raised plaques with silvery white scale, often mistaken for seborrheic dermatitis. The scales are slivery white and the plaque extends beyond the hair margin where as in seborrheic dermatitis, the scales are greasy and the patch is limited to the hair bearing area **(Figs. 47 to 52)**.

Flexural Psoriasis/Inverse Psoriasis

This is a variant of psoriasis that spares the typical extensor surfaces and affects intertriginous (i.e., axillae, inguinal folds, inframammary creases) areas with minimal scale. It is characterized by smooth, inflamed lesions without scaling due to the moist nature of the area where this type of psoriasis is located **(Figs. 53 to 56)**.

Candida intertrigo should be considered and there can be candida overgrowth in flexural psoriasis. Flexural psoriasis was observed in nearly 10% of childhood psoriasis. Localization of erythematous, sometimes macerated thick plaques to the folds of the skin, including axillae and groin,

CHAPTER 4 Clinical Aspects

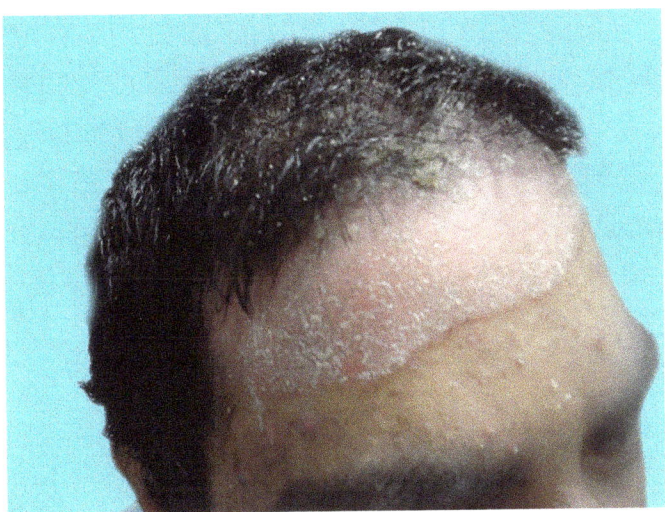

Fig. 47: Scalp psoriasis showing psoriatic corona.

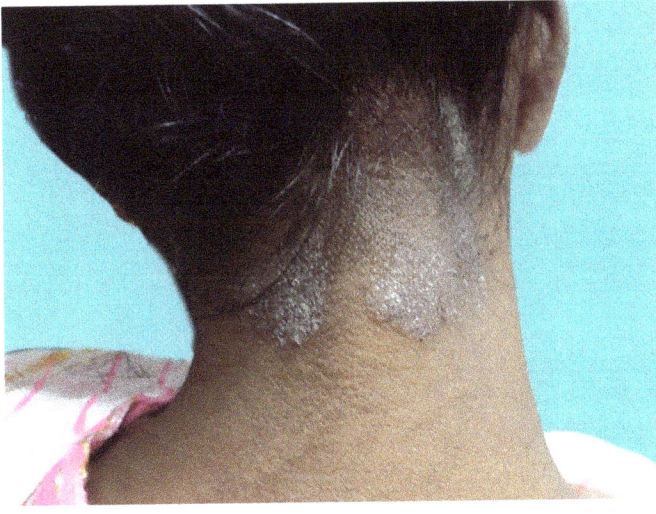

Fig. 50: Scalp psoriasis mimicking lichen simplex chronicus.

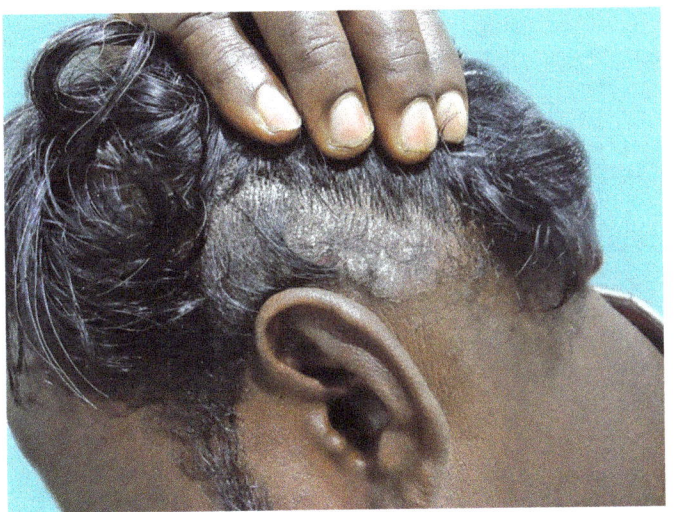

Fig. 48: Scalp psoriasis showing Auspitz sign.

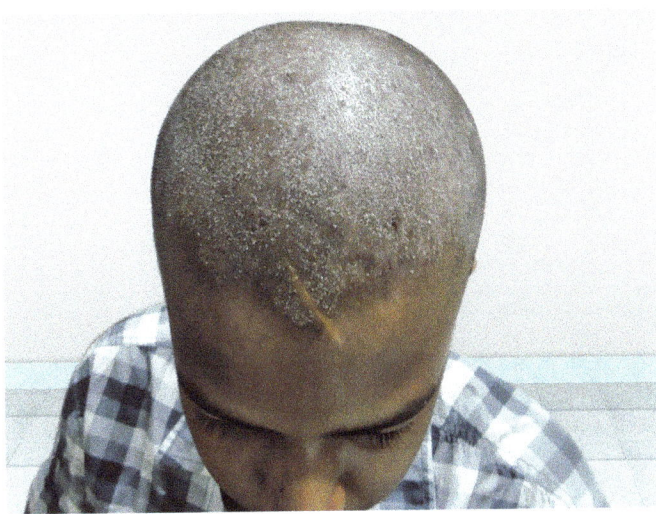

Fig. 51: Psoriasis of the scalp mimicking seborrheic dermatitis. Note the silvery white dry scale as against greasy scales of seborrheic dermatitis.

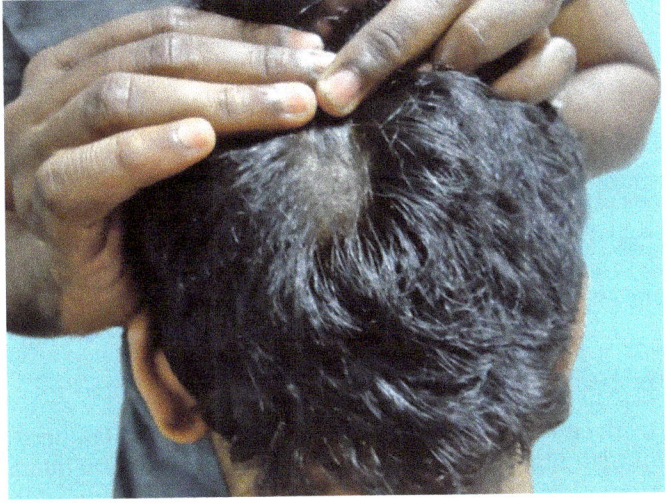

Fig. 49: Scalp psoriasis which can be easily missed as seborrheic dermatitis in a hairy scalp if thorough examination is not carried out.

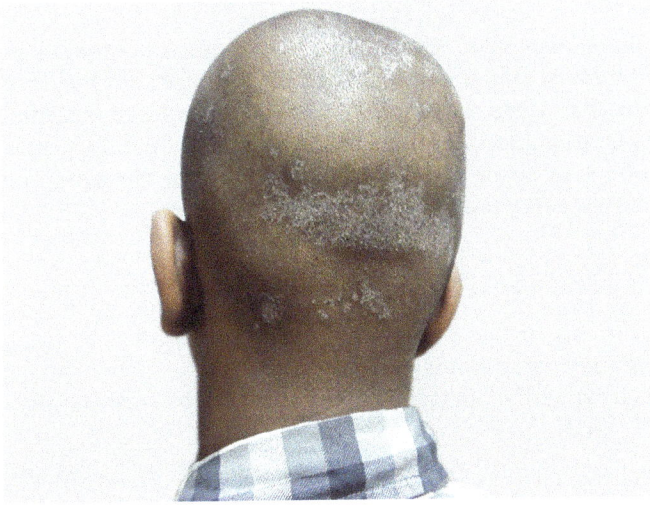

Fig. 52: Posterior view of patient in **Figure 51**.

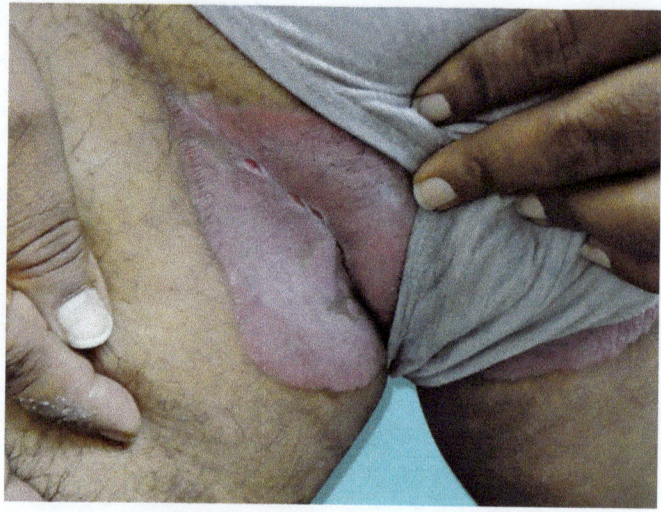

Fig. 53: Note the sharply marginated erythema with deep fissures in flexural psoriasis; candidal infection should be ruled out.

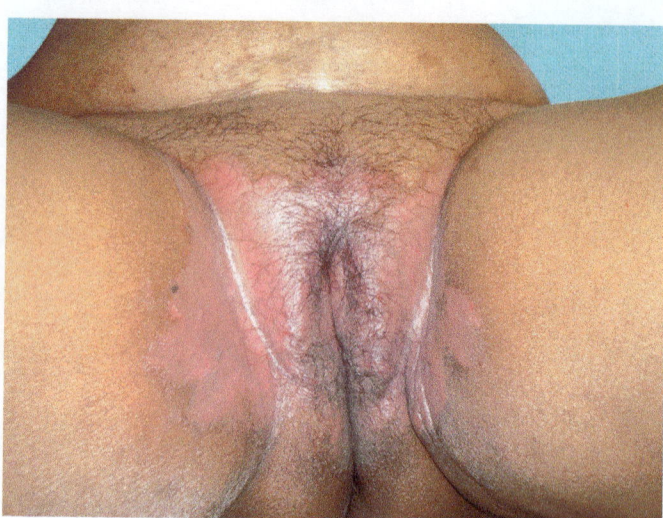

Fig. 55: Flexural psoriasis—female.

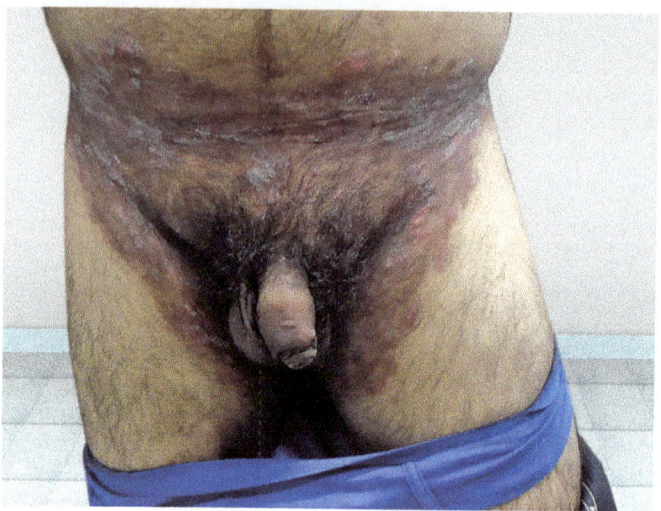

Fig. 54: Flexural psoriasis—male.

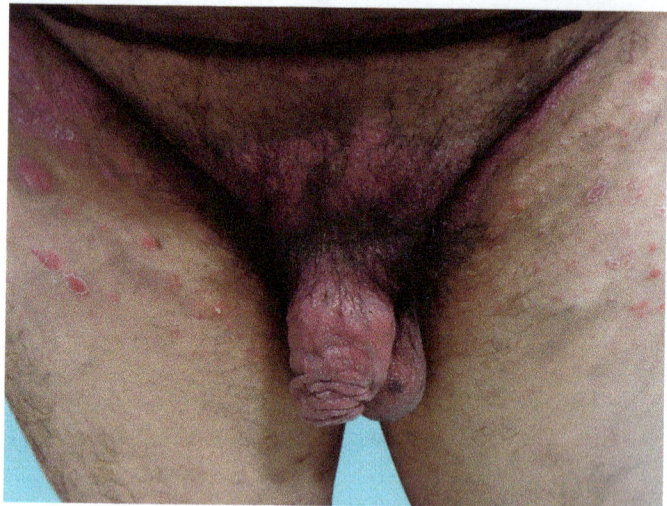

Fig. 56: Flexural psoriasis with psoriasis vulgaris.

can be associated with plaque type psoriasis in other sites. In infants, diaper dermatitis may be mistaken for psoriasis and vice versa. Dissemination with widespread eruption of erythemato squamous lesions on the whole body may follow. In obese adults, flexural psoriasis of the groin and axilla is easily mistaken for candida intertrigo.

Palmoplantar Psoriasis

Psoriasis of the palms and soles can manifest in three different ways, namely:
1. Typical scaly red patches similar to psoriasis elsewhere
2. Generalized thickening and scaling of the palms and soles (keratoderma)
3. Sheets of tiny yellow-brown pustules (PPP).

Palmoplantar psoriasis tends to be a chronic recurrent condition. In many patients, palmoplantar psoriasis is a painful condition, limiting day-to-day activities, resulting in poor job performance.

Palmoplantar psoriasis, the one with highest discomfort, was observed in about 12.8% of children with psoriasis in an Indian study. Tinea pedes, eczema and keratoderma due to other causes are to be excluded before contemplating antimitotic agents as treatment **(Figs. 57 to 70)**.

Mucosal Psoriasis

Involvement of mucosa is seen in up to 7% of children. Annular plaques on the tongue may be noted in patients with psoriasis. Geographic tongue is a common presentation of pustular psoriasis **(Fig. 71)**.

CHAPTER 4 Clinical Aspects

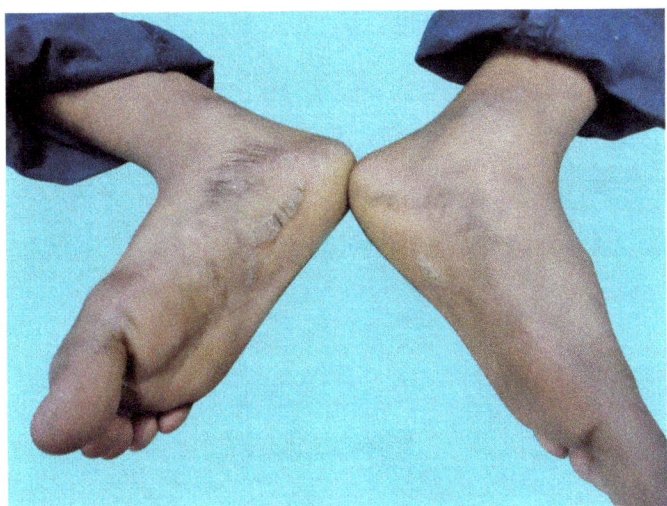

Fig. 57: Early stage of palmoplantar psoriasis.

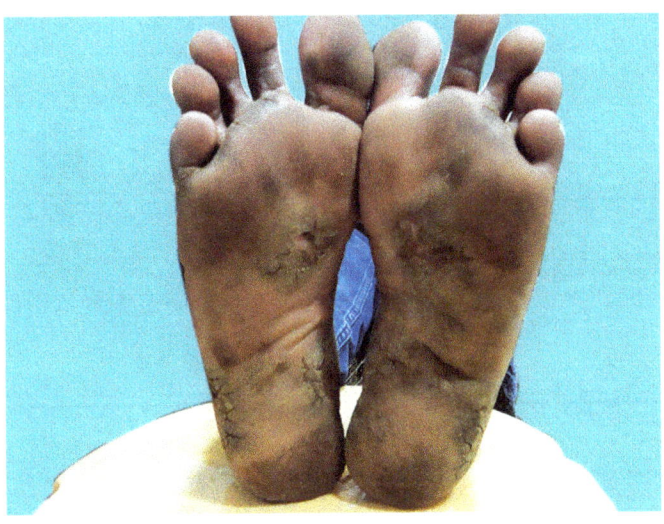

Fig. 60: Palmoplantar psoriasis affecting the instep and the heel. This type will need systemic therapy, even if there are no lesions elsewhere.

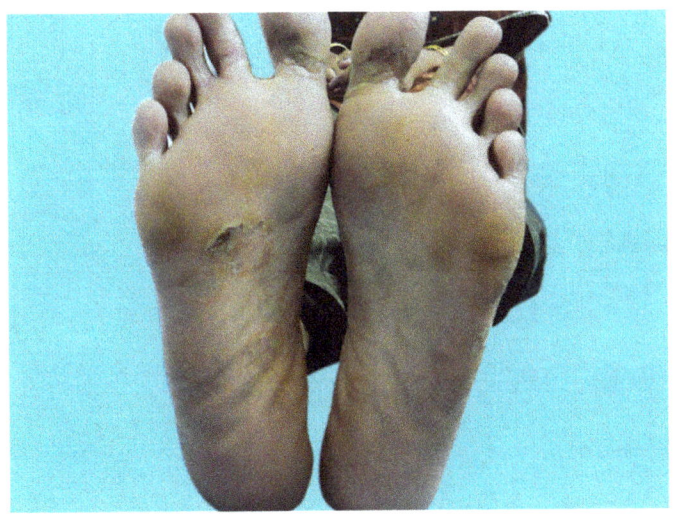

Fig. 58: Palmoplantar psoriasis.

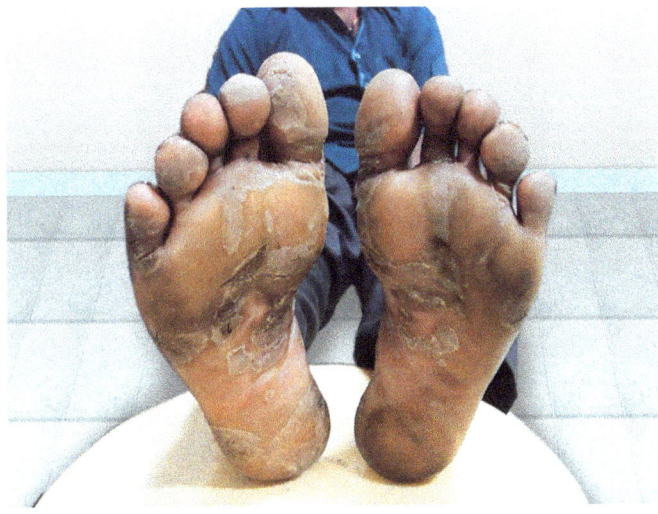

Fig. 61: Palmoplantar psoriasis affecting the entire sole.

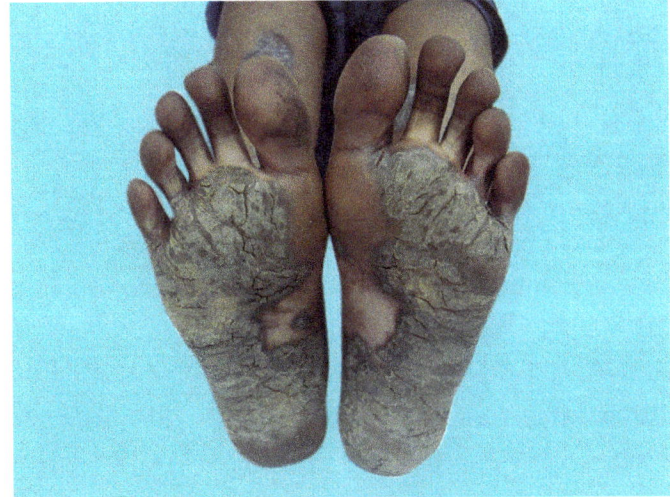

Fig. 59: Palmoplantar psoriasis—severe form.

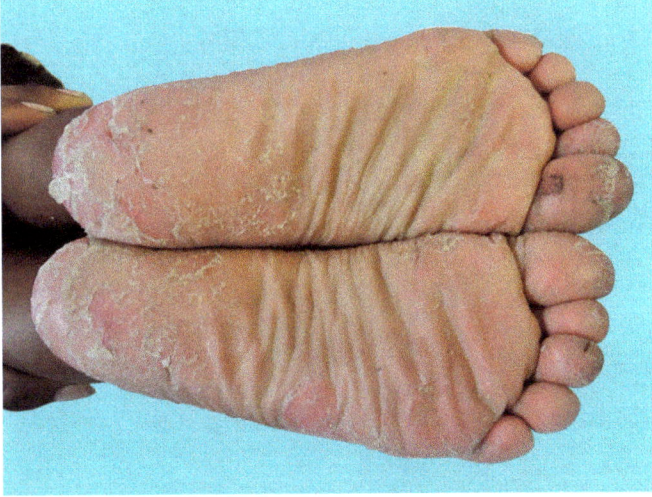

Fig. 62: Palmoplantar psoriasis mimicking tinea pedes.

CHAPTER 4 Clinical Aspects

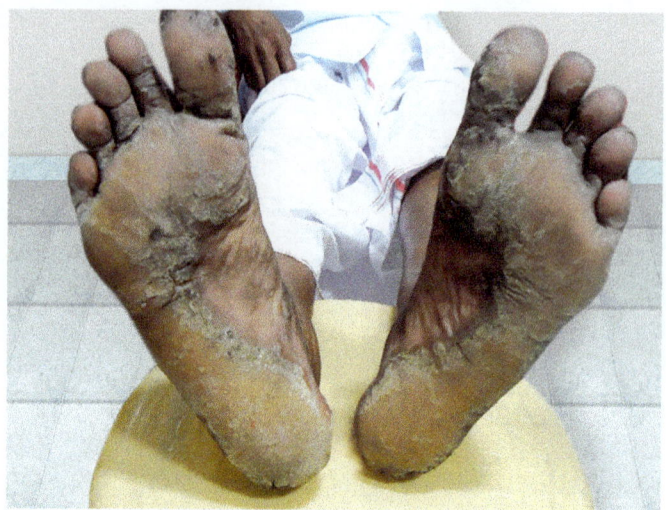

Fig. 63: Palmoplantar psoriasis sparing the instep.

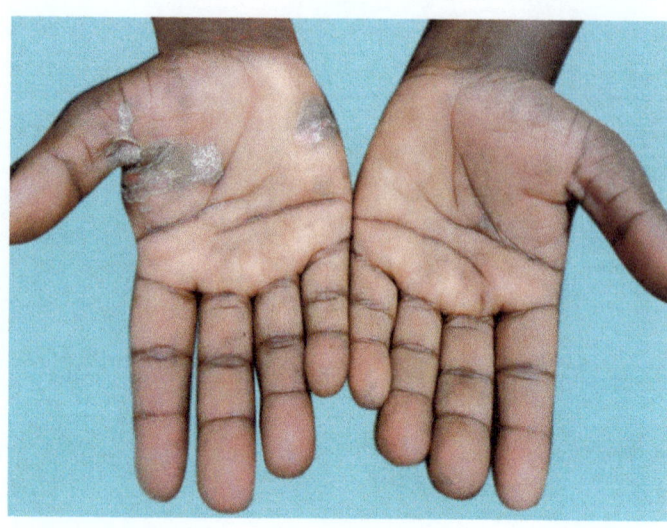

Fig. 66: Psoriasis of the palm—classical plaque with fissuring and scaling.

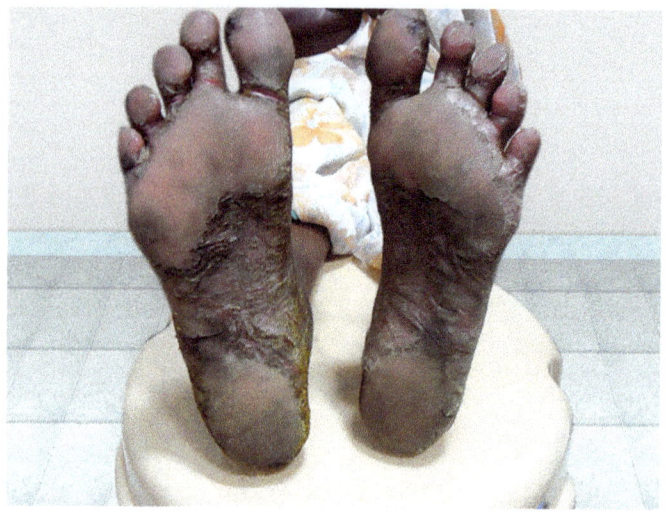

Fig. 64: Palmoplantar psoriasis with clean deep fissures in an agricultural worker.

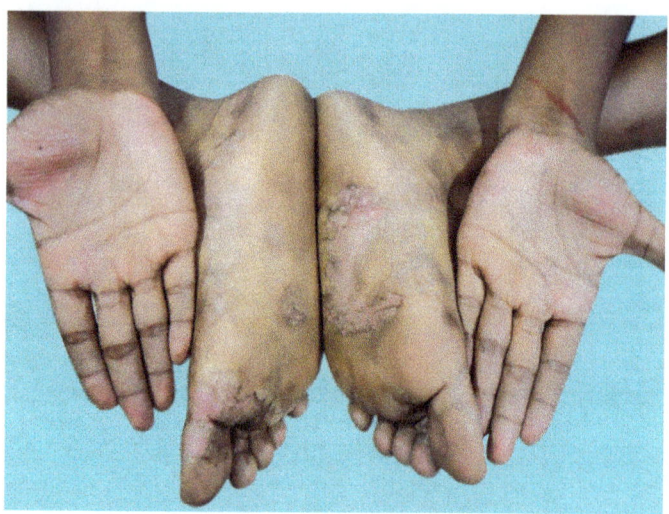

Fig. 67: Psoriasis of the palms and soles.

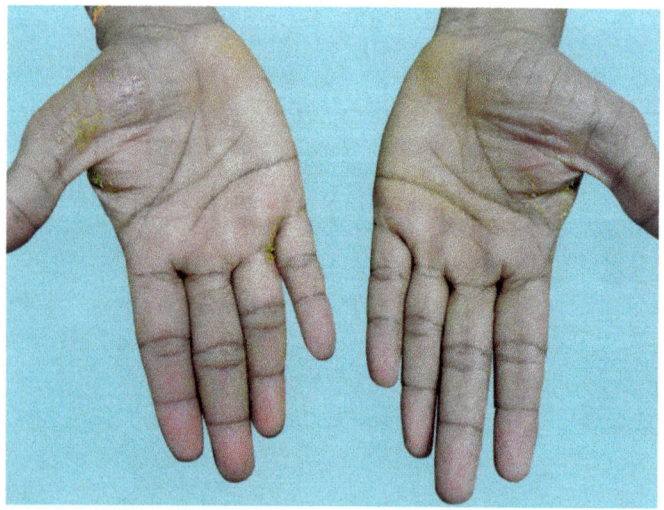

Fig. 65: Psoriasis of the palm—mild form.

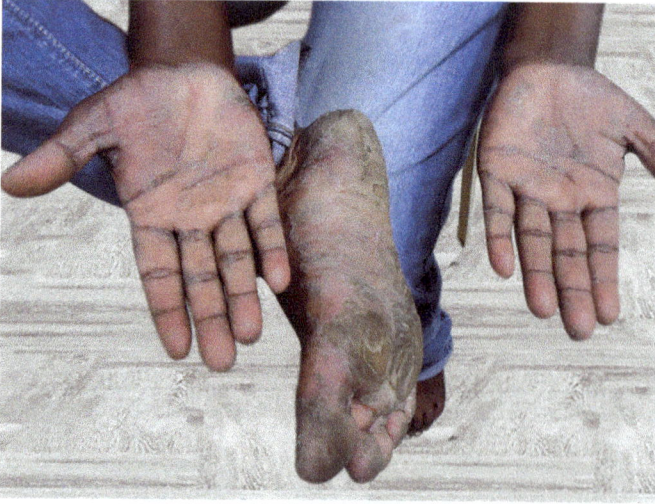

Fig. 68: Psoriasis of the palms and soles severe form warranting photo or systemic therapy.

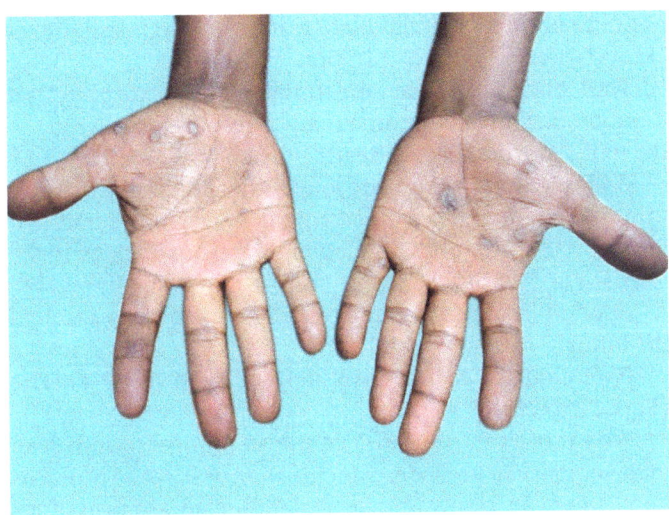

Fig. 69: Psoriasis mimicking secondary syphilis.

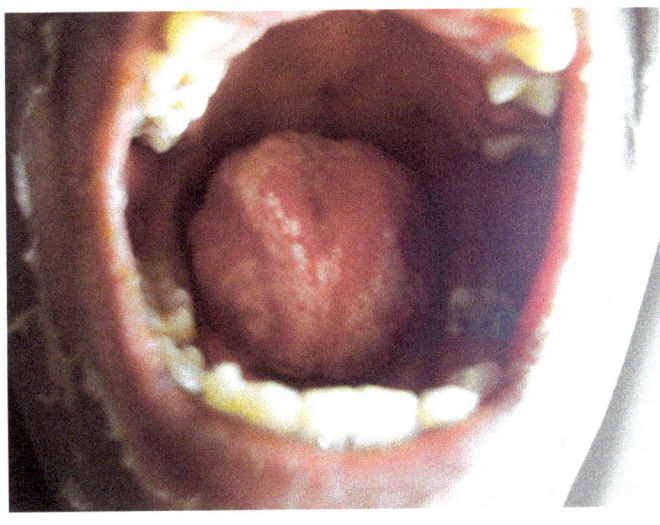

Fig. 71: Geographic tongue as oral mucosal involvement in psoriasis.

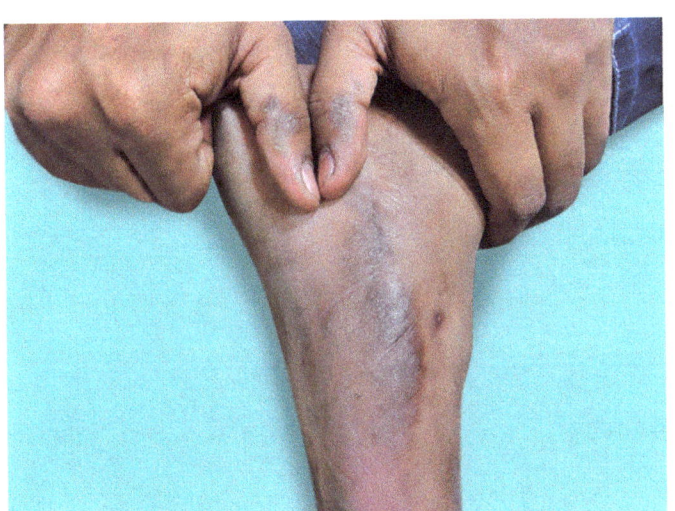

Fig. 70: Psoriasis resembling eczema.

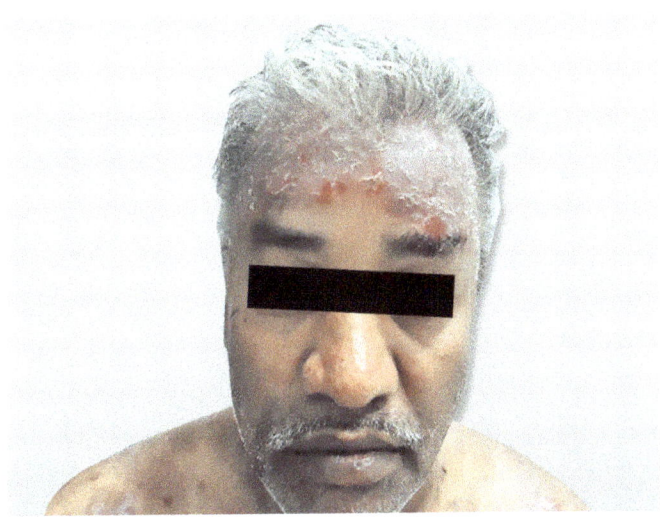

Fig. 72: Ocular manifestation in unstable psoriasis.

Fissured tongue is yet another manifestation of pustular psoriasis.

Ocular Psoriasis (Eye Involvement)

Ocular symptoms may occur in approximately 10% of psoriasis patients **(Fig. 72)**.

Ocular involvement is more common in men than in women. It is rare to have involvement of the eye prior to skin involvement of psoriasis. The incidence of ocular psoriasis can vary widely and may include such ocular conditions as, xerosis, symblepharon, trichiasis, blepharitis, conjunctivitis, uveitis and iritis, as well as reported cases of secondary corneal involvement resulting in keratitis. Chronic uveitis has been found,[36] particularly in patients with PsA. Eye problems may be directly related to flare-ups around the eyes or due to the disease affecting the eye, which can also lead to problems within the eye itself that when left untreated, can cause permanent vision loss. Psoriasis has early and extensive ocular involvement, sometimes earlier than joints.

Nail Psoriasis

The clinical findings associated with psoriatic nail disease correlate with the anatomical location of the nail unit that is affected by the disease **(Box 5)**.

Oil drop or salmon patch of the nail bed is a translucent, yellow-red discoloration in the nail bed resembling a drop of oil beneath the nail plate. This patch is the most diagnostic sign of nail psoriasis.

Pitting is a result of the loss of parakeratotic cells from the surface of the nail plate.

Beau's lines are transverse lines in the nails due to intermittent inflammation causing growth arrest lines.

Leukonychia or white nail plate is due to foci of parakeratosis within the body of the nail plate.

Subungual hyperkeratosis affects the nail bed and the hyponychium. Excessive proliferation of the nail bed can lead to onycholysis.

Onycholysis is functional distal separation of the nail plate from its underlying nail bed. It causes traumatic uplifting of the distal nail plate leading to the possibility of secondary microbial colonization.

Nail plate may become, thickened, dystrophic and discolored. Nail plate crumbling is a result of weakening of the nail plate, due to disease process.

Splinter hemorrhages are longitudinal black lines due to minute foci of capillary hemorrhage between the nail bed and the nail plate. This is analogous to the Auspitz sign in the skin.

Spotted lunula is nothing but an erythematous patch of the lunula.

Nail changes in psoriasis may be seen in up to 40% **(Figs. 73 to 79)**.

Nail pitting is the most common manifestation. Nail involvement can precede, coincide with, or succeed psoriasis and may even rarely appear isolated. Nail abnormalities are more frequent in PsA and in digital skin involvement. Psoriasis of the nails occurs in about three quarters of psoriatic patients with arthritis, but only in about one-third of those with skin lesions alone.

> **BOX 5: Nail involvement in psoriasis corresponding to anatomical site.**
>
> - *Oil drop sign*: Nail bed
> - *Pitting, beau lines*: Proximal nail matrix
> - *Leukonychia*: Mid-matrix
> - *Subungual hyperkeratosis*: Hyponychium
> - *Onycholysis*: Nail bed and nail hyponychium
> - *Dystrophy, crumbling*: Nail plate
> - *Splinter hemorrhage*: Papillary capillary
> - *Spotted lunula*: Distal matrix

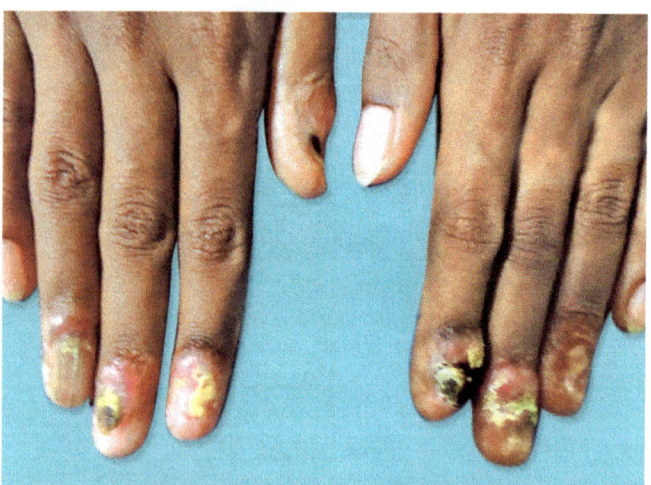

Fig. 73: Nail involvement in psoriasis showing frequent changes—pitting, yellow discoloration, subungual keratosis and onycholysis.

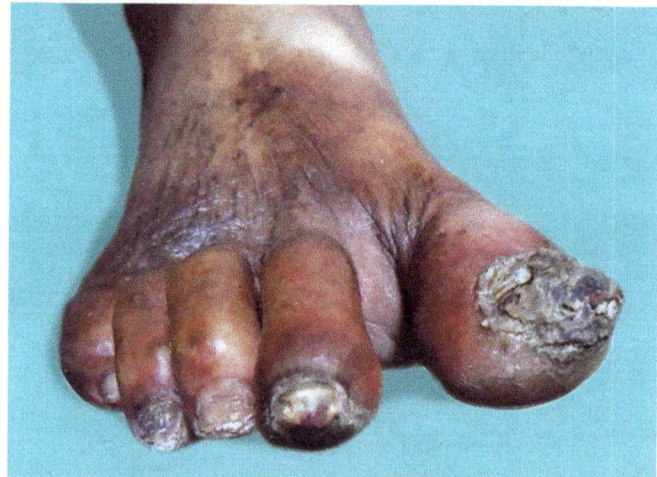

Fig. 75: Severe involvement of nail in psoriasis.

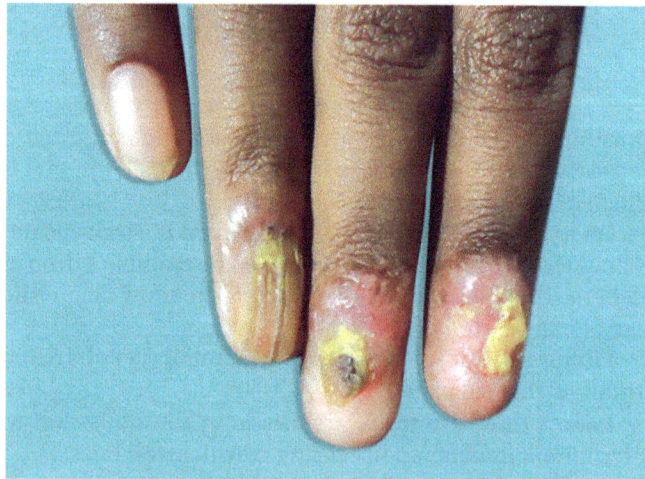

Fig. 74: Note the yellowish discoloration and subungual hyperkeratosis and the normal little finger nail.

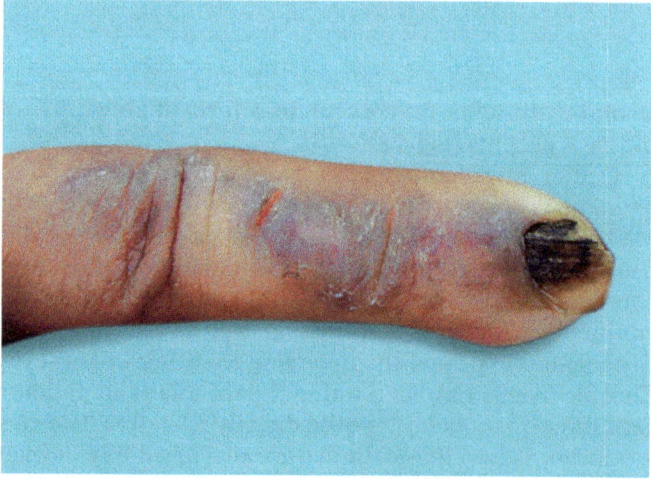

Fig. 76: Nail dystrophy in psoriasis; note the linear plaque that simulates lichen planus.

CHAPTER 4 Clinical Aspects

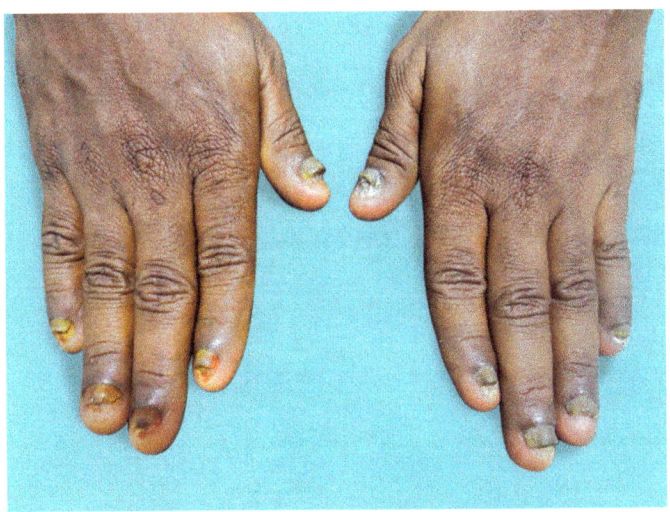

Fig. 77: Psoriasis nail with onychomycosis.

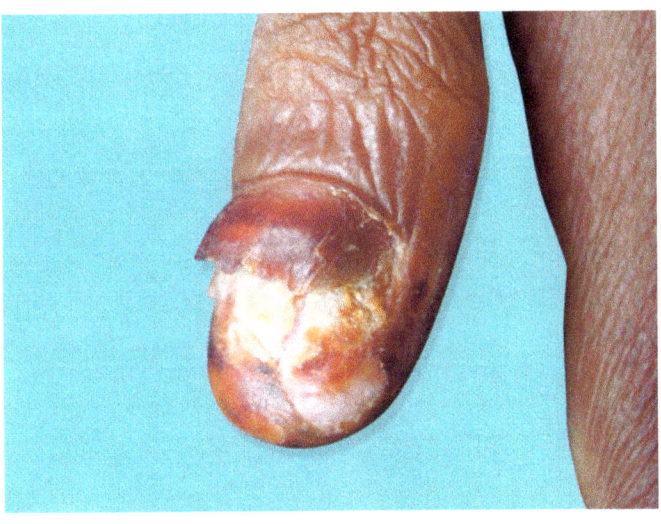

Fig. 79: Nail dystrophy in pustular psoriasis.

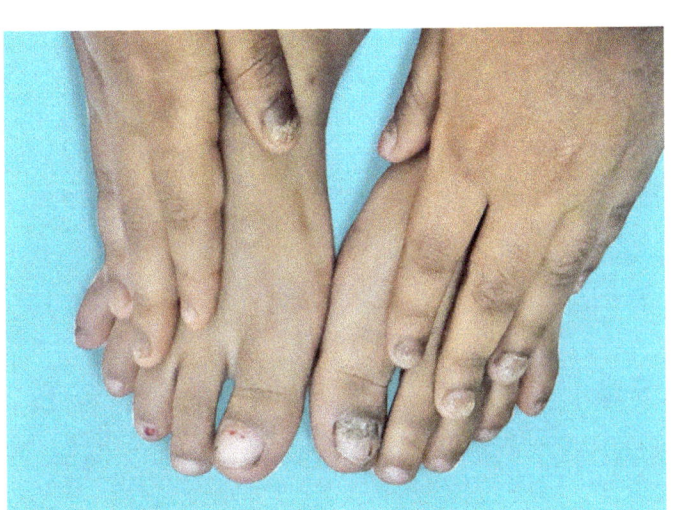

Fig. 78: Twenty nail dystrophy in psoriasis.

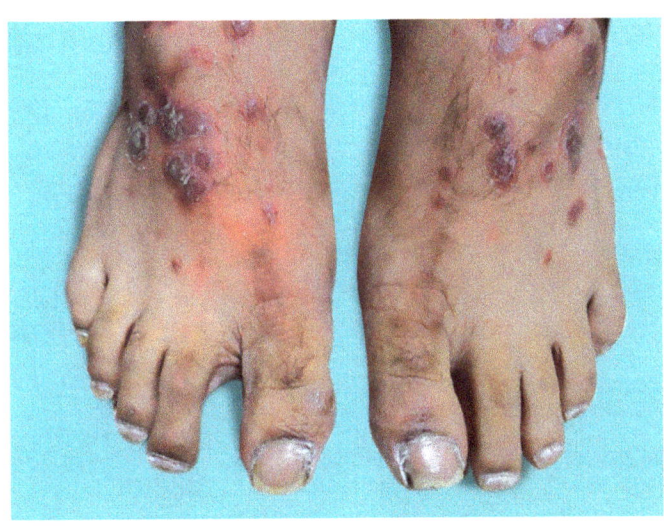

Fig. 80: Note the nail changes. This patient subsequently developed psoriatic arthropathy.

Arthropathic Psoriasis

Arthropathic psoriasis/PsA is an inflammatory "entheso-arthro-osteopathy" occurring in subjects with psoriasis or with a predisposition to psoriasis. It may involve peripheral and/or axial osteoarticular compartments and may be responsible for extra-articular manifestations. PsA develops in at least 5% of patients and is most commonly a seronegative oligoarthritis with less common but characteristic differentiating features of distal joint involvement and arthritis mutilans. Nearly half of patients with PsA have evidence of spondyloarthropathy and human leukocyte antigen B27 (HLA-B27) associated. Hence, it can be classified among the seronegative spondyloarthropathy. Peripheral joint disease occurs in 95% of patients with PsA, while in the other 5%, axial spine involvement occurs exclusively.

Up to 30% of people with psoriasis also develop PsA (**Figs. 80 to 88**).

In most cases, skin disease precedes joint affection, sometimes by many years. When arthritis symptoms occur with psoriasis, it is called PsA. About 20% of people who develop PsA will eventually have spinal involvement which is called psoriatic spondylitis. The inflammation in the spine can lead to complete fusion—as in ankylosing spondylitis—or skip areas where, e.g., only the lower back and neck are involved. Those with spinal involvement are most likely to test positive for the HLA-B27 genetic marker.

The correlation between severity of skin psoriasis and arthropathic involvement has not been consistent. Nor does the severity of the psoriasis relate to the pattern of joint involvement. But it is consistently reported that pustular psoriasis patients are more prone for joint involvement.

Onset of PsA in old age has a more severe onset and a more destructive outcome than PsA that affects younger subjects. The course of PsA is usually characterized by flares and remissions. Skin lesions were found to precede arthritis in nearly two-thirds of patients, arthritis antedated skin lesions in one-fifth and in nearly 16% skin and joint

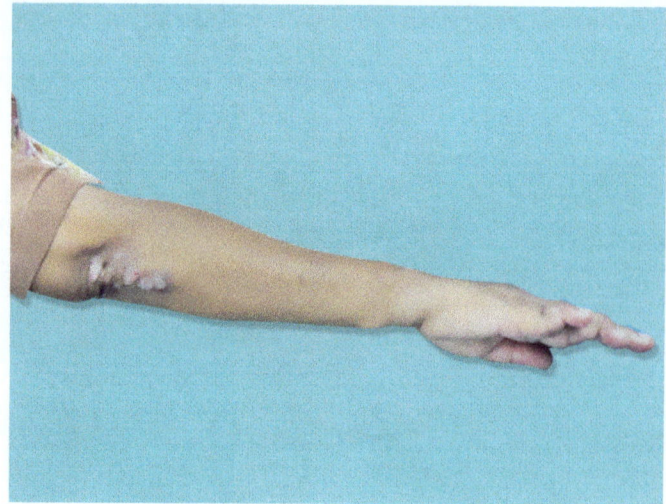

Fig. 81: Showing oligoarthritis.

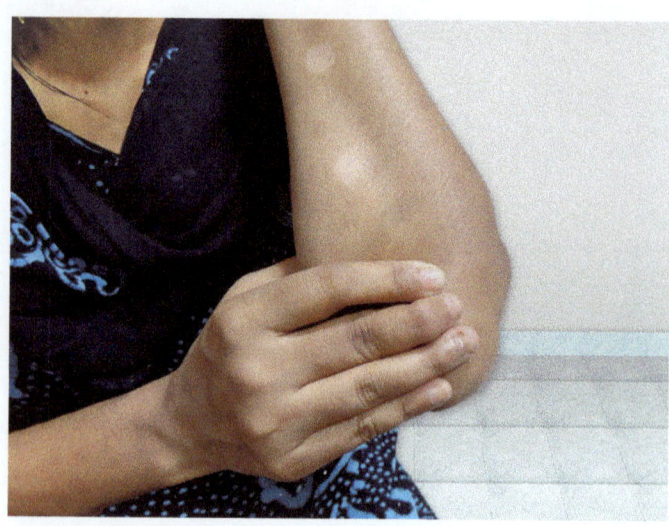

Fig. 84: This patient also had sacroiliitis.

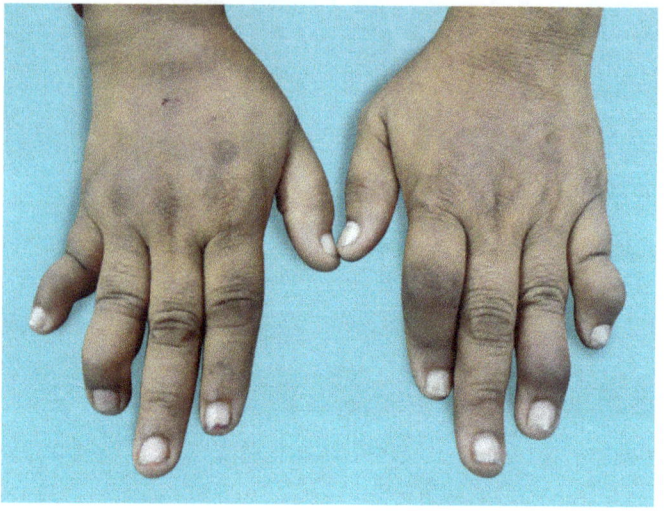

Fig. 82: Symmetrical arthropathy in a patient with no skin lesions of psoriasis.

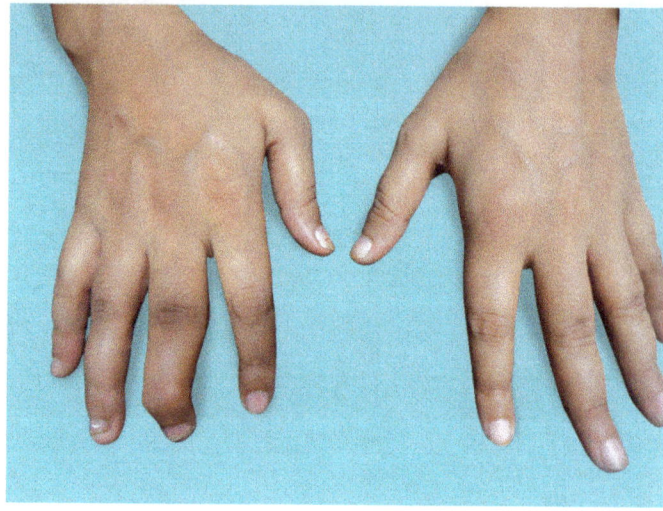

Fig. 85: Same patient as in **Figure 84** with asymmetrical psoriatic arthritis.

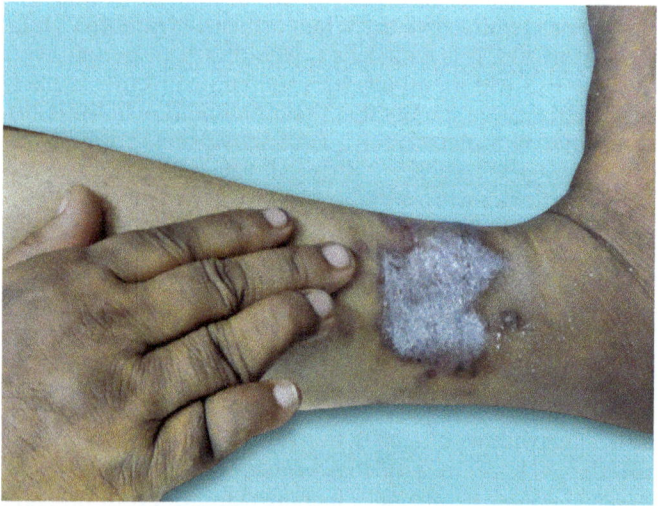

Fig. 83: Symmetrical arthropathy.

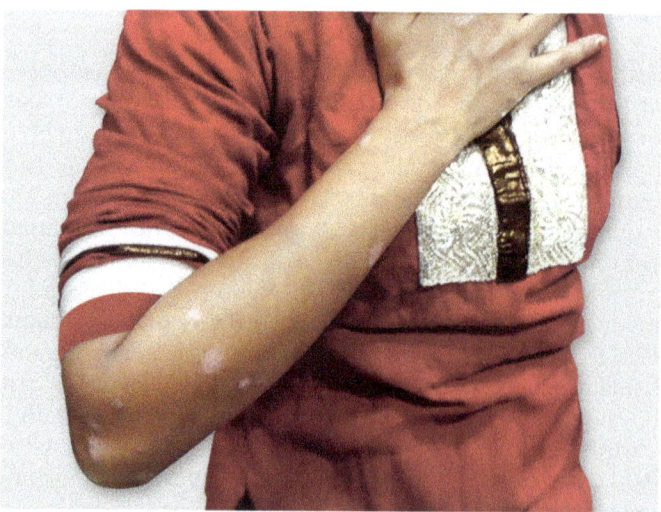

Fig. 86: Note the fusiform swelling. She was seronegative with a positive family history.

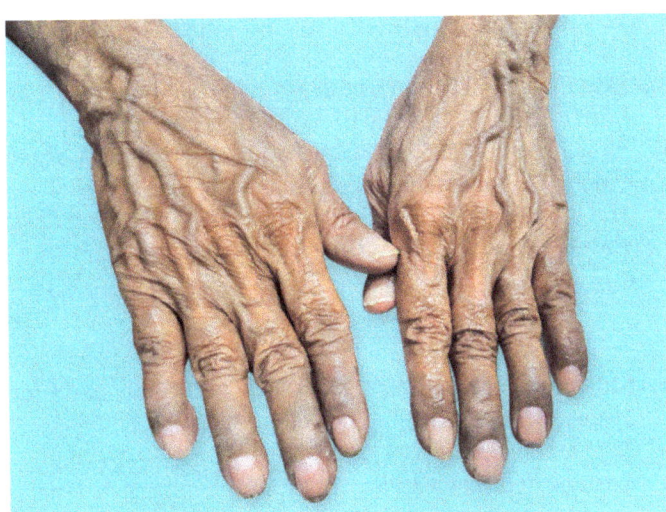

Fig. 87: Involvement of both peripheral and axial joints.

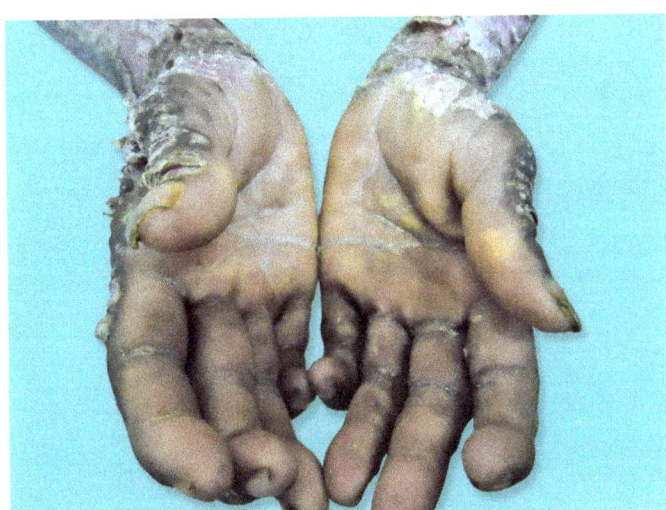

Fig. 88: Pustular psoriasis with arthropathy.

involvement occurred almost simultaneously. The peak age of onset of arthritis in this series was 40–60 years.

The patterns of PsA involvement are as follows:
- Asymmetrical oligoarticular arthritis
- Symmetrical polyarthritis
- Distal interphalangeal arthropathy
- Arthritis mutilans
- Spondylitis with or without sacroiliitis.

Arthritis mutilans is the least common but most severe type of psoriasis, occurring in about 5% patients with PsA. This form of the disease results in widespread destruction of the joints. When this affects the hands, it can cause a phenomenon sometimes referred to as "telescoping fingers." Similar changes can occur in the feet.

For a simpler approach, PsA can be classified into three main groups:
1. Asymmetrical arthritis, usually, but not always involving a small number of joints with few erosions, infrequent deformity and good preservation of function.
2. Symmetrical polyarthritis, frequently erosive, deforming and functionally disabling but distinguished from rheumatoid arthritis by association with distal interphalangeal joint involvement, spondylitis and negative rheumatoid factor (RF) (titer < 1:80).
3. Predominant spondylitis, similar to ankylosing spondylitis, possibly accompanied by peripheral arthritis but behaving independently of it.

Cervical spine, temporomandibular joint, sternal joint are other rare joints involved in psoriasis. Extra-articular features like subcutaneous nodule, as in rheumatoid arthritis, are not seen in PsA. In contrast, inflammatory eye lesions like Reiter's disease and cardiac involvement similar to that seen in ankylosing spondylitis has been reported.

The Classification Criteria for Psoriatic Arthritis (CASPAR) consist of established inflammatory articular disease with at least 3 points from the following features:

Current psoriasis: 2
A history of psoriasis (in the absence of current psoriasis): 1
Family history of psoriasis (in the absence of current or history of psoriasis): 1

Dactylitis: 1
Juxta-articular new bone formation: 1
RF negativity: 1
Nail dystrophy: 1

Arthropathic psoriasis in children: Psoriatic arthritis is relatively uncommon in children; it may occur with either plaque or guttate psoriasis and may precede skin involvement. The estimated prevalence of PsA in all patients with psoriasis differs from 5 to 30%.[37,38] The age of onset of findings in childhood ranges from 9 to 12 years of age.

Based on Disease Manifestation

Based on disease manifestation, psoriasis can be graded in order to select or modify therapy and for assessing the disease outcome. This working classification of psoriasis into six stages of clinical presentation will help both the clinician and the patient well informed of the disease status, which will enable planned investigations and treatment, effectively **(Box 6)**.[39,40]

> **BOX 6: Classification of psoriasis based on disease manifestation.**
>
> *Based on disease manifestation:*
> - Latent psoriasis
> - Mild psoriasis
> - Moderate psoriasis
> - Moderate-to-severe psoriasis
> - Severe psoriasis
> - Psoriasis with guarded prognosis

Latent Psoriasis

- In-remission and minimal psoriasis
- Stable remission with no psoriatic lesions
- Signs of borderline psoriasis (e.g., nail pitting, severe dandruff)
- A few isolated lesions negligible to patient.

Mild Psoriasis (Fig. 89)

- Involving <10% of BSA
- Surface area (or PASI <10)
- Good control of lesions with topical therapy.

Moderate Psoriasis (Figs. 90 and 91)

- Skin involvement >10% of BSA
- Topical therapy still possible without having the need for systemic therapy.

Moderate-to-severe Psoriasis (Figs. 92 to 94)

- Skin involvement >10% of BSA
- Surface area and topical therapy fail to control disease
- Skin involvement <10% but lesions in difficult areas (such as involvement of face, hands, or feet)
- Having distressing/disabling effects incapacitating daily routine/day-to-day work.

Severe Psoriasis (Figs. 95 and 96)

- Skin involvement >20% (or PASI > 20) with need for systemic treatment
- Skin involvement (10–20%)
- Lesions in difficult areas
- Distressing/disabling effects
- Unstable psoriasis
- PsA.

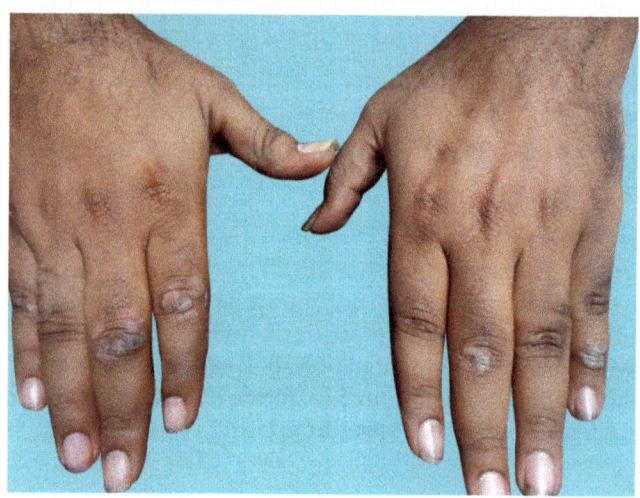

Fig. 89: Mild psoriasis with <10% body surface area (BSA) involvement.

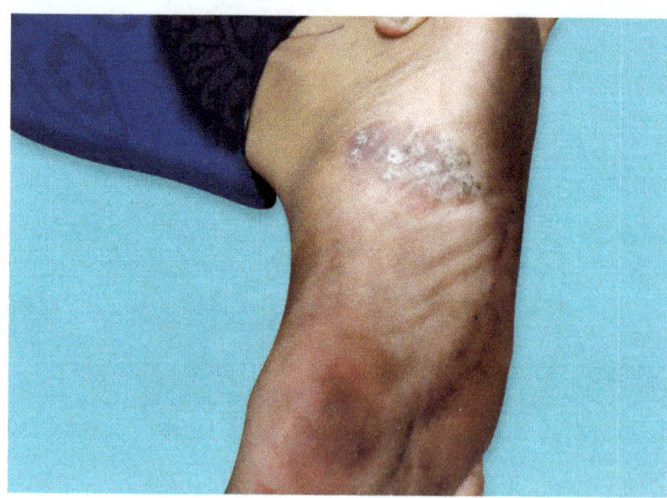

Fig. 91: Moderate psoriasis to be considered as severe since the plantar involvement is affecting the routine work of the patient and hence warrants systemic therapy.

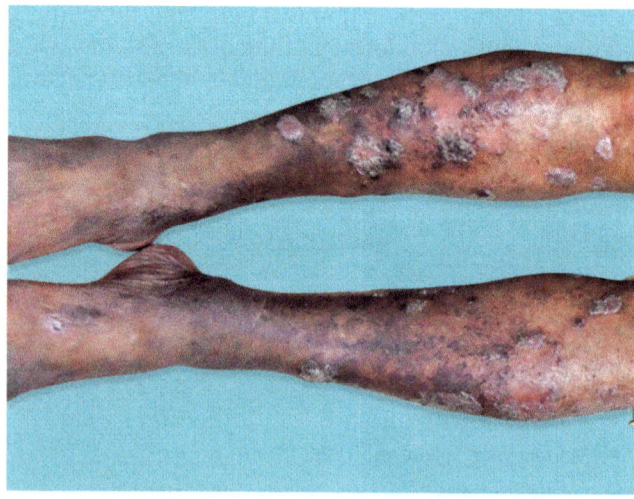

Fig. 90: Moderate psoriasis.

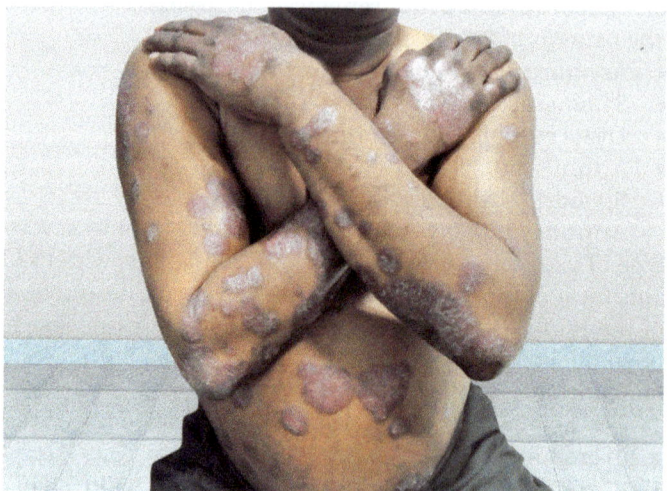

Fig. 92: Moderate-to-severe psoriasis where early initiation of systemic therapy will help control the disease and prevent other complications.

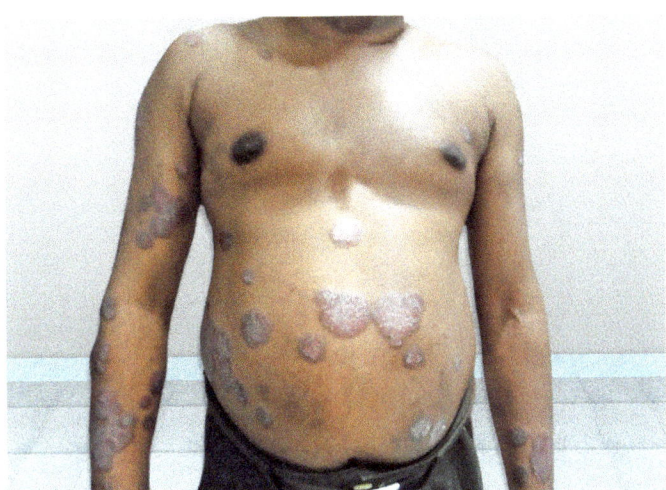

Fig. 93: Moderate-to-severe psoriasis where early initiation of systemic therapy will help control the disease and prevent other complications.

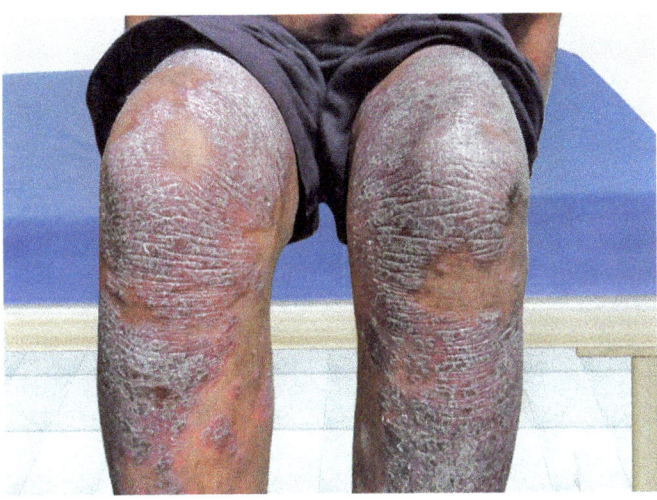

Fig. 95: Severe psoriasis which needs systemic therapy.

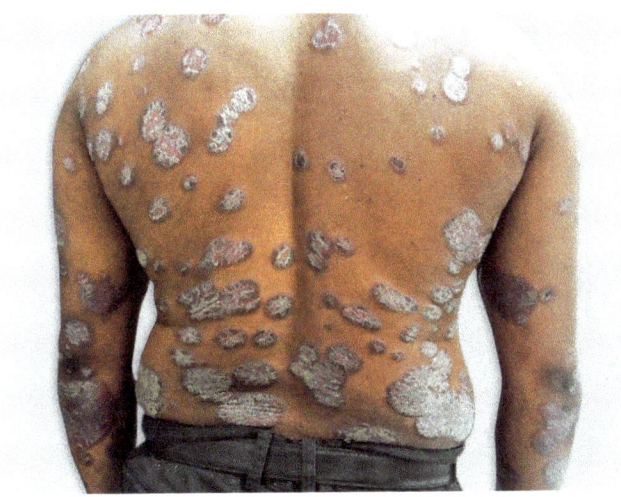

Fig. 94: Moderate-to-severe psoriasis where early initiation of systemic therapy will help control the disease and prevent other complications.

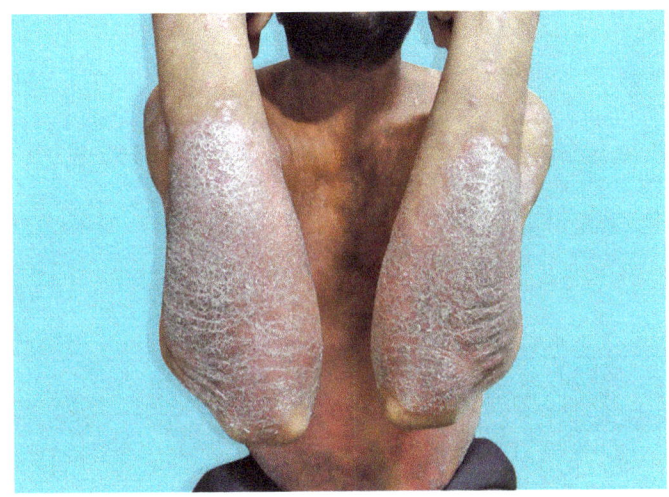

Fig. 96: Severe psoriasis which needs systemic therapy.

Psoriasis with Guarded Prognosis (Fig. 97)

- Impending skin failure
- GPP (von Zumbusch type)
- Psoriatic erythroderma.

The different configurations of psoriasis are:
- *Psoriasis gyrata*: In which curved linear patterns predominate **(Figs. 98 and 99)**
- *Annular psoriasis*: In which ring-like lesions develop secondary to central clearing **(Fig. 100)**
- *Psoriasis follicularis*: In which minute scaly papules are present at the openings of pilosebaceous follicles **(Fig. 101)**
- *Rupioid psoriasis*: Are small plaques (2–5 cm in diameter) and highly hyperkeratotic, resembling limpet shells **(Fig. 102)**
- *Ostraceous psoriasis*: Psoriasis refering to hyperkeratotic plaques with relatively concave centers, similar in shape to oyster shells **(Fig. 103)**
- Rarely zebra like manifestations are observed in erythrodermic psoriasis which will need constant and regular follow-up **(Fig. 104)**.

DISEASE ASSOCIATION

Studies have reported association between psoriasis and many other diseases, both cutaneous and systemic **(Figs. 105 to 108)**.

The common etiological factor involved in psoriasis and atopy being the T-cell, the association between psoriasis and atopy has been well documented. Lichen

CHAPTER 4 Clinical Aspects

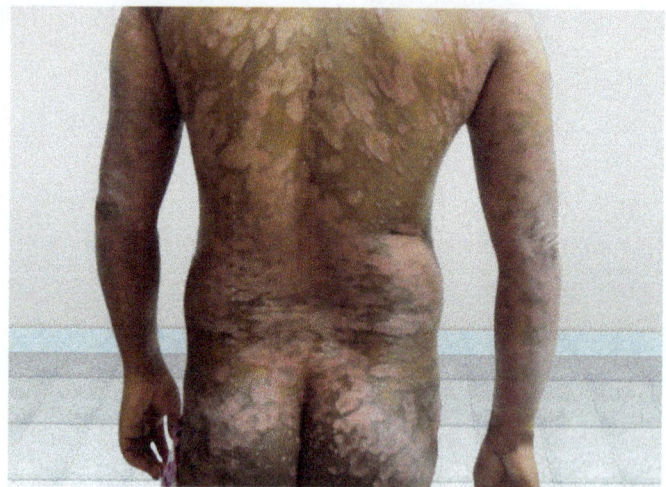

Fig. 97: Severe psoriasis that is unstable whose prognosis is guarded.

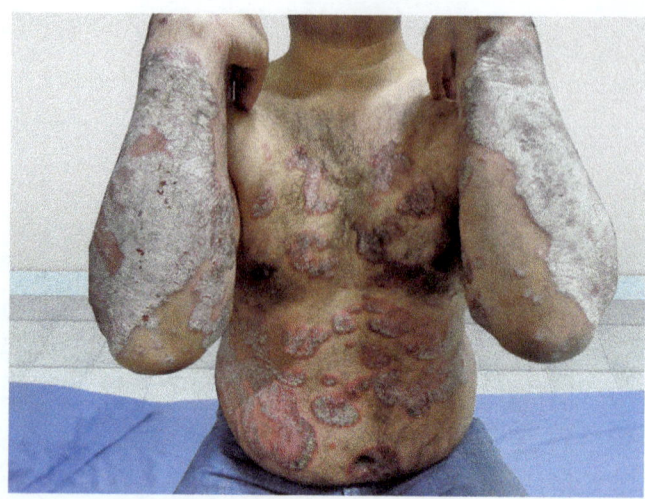

Fig. 100: Annular psoriasis with large plaque type psoriasis.

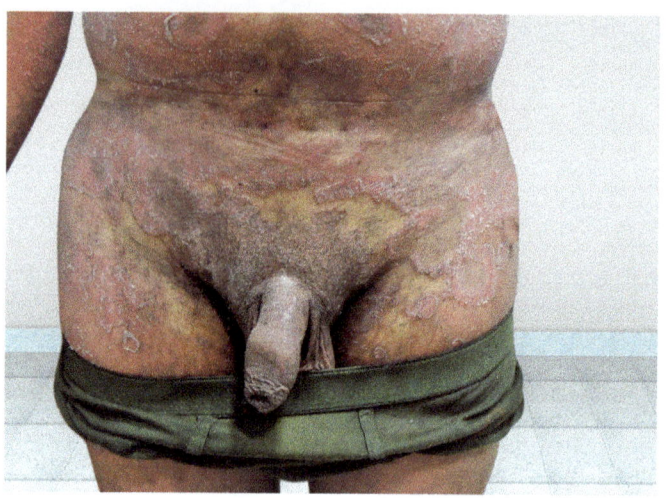

Fig. 98: Annular plaques with few gyrate lesions in a severe form of psoriasis.

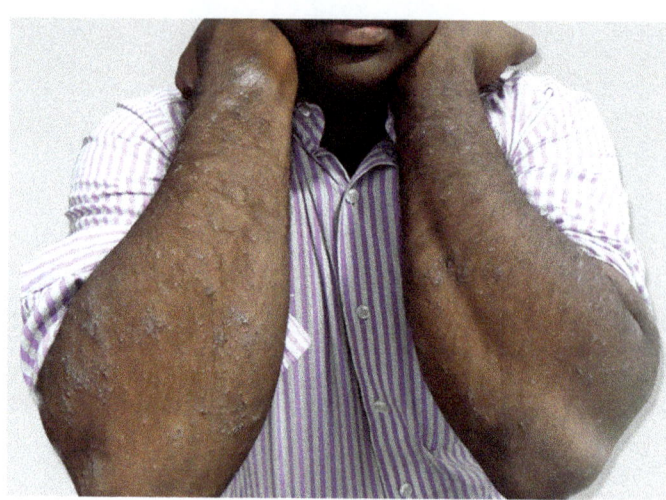

Fig. 101: Follicular psoriasis.

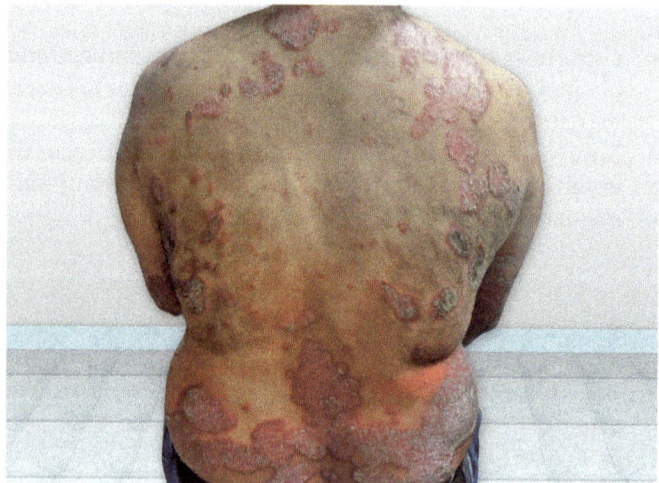

Fig. 99: Annular psoriasis showing ring like lesions.

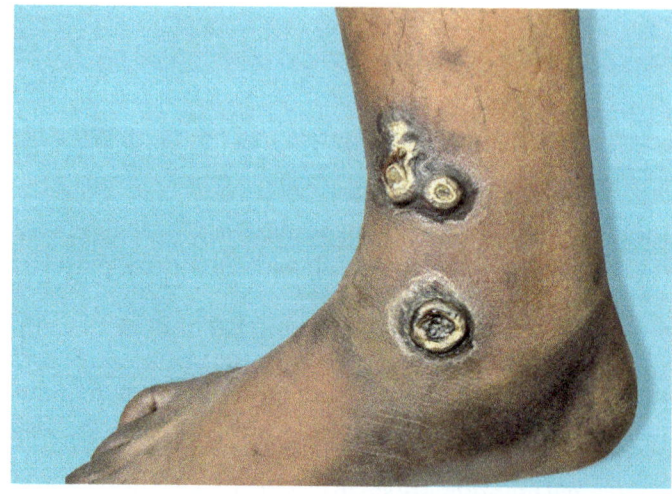

Fig. 102: Rupioid lesions in a patient with Reiter's syndrome.

CHAPTER 4 Clinical Aspects

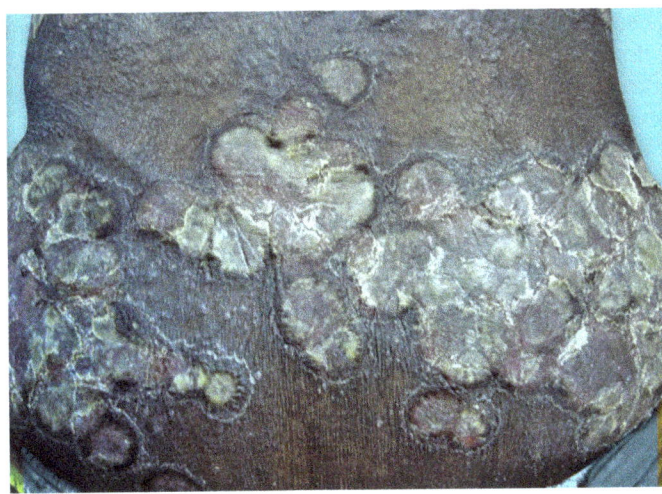

Fig. 103: Note hyperkeratotic plaques with concave center resembling oyster shell.

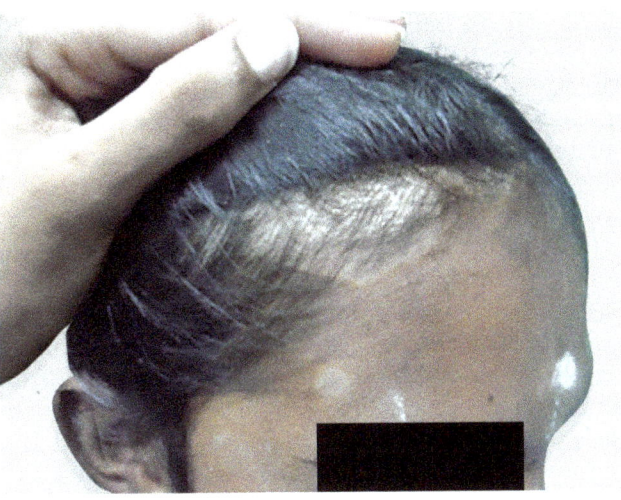

Fig. 106: Psoriasis occurring over a vitiliginous patch.

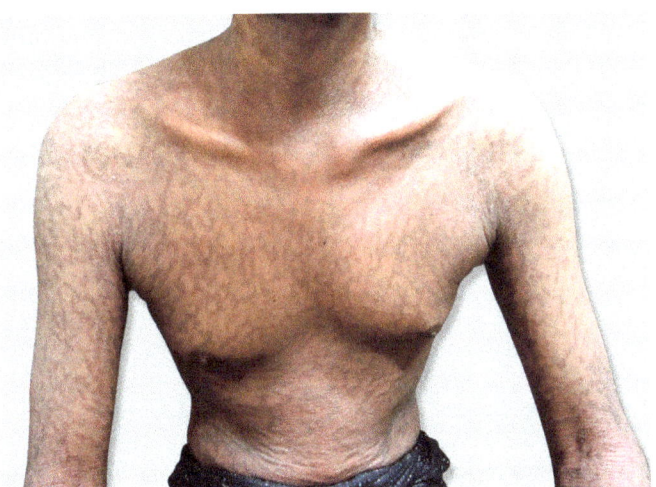

Fig. 104: Unusual presentation of erythrodermic psoriasis.

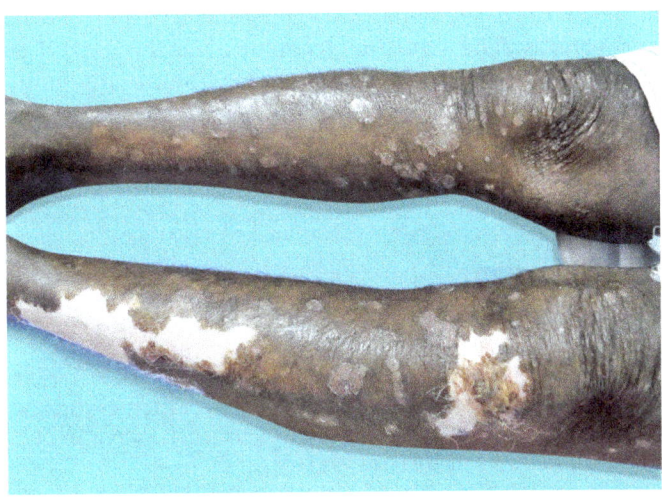

Fig. 107: Psoriasis with vitiligo.

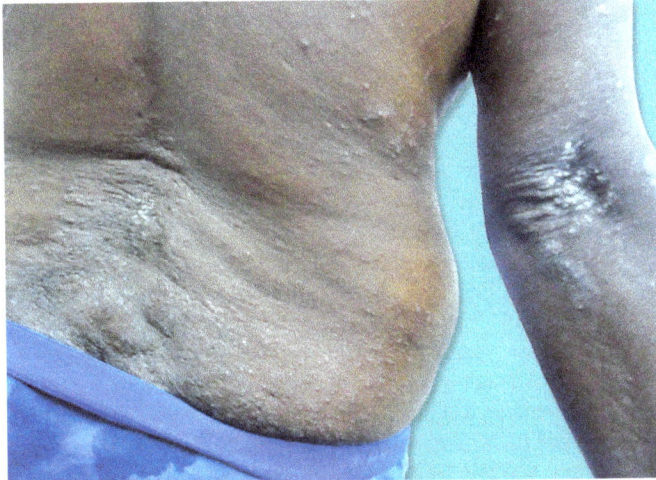

Fig. 105: Psoriasis in association with atopic dermatitis. Note the oozing plaque over the lower back and keratotic scaly plaque over the elbow.

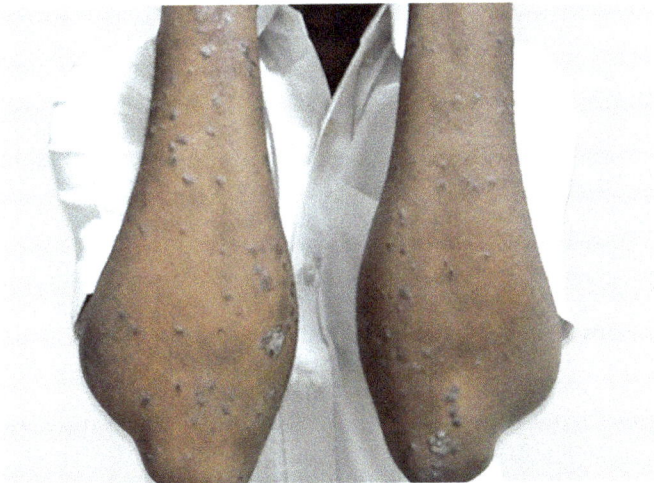

Fig. 108: Psoriasis with lichen planus.

planus, vitiligo, bullous pemphigoid are known to be associated with psoriasis. Infections due to bacteria, fungi; especially dermatophytes, virus including human immunodeficiency virus (HIV) are well documented to be occurring in increased frequency in psoriasis. Gout and hypocalcemia are documented metabolic associations of psoriasis.

Pustular psoriasis is associated with many diseases like Crohn's disease, apart from various arthritis/arthropathies including chronic recurrent multifocal osteomyelitis, pustular arthro-osteitis, axial and peripheral arthritis. A significant incidence of hyper- and hypothyroidism, and the presence of thyroid antibodies has been found in association with pustular psoriasis. The association and increased incidence of diabetes other comorbidities and malignancies is dealt with later.

Synovitis, acne, pustulosis palmaris, hyperostosis and osteomyelitis (SAPHO) syndrome is a chronic disorder that involves the skin, bone and joints, first described by Chamot et al. in 1987, synovitis, acne, pustulosis, hyperostosis, and osteitis. The joint involvement is closely linked to PsA. SAPHO syndrome is characterized by variable bone changes (hyperostosis, arthritis, aseptic osteomyelitis) of the chest wall, sacroiliac joints and long bones. Dermatologic manifestations include PPP, hidradenitis suppurativa, and pustular psoriasis, dissecting cellulitis of the scalp, sweet syndrome and Sneddon-Wilkinson disease. Skin and osseous involvement may occur simultaneously or be separated by as long as 20 years.

SUMMARY

Psoriasis, which is now accepted as a systemic disease affecting mainly the skin and joint, with a potential to affect almost all other systems, should be meticulously examined and carefully assessed. It is essential that the time of first onset, whether early or late; the morphologic aspects of elementary lesions; degree of inflammation, whether mainly inflammatory or hyperkeratotic; extent of disease, whether involves single site, many sites or generalized; presence or not of joint involvement; velocity of propagation as stable; unstable or eruptive; associated comorbidities and other conditions like HIV infection will all have to be assessed before completing the diagnosis.

REFERENCES

1. Henseler T. The genetics of psoriasis. J Am Acad Dermatol. 1997;37:S1-11.
2. Riveira-Munoz E, He SM, Escaramís G, et al. Meta-analysis confirms the Ice3c_Ice3b deletion as a risk factor for psoriasis in several ethnic groups and finds interaction with HLA-Cw6. J Invest Dermatol. 2011;131(5):1105-9.
3. Seyhan M, Cos, Kun BK, et al. Psoriasis in childhood and adolescence: evaluation of demographic and clinical features. Pediatr Int. 2006;48:525-30.
4. Morris A, Rogers M, Fischer G, et al. Childhood psoriasis: a clinical review of 1262 cases. Pediatr Dermatol. 2001;18:188-98.
5. Grjibovski AM, Olsen AO, Magnus P, et al. Psoriasis in Norwegian twins: contribution of genetic and environmental effects. J Eur Acad Dermatol Venereol. 2007;21:1337-43.
6. Henseler T, Christophers E. Psoriasis of early and late onset: characterization of two types of psoriasis vulgaris. J Am Acad Dermatol.1985;13:450-6.
7. al-Fouzan AS, Nanda A. A Survey of Childhood Psoriasis in Kuwait. Pediatric Dermatol. 1994;11:116-9.
8. Altobelli E, Petrocelli R, Marziliano C, et al. Family history of psoriasis and age at disease onset in Italian patients with psoriasis. Br J Dermatol. 2007;156:1400-1.
9. Honig PJ. Guttate psoriasis associated with perianal streptococcal disease. J Pediatr. 1988;113:1037-9.
10. Cassandra M, Conte E, Cortez B. Childhood pustular psoriasis elicited by the streptococcal antigen: a case report and review of the literature. Pediatr Dermatol. 2003;20:506-10.
11. Lazar AP, Roenigk HH. Acquired immunodeficiency syndrome (AIDS) can exacerbate psoriasis. J Am Acad Dermatol. 1988;18:144.
12. Tsankov N, Angelova I, Kazandjieva J. Drug-induced psoriasis. Recognition and management. Am J Clin Dermatol. 2000;1: 159-65.
13. Wolf R, Ruocco V. Triggered psoriasis. Adv Exp Med Biol. 1999;455:221-5.
14. O'Brien M, Koo J. The mechanism of lithium and beta-blocking agents in inducing and exacerbating psoriasis. J Drugs Dermatol. 2006;5:426-32.
15. Benoit S, Hamm H. Childhood psoriasis. Clinics in Dermatology. 2007;25:555-62.
16. Barisic-Drusko V, Rucevic I. Psoriasis in childhood. Coll Antropol. 2004;1:211-85.
17. Naldi L, Gambini D. The clinical spectrum of psoriasis. Clin Dermatol. 2007;25:510-8.
18. Nanda A, Kaur S, Kaur I, et al. Childhood psoriasis: an epidemiological survey of 112 patients. Pediatr Dermatol. 1990;7:19-21.
19. Stern RS, Wu J. Psoriasis. In: Arndt KA, LeBoit PE, Robinson JK, et al. (Eds). Cutaneous Medicine and Surgery. Philadelphia: WB Saunders; 1996.
20. Gottlieb AB, Chaudhari U, Baker DG, et al. The natural psoriasis foundation score (NPF-PS) system versus the psoriasis area severity index (PASI) and physicians global assessment (PGA): a comparison. J Drugs Dermatol. 2003; 2:260-6.
21. Langley RB, Krueger GG, Griffiths CE. Psoriasis: epidemiology, clinical features, and quality of life. Ann Rheum Dis. 2005;64: ii18-23.
22. Dhar S, Banerjee R, Agrawal N, et al. Psoriasis in children: an insight. Indian J Dermatol. 2011;56(3):262-5.

23. Han MH, Jang KA, Sung KJ, et al. A case of guttate psoriasis following Kawasaki disease. Br J Dermatol. 2000;142:548-50.
24. Li W, Man XY. Linear psoriasis. CMAJ. 2012;184:789.
25. Chien P, Rosenman K, Cheung W, et al. Linear psoriasis. Dermatol Online J. 2009;15(8):4.
26. Ashurst PJ. Relapsing pustular eruptions of the hands and feet. Br J Dermatol. 1964;76:169-80.
27. Reitamo S, Erkko P, Remitz A. Palmoplantar pustulosis. Eur J Dermatol. 1992; 2: 311-4.
28. O'Doherty CJ, MacIntyre C. Palmoplantar pustulosis and smoking. Br Med J. 1985;291:861-4.
29. Iria N, Navarini AA, Yawalkar N. Alitretinoin abrogates innate inflammation in palmoplantar pustular psoriasis. Br J Dermatol. 2012:167;1170-4.
30. Pandhi D, Chowdhry S, Grover C, et al. Parakeratosis pustulosa—a distinct but less familiar disease. Indian J Dermatol Venereol Leprol. 2003;69:48-50.
31. Baker H, Ryan TJ. Generalized pustular psoriasis. Br J Dermatol. 1968;80:771-93.
32. Dawson TA. Tongue lesions in generalized pustular psoriasis. Br J Dermatol. 1974;91:419-24.
33. de Oliveira ST, Maragno L, Arnone M, Fonseca Takahashi MD, Romiti R. Generalized Pustular Psoriasis in Childhood. Pediatr Dermatol. 2010;27(4):349-54.
34. Burden AD. Management of psoriasis in childhood. Clin Exp Dermatol. 1999;24:341-5.
35. Liao P, Rubinson R, Howard R, et al. Annular pustular psoriasis—most common form of pustular psoriasis in children: report of three cases and review of the literature. Pediatr Dermatol. 2002;19:19-25.
36. Zelickson BD, Muller SA. Generalized pustular psoriasis in childhood. J Am Acad Dermatol. 1990;24:186-94.
37. Xiao T, Li B, He CD, et al. Juvenile generalized pustular psoriasis. J Dermatol. 2007;34:573-6.
38. Catsarou-Catsari A, Katsambos A, Theodoropoulus P, et al. Ophthalmological manifestations in patients with psoriasis. Acta Derm Venereol (Stockh). 1984;64:557-9.
39. Espinoza LR, Cuellar ML, Silveira LH. Psoriatic arthritis. Curr Opin Rheumatol. 1992;4:470-8.
40. Zachariae H. Prevalence of joint disease in patients with psoriasis: implications for therapy. Am J Clin Dermatol. 2003;4:441-7.

Pediatric Psoriasis

INTRODUCTION

Psoriasis is a T-cell mediated chronic inflammatory disorder of the skin seen in about 3.5% of the population.[1] One-third of psoriasis cases in a dermatology center are seen in pediatric age group.[2] Pediatric psoriasis consists broadly of 3 age groups of psoriatic patients: infantile psoriasis, a self-limited disease of infancy, psoriasis with early-onset, and pediatric psoriasis with psoriatic arthritis.[3] Timely diagnosis and appropriate management cannot only arrest progression but also minimize the psychosocial burden imposed by this illness. Thereby disfiguring states and its evolution into a metabolic syndrome requiring extensive treatment can well be averted. This review will cover almost all aspects of psoriasis including the rare clinical forms like impetigo herpetiformis and congenital erythrodermic psoriasis (CEP) and present the latest update especially on the etiopathogenesis and treatment options.

EPIDEMIOLOGY

One-third of adults with psoriasis report onset in childhood. Ethnic variation is not clear, with some studies quoting incidence highest in caucasians, black then Asian populations.[4] It is alarming to note that 40,000 children under 10 years were afflicted by psoriasis.[5] The distribution of psoriasis is almost equal in boys and girls. However, female preponderance has been observed by some authors.[4] The occurrence of psoriatic diaper rash in younger children and its inclusion increases incidence of psoriasis in children under two.[4] The exact age distribution is not clear though literature states that nearly 30% of patients with psoriasis develop the disease before the age of 18.[6] It is of interest to note that in the age group <20 years the frequency of psoriasis was 20% higher in girls than in boys, in contrast to adults.[7] Compared with 37% in adult-onset patients, 49% of pediatric-onset patients had first-degree family members affected with psoriasis.[2] Some studies have reported familial incidence in childhood cases of psoriasis as high as 89%.[8] Nearly two-thirds of children manifest with plaque-type psoriasis vulgaris.[3] Involvement of joints with psoriatic arthritis is less prevalent in younger patients; however, it does occur in childhood disease and should be considered in the differential of pediatric arthritis.[9]

ETIOPATHOGENESIS

Psoriasis is a systemic, immune-mediated disorder, characterized by inflammatory skin and joint manifestations. The exact pathogenesis of psoriasis has not been completely elucidated. However, it is known to have a genetic basis, as 23.4–71% of children will have a family history of psoriasis[3] and psoriasis is more common in identical than fraternal twins (65–72% vs. 15–30%). Human leukocyte antigen (HLA)-Cw6 has been known to be a susceptibility gene in psoriasis.[10]

Major gene for psoriasis susceptibility is thought mainly to be located on chromosome 6, the site of HLA class I (associated with early-onset disease) and II (late-onset disease) antigens which are thought to produce differing subtypes of the disease. Individuals with the Cw0602 allele are four times more likely to develop guttate psoriasis.[4] A series of genes have been isolated in which mutations have been associated with psoriatic disease, including interleukin (IL)-12-B9 (1p31.3), IL-13 (5q31.1), IL-23R (1p31.3); HLA-Bw6 psoriasis susceptibility locus (PSORS)-6 signal transducer and activator of transcription (STAT)-2/IL-23A (12q13.2); tumor necrosis factor (TNF), alpha-induced protein (TNFAIP)-3 (6q23.3); and TNFAIP3 interacting protein (TNIP)-1 (5q33.1). These genes play a role in Th2 cell and Th17 cell activity which have been noted in psoriatic lesions.[11,12]

Several attempts have been made to detect psoriasis susceptibility loci by linkage studies. Up to now, at least nine loci are known "PSORS1-9".[13] Interestingly, a strong association exists in early-onset psoriasis for the HLA-Cw6 allele.[14]

Precipitating factors are more important in pediatric than in adult-onset psoriasis.[2] They largely include trauma, infections, drugs, and stress. Streptococcal pharyngitis or perianal streptococcal dermatitis typically provokes guttate psoriasis. Infection with human immunodeficiency virus can induce or exacerbate psoriasis.[15]

Children with obesity and overweight get more adipose tissue. The tissue is a vigorous endocrine organ capable of secreting multiple proinflammatory adipocytokines, such as IL-6, IL-1, TNF-α11 and adiponectin[7] which play an important role in the pathogenesis of psoriasis. Serum and skin levels of TNF-α and IL-6 are increased in psoriasis and are positively correlated with disease severity. Obesity is a risk factor for psoriasis and can increase the severity of psoriasis.[16,17] There is a strong correlation between psoriasis and autoimmune disease and atopy. Coexistence of psoriasis with any of the above been reported.

Expression of the disease clinically depends on the capacity of the child's epidermis to express the same. This is a complex process, linked to interaction of cells of the epidermis, dermis, immune system, and humoral elements. The inherent phenotype has a capacity of the keratinocyte for hyperproliferation and altered differentiation, both of which are genetically controlled. A genetic aberration can therefore trigger the cascade of inflammatory events in the evolution of the disease.

PATHOLOGY

From a histological point of view, psoriasis is a dynamic dermatosis that changes during the evolution of an individual lesion. Lesions are usually diagnostic only in early stages or near the margin of advancing plaques. Hyperkeratosis, parakeratosis, Munro microabscesses, spongiform pustule of Kogoj, diminished or absent granular layer, regular acanthosis, papillomatosis, tortuosity and dilatation of papillary capillaries, and chronic inflammation in the upper dermis are the common features seen in psoriasis. However, Munro microabscesses and Kogoj's micropustules are diagnostic clues of psoriasis, but they are not always present in all cases at all stages. All other features can be found in various types of eczemas and other dermatoses.[18] Depending on type, site and stage of the disease histological features tend to differ. Leclerc-Mercier et al. have studied various histological patterns in infantile erythroderma, and classified them into psoriasiform, spongiform and ichthyosiform.[19] The psoriasiform pattern included:
- Psoriasiform epidermal hyperplasia
- Parakeratosis
- None or mild spongiosis.

Psoriasiform epidermal hyperplasia comprised confluent parakeratosis, hyperkeratosis, hypogranulosis, and suprapapillary thinning of the epidermis, regular acanthosis often with clubbed rete ridges. According to Walsh et al., the mean accuracy of the histopathological diagnoses was <55%, even in adult erythroderma.[20] In the case of psoriatic erythroderma particularly in infants, Netherton syndrome (NS) was the closest histological mimicker. Prior to the availability of lymphoepithelial Kazal-type inhibitor (LEKTI) antibody nearly one-fifth of the cases of NS being misdiagnosed as psoriasis most often.[21] Determination of the underlying cause is usually a challenge for clinicians, considering the poor specificity of clinical signs. Consequently, the diagnosis is often delayed by 11 months.[22]

The most consistent feature of CEP according to the authors was acanthosis and dilatation of papillary capillaries with neutrophilic squirting into the epidermis.

Psoriasis and atopic dermatitis (AD) were once believed to be mutually exclusive. In a prospective study undertaken by Beer et al. 16.7% of AD patients had psoriasis and 9.5% of psoriasis patients had AD. In consecutive occurrences, psoriasis generally followed AD. The ratio of concurrent to consecutive incidence was 3:1. The two diseases are shown not to be mutually exclusive and may coexist in the same individual.[23] Distinct populations of T cells are defined by their unique patterns of cytokine production.[24] Keratinocytes of patients with AD and psoriasis show an intrinsically abnormal and different chemokine production profile and favor the recruitment of distinct leukocyte subsets into the skin.[25] However, in spite of their differences, both AD and psoriasis share epidermal hyperplasia, aberrant immunity, and skin barrier anomalies.

Genetic studies of both psoriasis and AD suggest that defects affecting cells of the skin need to be as seriously considered as defects in adaptive immunity. The epidermal differentiation complex has been implicated in both AD and psoriasis.[26] It transcribes within terminally differentiating keratinocytes and contains many genes that may modify immune processes in the epithelium. The colocalization of AD to psoriasis loci indicates that AD is influenced by genes that modulate dermal responses independently from atopic mechanisms. The histological findings of both diseases occurring simultaneously as early as in infancy definitely adds further evidence to the association between psoriasis and AD.[27]

Histological confirmation of psoriasis is not always mandatory as most of the cases are clinically diagnosed even in children. However, early skin biopsy is helpful in the diagnosis of neonatal and infantile erythroderma where the etiology of erythroderma can be many and timely diagnosis will help to manage the child better.

CLINICAL ASPECTS

Psoriasis in children is not uncommon. A positive family history, precipitating trigger factors and age of onset can all to some extent predict the prognosis of the disease in children. A positive family history has been reported in 23.4–71% of children with psoriasis.[28,29] Identical twins have more chances of manifesting psoriasis than fraternal twins.[30]

Age of Onset

Variations exist between studies regarding the age of onset of childhood psoriasis. According to Stefanaki et al. majority of the children were 9–10 years as they represented 40% of their study population.[31] According to Stefanaki, the peak age of onset is between 8 and 12 years which they compared and stated to be the same with studies from China, Denmark and India, in which most of the children had an onset of disease at 8–12 years of age, contrary to the reports from Middle East and Australia where the onset was before 5 years of age.[32] Such differences may be attributable to the referral pattern, and also due to inadequate documentation and statistics as children are being treated by neonatologists, pediatricians and family and adolescent physicians apart from dermatologists, in various set ups. A positive family history was obtained in only 16% of study conducted by Stefanaki et al. Family history of psoriasis predicts early disease onset.[33]

Triggering and Exacerbating Factors

Precipitating factors are more important in pediatric, than in adult-onset psoriasis.[2] They largely include trauma, infections, drugs, and stress. The appearance of psoriatic lesions in uninvolved skin at sites of former trauma is known as isomorphic response or Koebner phenomenon. Any form of trauma including physical, chemical, thermal, surgical, or inflammatory trauma can result in exacerbation of psoriasis. Streptococcal pharyngitis or perianal streptococcal dermatitis typically provokes guttate psoriasis and childhood pustular psoriasis can be elicited by the streptococcal antigen.[34,35] Infection with human immunodeficiency virus can induce or exacerbate psoriasis.[36] Whereas the use of β-blocking agents and lithium is a well-known trigger of psoriasis in adult patients, antimalarials and withdrawal of oral or topical corticosteroids play a more important role in rebound or induction of childhood psoriasis.[37-39] In addition, several studies emphasize the influence of psychological and psychosomatic factors like stress or lack of social support in the course of psoriasis.[15] Inflammatory focus was the most frequent trigger factor observed by Barisic-Drusko and Rucevic.[40]

Type I psoriasis has an early onset and therefore, it may be appropriate to group all children under type I psoriasis and consider those children with a positive family history and who are positive for HLAs Cw6, B57, DR7 to have severe presentation and course.[14] According to Morris et al. no gender difference has been observed in childhood psoriasis, whereas Stefanaki et al. have observed a female to male ratio of 1.4: 1 in a study of 125 children.[31] Many authors have observed girls to be affected more than boys.[6,15,41] The clinical types of psoriasis are more or less the same as in adults with some variation in the incidence of different types. Plaque type psoriasis, scalp psoriasis, guttate psoriasis, nail psoriasis, flexural psoriasis, napkin psoriasis, unstable psoriasis, pustular psoriasis are the types of psoriasis commonly encountered in children. Congenital psoriasis, congenital psoriatic erythroderma and infantile psoriasis are rare forms of psoriasis seen in the first year of life. Erythrodermic psoriasis and psoriatic arthritis are less frequent when compared to adulthood psoriasis. Mucosal involvement has been rare in Indian children.[42] Psoriasis can now be considered as a disease manifesting from "womb to tomb".

The disease in children is more pruritic, and the lesions are relatively thinner, softer, and less scaly.[15] The classical erythematous scaly papule or plaque will mostly give a clue to diagnosis. The following features are pertinent and helpful in the clinical diagnosis of psoriasis:[43]
- The isomorphic response or Koebner phenomenon, which is occurrence of lesions in areas of trauma
- The Auspitz sign—pinpoint bleeding at the base of scale that has been removed
- Presence of nail pitting, which can aid in diagnosis of the disease
- Altered pigmentation with lesional clearance.

The first two findings are useful to assess the disease activity.

Grading

Severity grading for psoriasis is usually based on surface area and severity.

Psoriasis area and severity index (PASI) is the most widely used tool for the measurement of severity of psoriasis. PASI combines the assessment of the severity of lesions and the area affected into a single score in the range 0 (no disease) to 72 (maximal disease).

Within each area, the severity is estimated by three clinical signs: erythema (redness), induration (thickness) and desquamation (scaling). Severity parameters are measured on a scale of 0–4, from none to maximum.

The sum of all three severity parameters is then calculated for each section of skin, multiplied by the area score for that area and multiplied by weight of respective section (0.1 for head, 0.2 for arms, 0.3 for body and 0.4 for legs).

A simpler way to assess the severity would be mild, moderate and severe which are represented as <3%, 3–10%, and >10% body surface area (BSA) respectively.[44]

CLINICAL ASPECTS

Plaque Psoriasis

Plaque-type psoriasis is by far the most common clinical type of psoriasis in children accounting from 30 to 60% of the total pediatric cases studied 56.8% **(Figs. 1 to 10)**.[31]

Classical plaque is characterized by erythema and silvery white scales. However, in dark skinned children, both erythema and scaling are not so obvious. The common sites involved include, scalp, postauricular area, elbows, knees, umbilical region and buttocks. Scalp was the most common initial site affected (50.3%).[41] In an Indian study, leg was the most frequently affected site than the scalp involvement.[45] Facial involvement in children is a frequent observation in majority of the reports which varies from 18 to 46%.[29,46]

CHAPTER 5 Pediatric Psoriasis

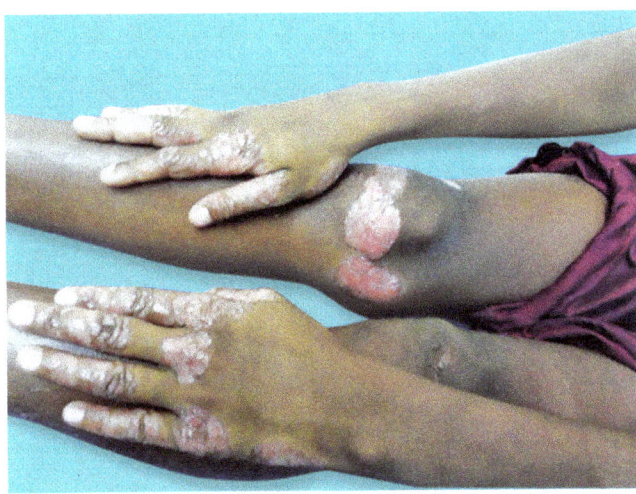

Fig. 1: Classical erythematous plaque with silvery white scales over the extensor aspect of the knees and hands in a boy having psoriasis vulgaris.

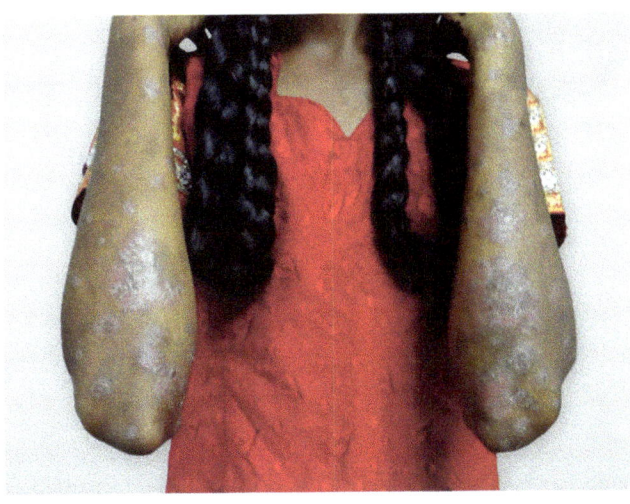

Fig. 4: Girl with plaque psoriasis involving >20% body surface area (BSA).

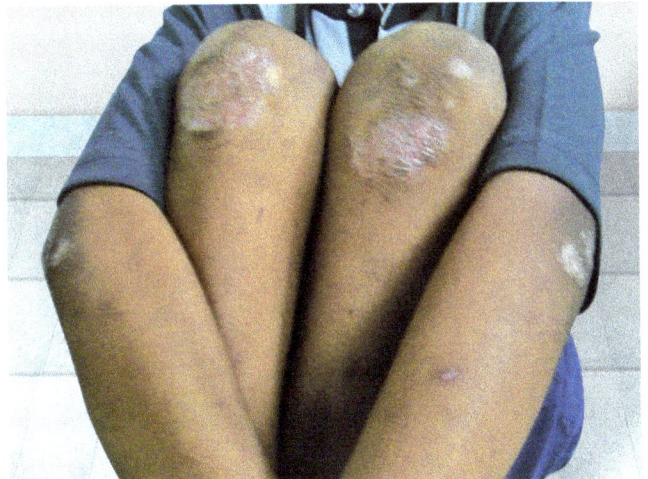

Fig. 2: Knees and elbows showing silvery white psoriatic plaques.

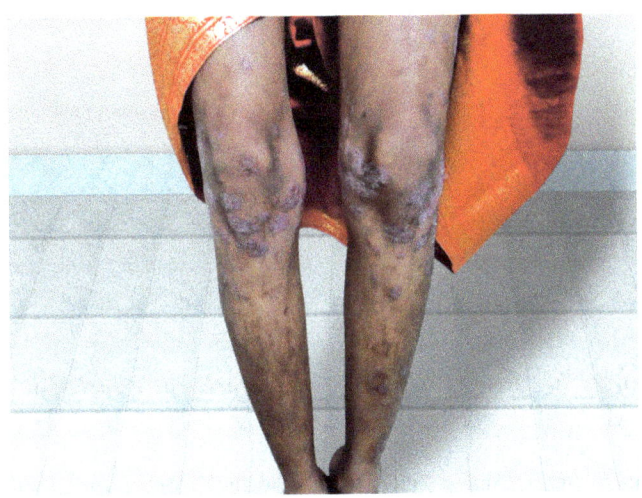

Fig. 5: This child (same girl as in **Fig. 4**) will require systemic therapy avoid psoralen and ultraviolet light A (PUVA).

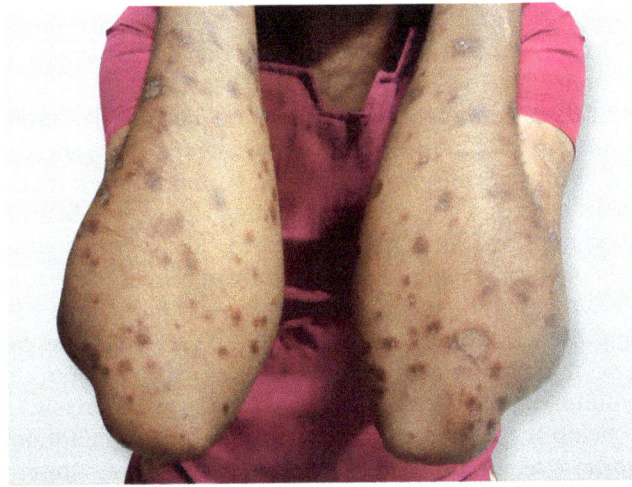

Fig. 3: Multiple erythematous plaques with silvery scales.

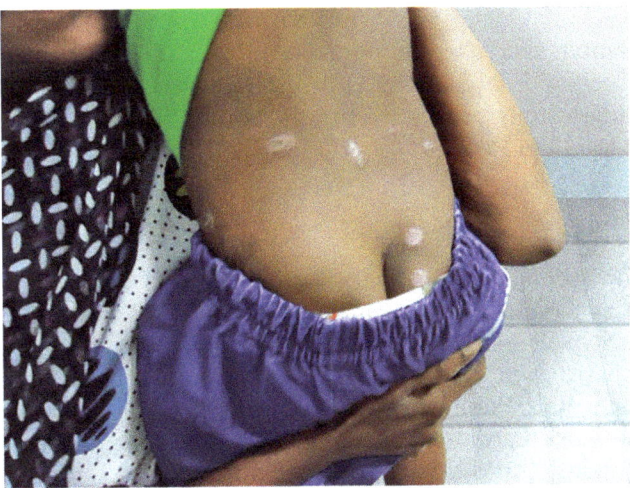

Fig. 6: Infant with plaque lesions.

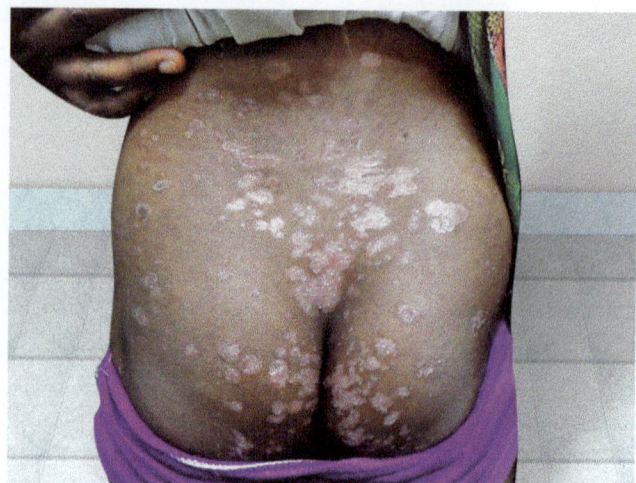

Fig. 7: The lower back is another oft-affected area in psoriasis as seen in this picture.

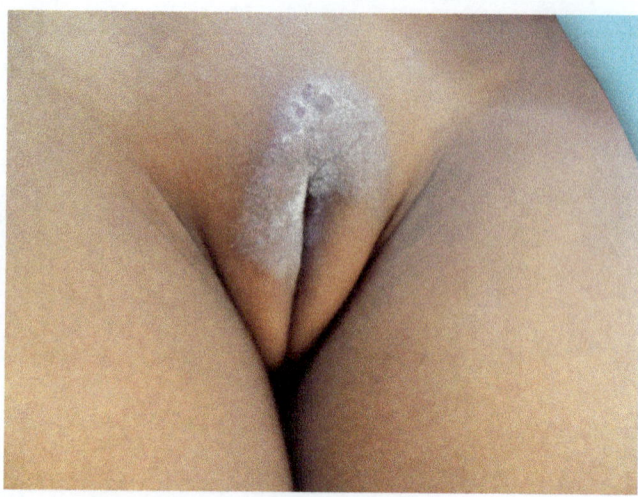

Fig. 9: Odd site of plaque psoriasis where potent topical steroid should be avoided.

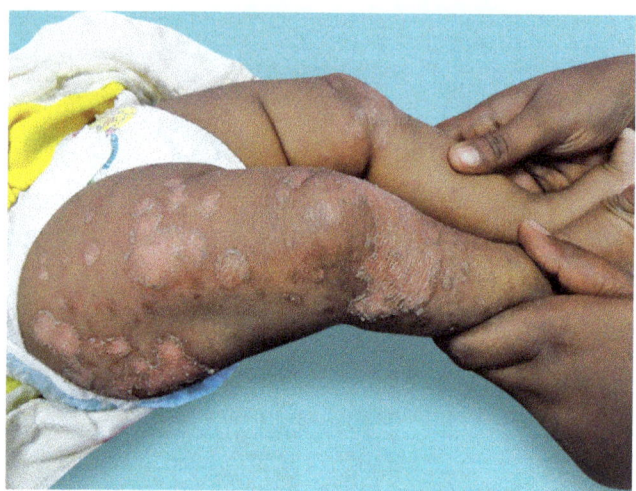

Fig. 8: Severe type of plaque psoriasis in an infant.

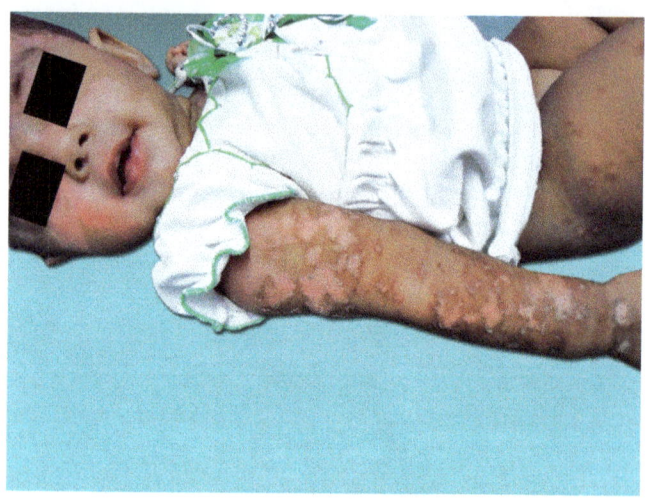

Fig. 10: Classical plaque type psoriasis in an infant who should be watched for evolution to erythrodermic psoriasis.

Plantar Psoriasis

Plantar psoriasis, the one with highest discomfort, was observed in about 12.8% of children with psoriasis in an Indian study conducted in 419 children by Kumar et al. **(Figs. 11 to 14)**.[9]

Guttate Psoriasis

Guttate psoriasis is characterized by eruption of small scaly papules in a widespread fashion involving the trunk, abdomen and back **(Figs. 15 to 17)**.

History of recent pharyngitis is invariably present in the majority of the children and in up to 85% of children, associated streptococcal infection could be proved.[29,32] Guttate psoriasis can evolve into plaque type psoriasis in some children.

Scalp Psoriasis

Scalp is the most common site involved in majority of children affected by psoriasis **(Figs. 18 to 25)**.[29,32]

Scalp can be involved either as an isolated site of affection or as part of plaque type psoriasis, pustular psoriasis and erythrodermic psoriasis. The scaling and erythema typically transgress the frontal hair line feature that helps in differentiating from seborrheic dermatitis. Circumscribed scaly plaques are sometimes the only presentation. Plaque of pityriasis amiantacea over the scalp is characterized by the presence of asbestos-like scales. Localized hair loss can be seen in children with pityriasis amiantacea.[14] There can be diffuse hair loss in those with erythrodermic psoriasis.

Scalp is the most common site involved in childhood psoriasis as in adults. Itching and hair loss are common symptoms though not a feature seen in all.

CHAPTER 5 Pediatric Psoriasis

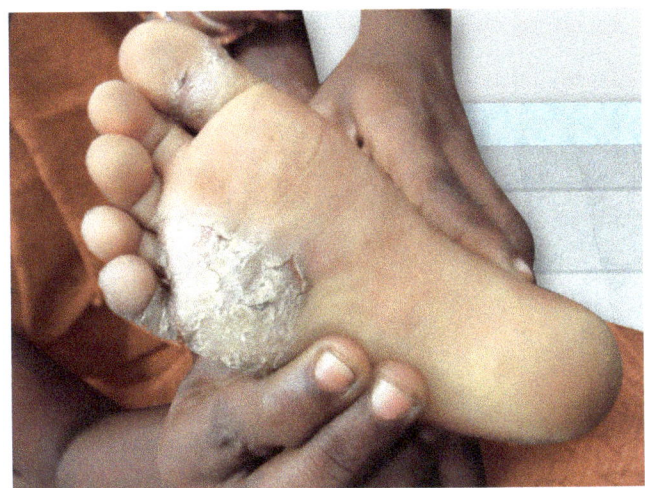
Fig. 11: Single plaque of plantar psoriasis in a child.

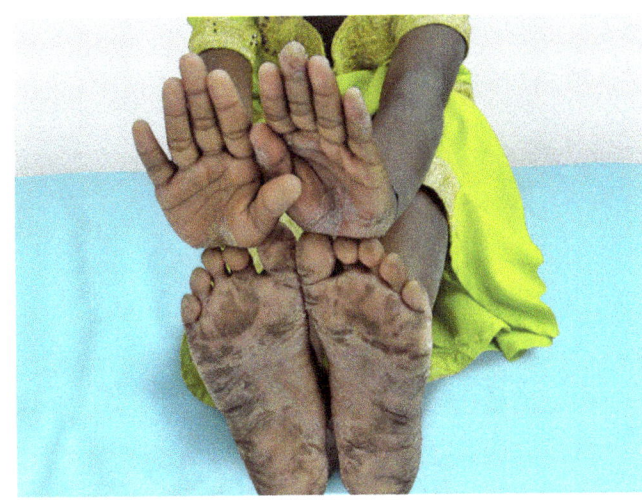
Fig. 14: Classical palmoplantar psoriasis in a child.

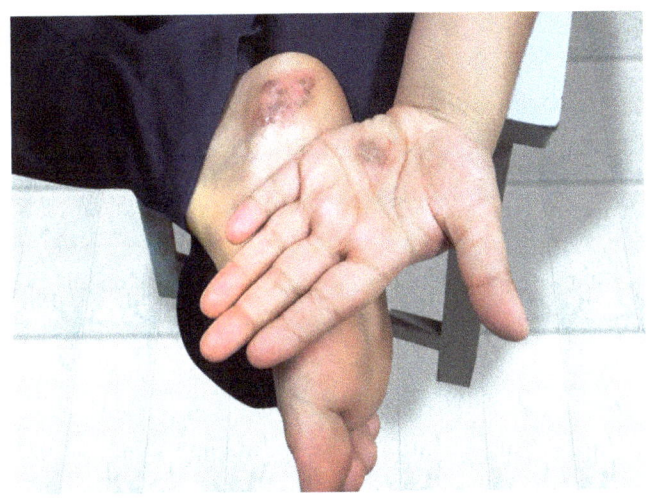
Fig. 12: Early lesions of palmoplantar psoriasis in a 12-year-old.

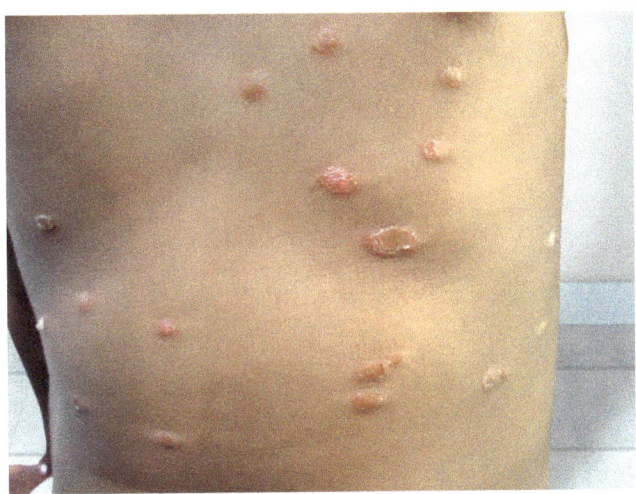
Fig. 15: Drop-like guttate psoriasis on the trunk.

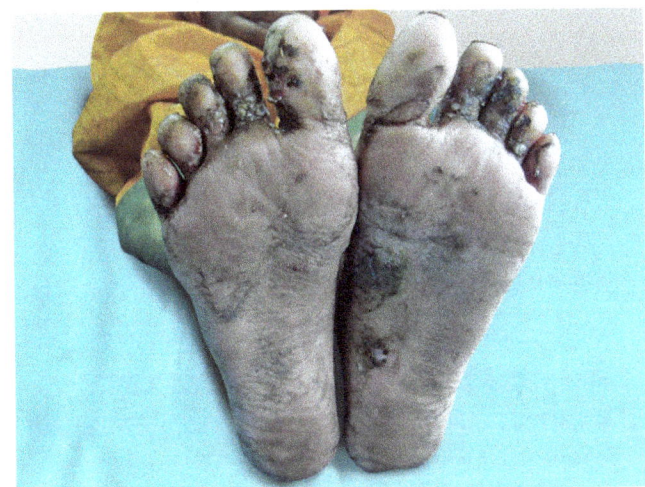
Fig. 13: Plantar psoriasis in a girl with no other lesion.

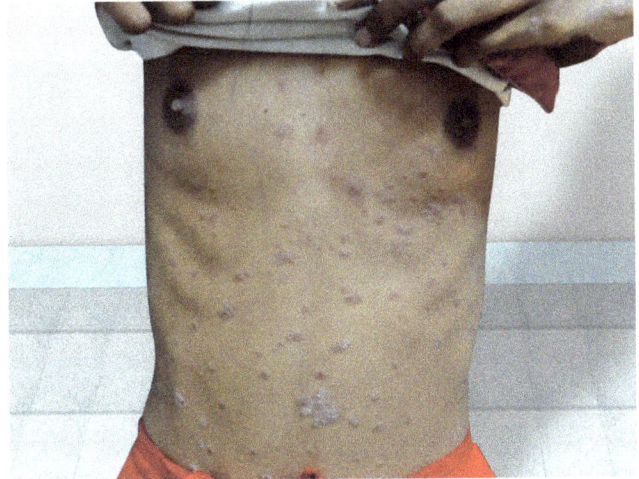
Fig. 16: Child with guttate psoriasis.

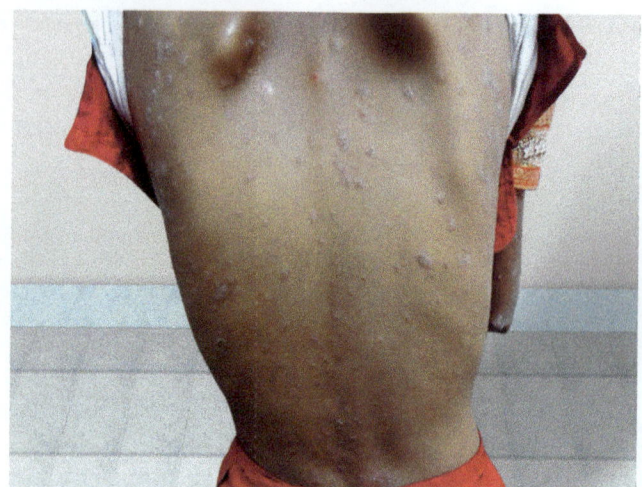

Fig. 17: Same child as in **Figure 16** who later developed psoriasis vulgaris.

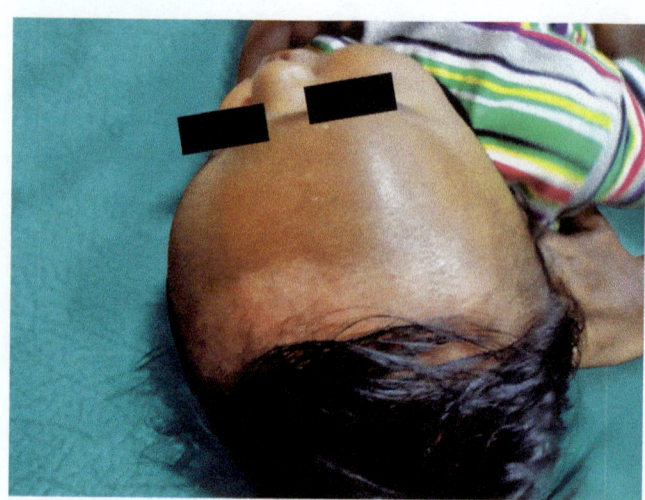

Fig. 20: Note extension of scales beyond the hairline.

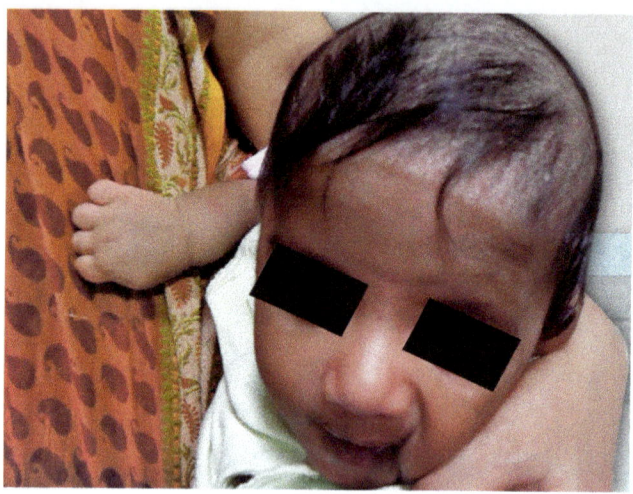

Fig. 18: Scalp psoriasis in an infant.

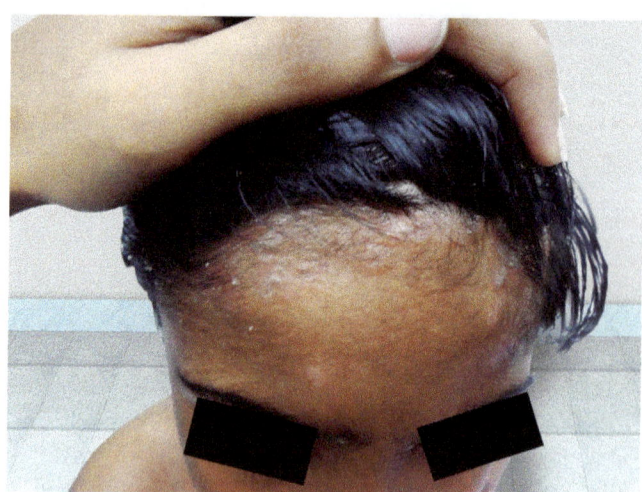

Fig. 21: Scalp psoriasis showing the "psoriatic corona".

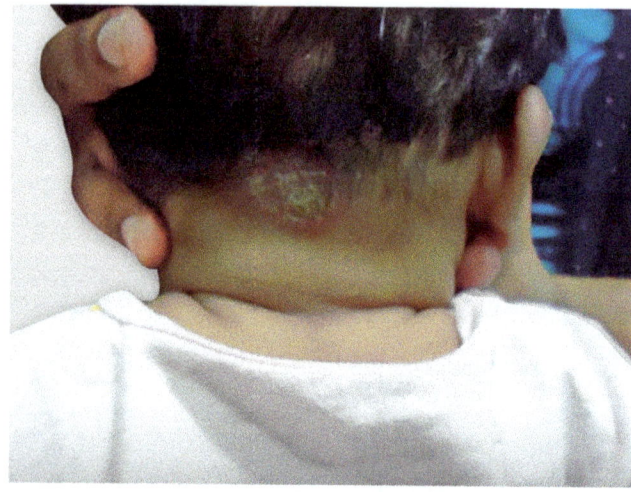

Fig. 19: Scalp scales that extend below the hairline is almost always suggestive of psoriasis.

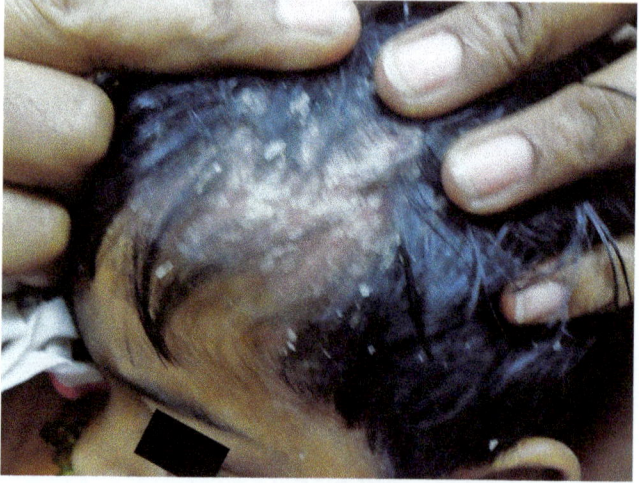

Fig. 22: Thick loose silvery scales as against greasy scales of seborrheic dermatitis.

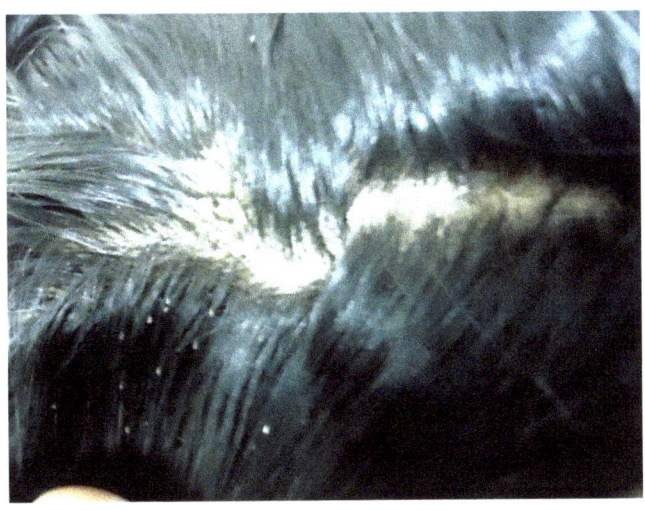
Fig. 23: Large obvious silvery scales of psoriasis on the scalp.

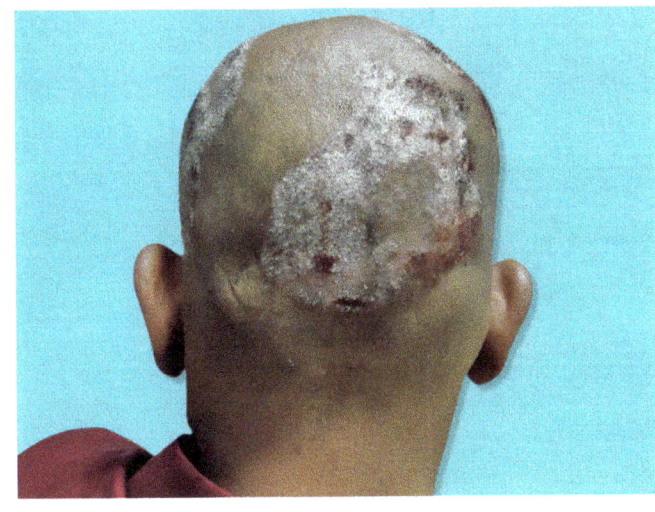
Fig. 25: Same boy as in **Figure 24**.

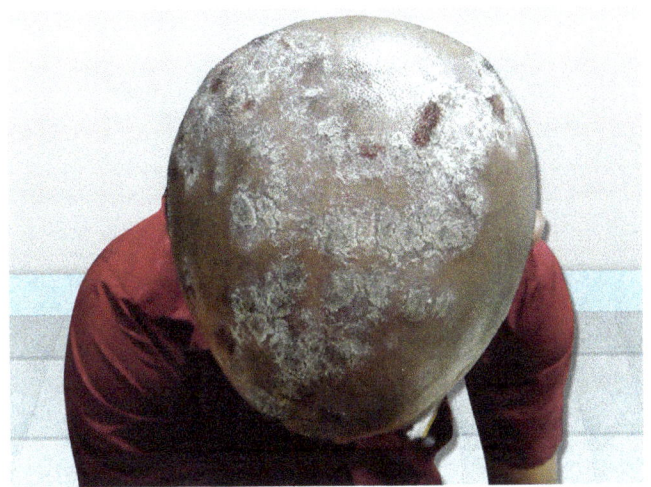
Fig. 24: Severe involvement of scalp in a grown-up boy.

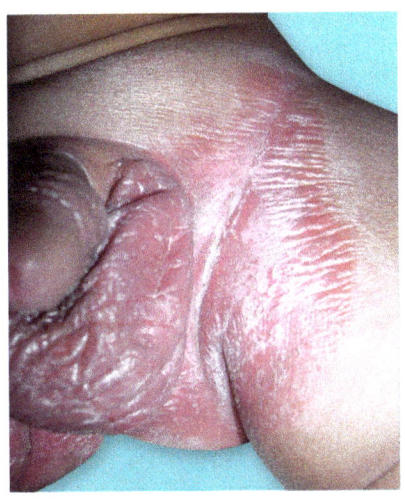
Fig. 26: Classical flexural psoriasis in the napkin area.

Flexural/Inverse/Napkin Psoriasis

Flexural psoriasis was observed in 12 out of 125 children studied by Stefanaki et al. Localization of erythematous, sometimes macerated thick plaques to the folds of the skin, including axillae and groin can be associated with plaque type psoriasis in other sites. Although clinical diagnosis is often possible, similarity to other diseases may require biopsy for differentiation. Secondary infection with *Candida* and/or *Streptococcus* may require cutaneous culture and usage of topical anti-infectives.

In contrast to irritant diaper dermatitis, it is sharply demarcated, brightly red, and involves the inguinal folds. Typically, symptoms respond poorly to conventional treatment of diaper dermatitis. Dissemination with widespread eruption of erythemato-squamous lesions on the whole body may follow. In the series of Morris et al. 13% of the children presented with diaper rash with dissemination and 4% with localized psoriatic diaper rash. A special clinical variant in young children is psoriatic diaper rash, which usually occurs until the age of 2 years. Macerated shiny erythema of the groin region including the folds and the genital skin with sharply demarcated, brightly red, erythema involving the inguinal folds will differentiate it from diaper dermatitis where the convexities are more affected sparing the folds (**Figs. 26 to 32**).[29]

Linear Psoriasis

Erythematous scaly papules or plaques following the lines of Blaschko are typically present since birth (**Figs. 33 to 36**).

Unlike inflammatory linear verrucous epidermal nevus, there is no or only mild pruritus. Presence of Koebner phenomenon and demonstration of Auspitz sign will help clinical diagnosis which can be further confirmed with biopsy, the histology of which will show psoriasiform features. Family history for psoriasis is often positive.[9]

CHAPTER 5 Pediatric Psoriasis

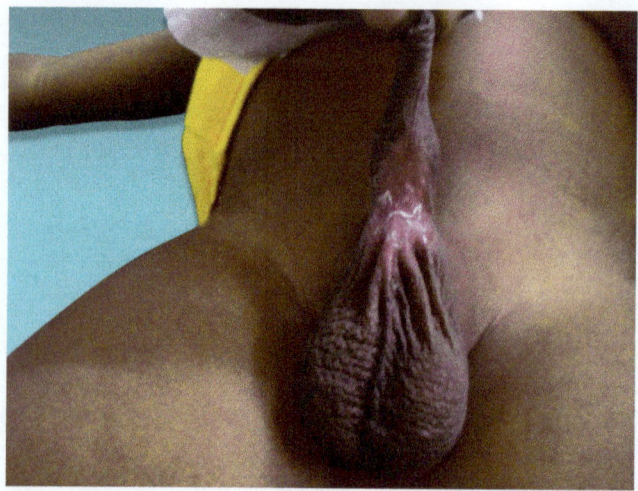

Fig. 27: Flexural psoriasis with no other suggestive lesions over the flexures.

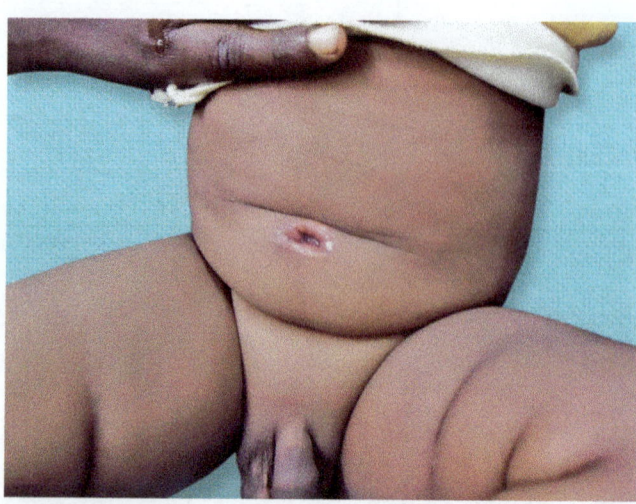

Fig. 30: Erythematous scaly plaque around umbilicus with loose scales signaling psoriasis infant.

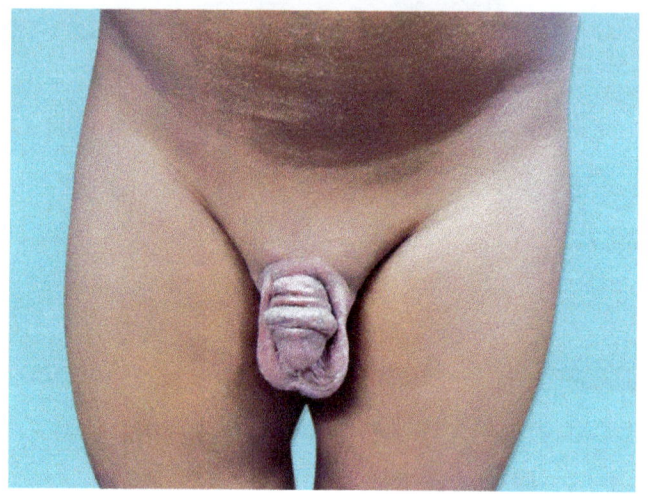

Fig. 28: Well-defined erythematous scaly plaque of psoriasis.

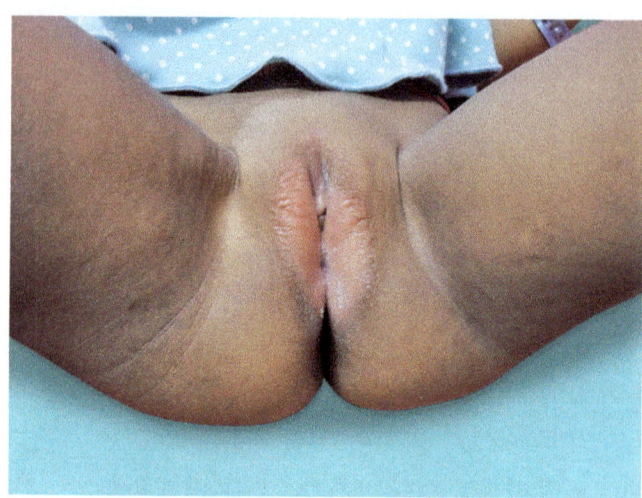

Fig. 31: Psoriasis of the napkin area in a girl child.

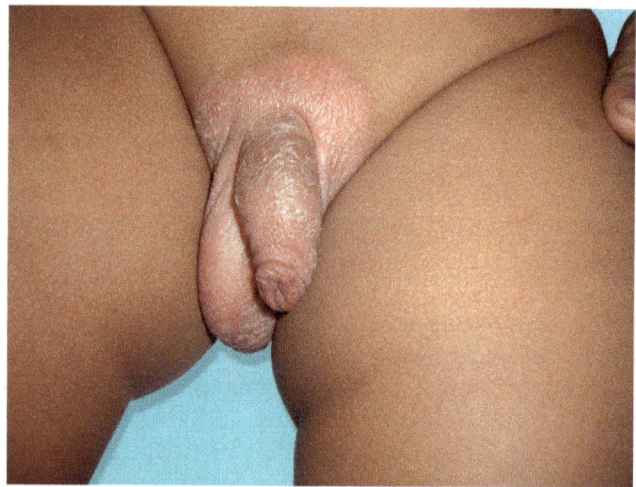

Fig. 29: Psoriasis affecting the genitals.

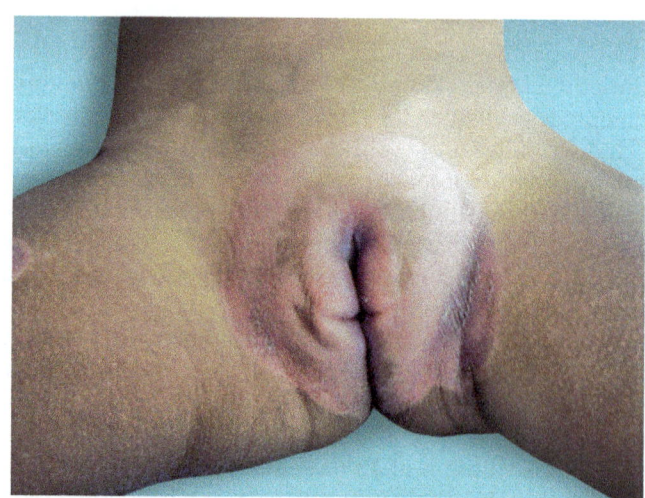

Fig. 32: Infant with napkin psoriasis.

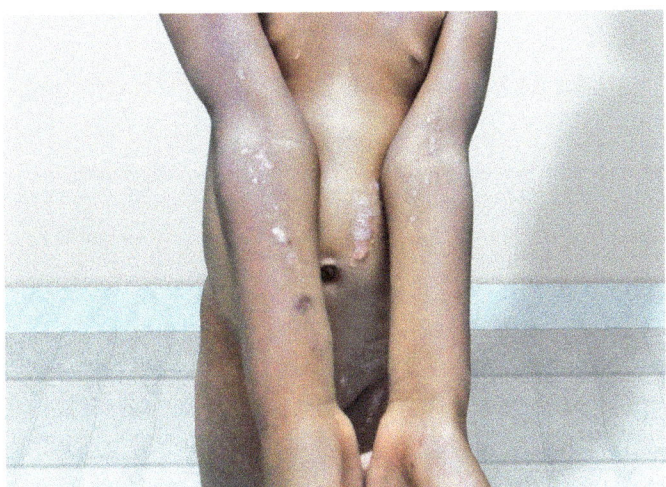

Fig. 33: Psoriasis along Blaschko's lines.

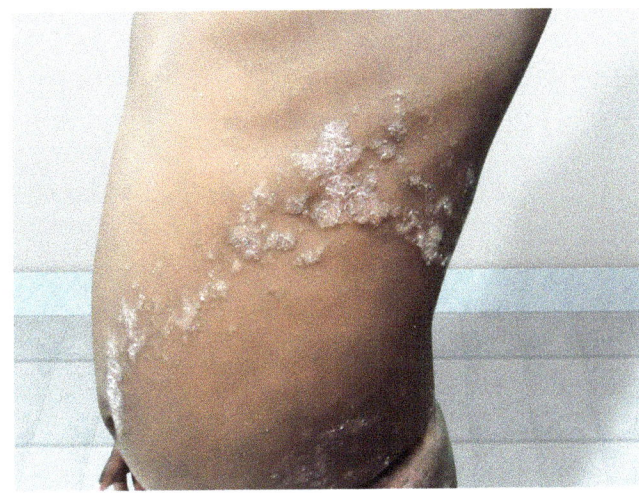

Fig. 35: Psoriasis along Blaschko's lines.

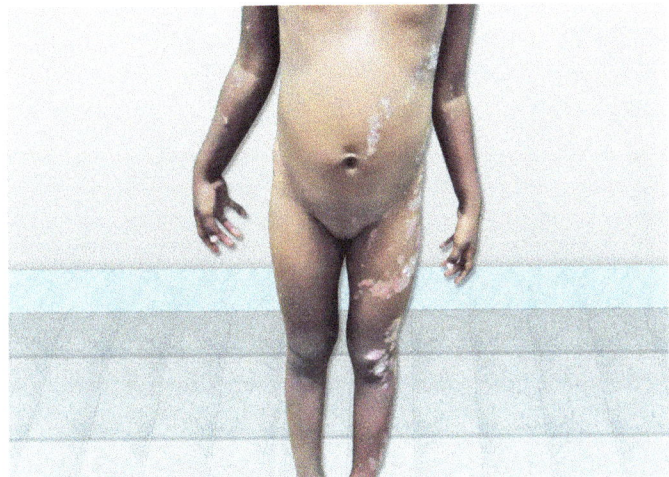

Fig. 34: Psoriasis along Blaschko's lines.

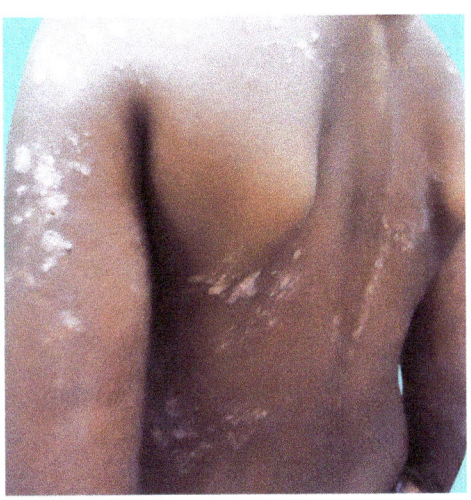

Fig. 36: Psoriasis along Blaschko's lines.

Nail Psoriasis

Stefanaki et al. have reported 10.4% of children to present with nail involvement **(Fig. 37)**.[4]

Nail changes in psoriasis may be seen in up to 40%.[9,32,42] Nail pitting is the most common manifestation. Oil drop sign, onycholysis, subungual hyperkeratosis, onychodystrophy, and splinter hemorrhages can also be observed. Nail involvement can precede, coincide with, or succeed psoriasis and may even rarely appear isolated. Nail abnormalities are more frequent in psoriatic arthritis and in digital skin involvement.[15]

Mucosal Psoriasis

Involvement of mucosa is seen in up to 7% of children in a study conducted by Alfonza and Nanda.[32] Annular plaques on the tongue may be noted in patients with psoriasis (**Fig. 38**). Geographic tongue is a common presentation of pustular psoriasis.

Erythrodermic Psoriasis

Psoriasis constituted about 18% of erythroderma in children in a study conducted by Sarkar and Garg.[47] Erythrodermic psoriasis is a rare clinical presentation in childhood psoriasis. It may arise from any type, commonly from the plaque type. It may arise from any type of psoriasis. Drugs, environmental, psychological, and metabolic factors can trigger the onset of erythrodermic form of the disease.[48,49] This spectrum of psoriasis is characterized by generalized erythema, edema, desquamation and systemic compromise. The child will present with fever, dehydration, malaise and malnutrition.[50] The overall presentation can range from mild to severe form. The erythrodermic form occurs in about 1.4% of psoriasis cases in children and

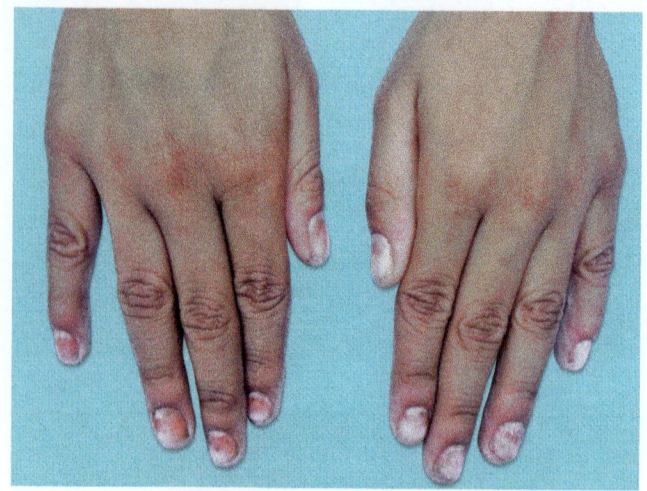

Fig. 37: Nail pitting in a boy with psoriasis.

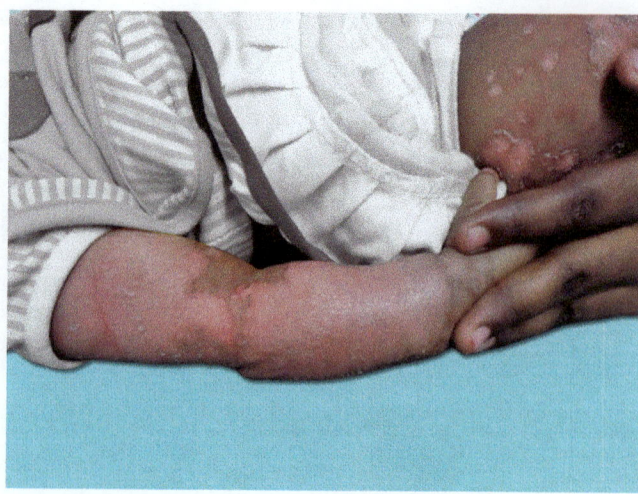

Fig. 39: Plaque psoriasis as in **Figure 8** evolving to erythrodermic psoriasis.

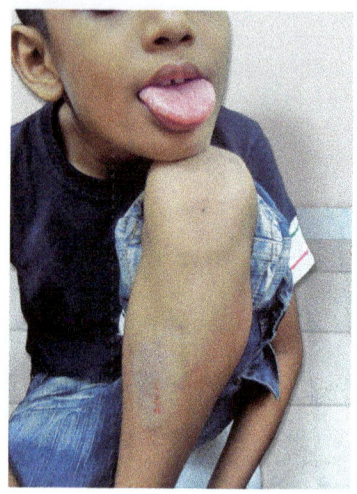

Fig. 38: Oral mucosal involvement in a boy with psoriasis.

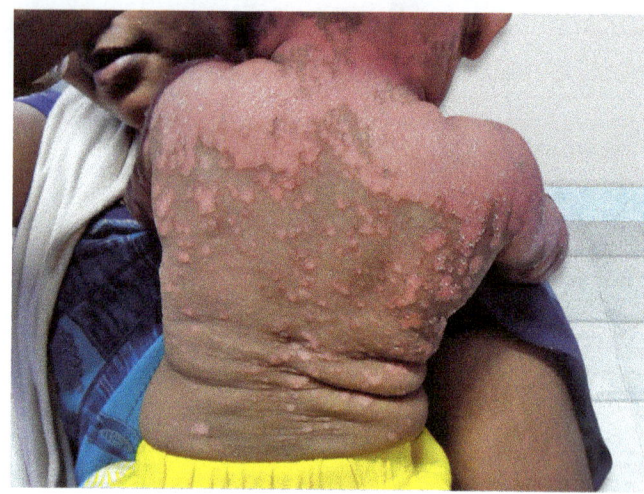

Fig. 40: Same child as in **Figure 39** with impending erythroderma.

adolescents.[3,6] Overall <3% of childhood psoriasis manifests with erythroderma **(Figs. 39 to 46)**.[51]

Congenital Psoriasis

Congenital psoriasis, meaning psoriasis present at birth or appearing during the neonatal period, is exceptional **(Figs. 47 to 51)**.

Congenital occurrence of psoriasis, defined as the development of any of its clinical variants at birth or during very first days of life is considered very rare.[52] The erythrodermic variant is exceptional. CEP is one of the most rare and severe forms of psoriasis. It was first described in 1966 by Frost and Van Scott who distinguished this entity from nonbullous ichthyosis form congenital erythroderma, with which it might be confused.[53] The neonates with erythroderma are at increased risk of hypernatremic dehydration, severe systemic infections, hypoalbuminemia and hyperpyrexia or hypothermia as a result of consequences of erythroderma. CEP is reported in as young as 5-day-old infant.[54]

Infantile Psoriasis

As high as 16% of childhood psoriasis were reported to have started during the first year of life **(Figs. 52 to 55)**.[29]

Psoriatic diaper rash, otherwise known as the napkin psoriasis and erythrodermic psoriasis are the two common manifestations during the first year of life. Scalp psoriasis is easily missed as cradle cap or seborrheic dermatitis.[55] The associated AD can sometimes pose a diagnostic dilemma in erythrodermic form in infants.[56]

Pustular Psoriasis

Pustular psoriasis appears at 2–10 years of age constituting <1% of childhood psoriasis **(Figs. 56 to 59)**.[15,56,57]

CHAPTER 5 Pediatric Psoriasis

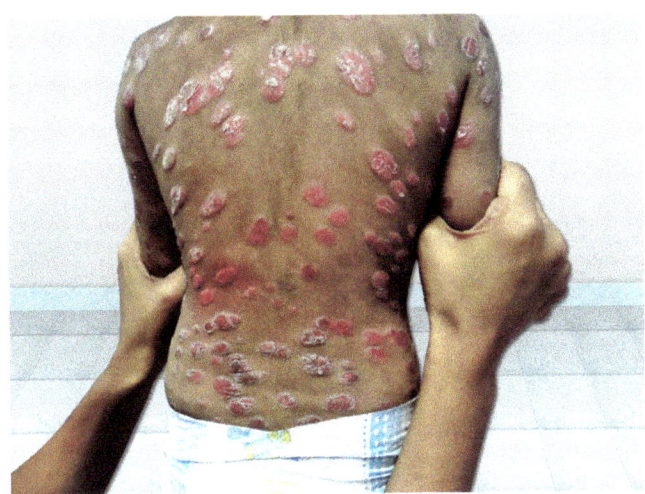

Fig. 41: Unstable psoriasis as seen by the fiery red plaques with irregular margins.

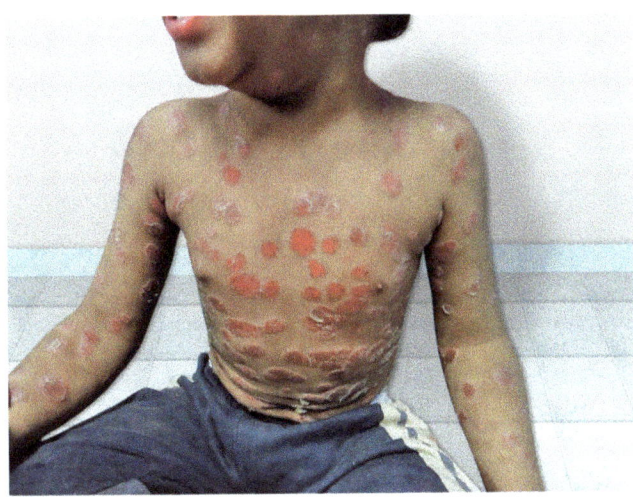

Fig. 44: Rapidly evolving severe plaque type psoriasis in an infant must think of unstable psoriasis.

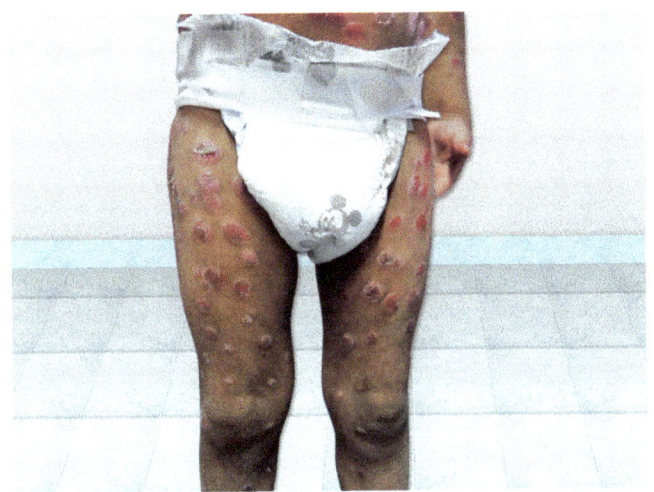

Fig. 42: Same child as in **Figure 40** with bright red plaques and irregular margins.

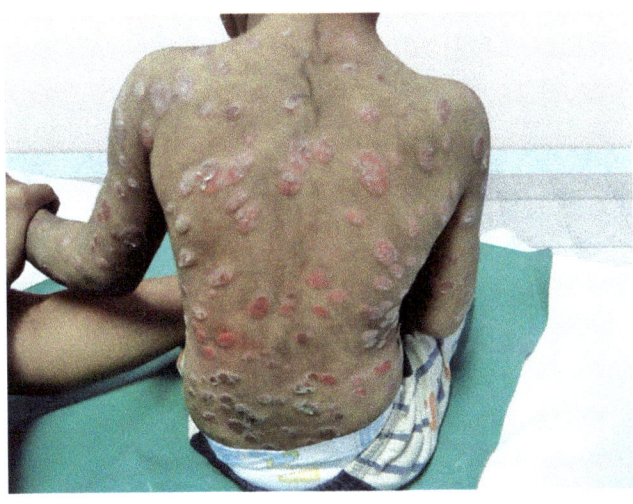

Fig. 45: Back of child seen in **Figure 44**.

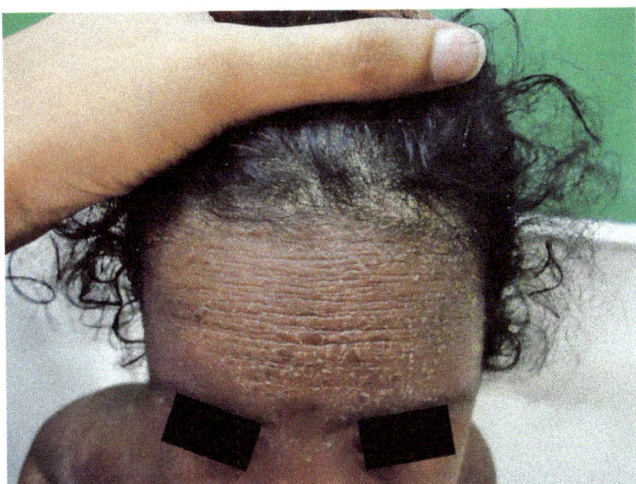

Fig. 43: Involvement of scalp in erythrodermic psoriasis.

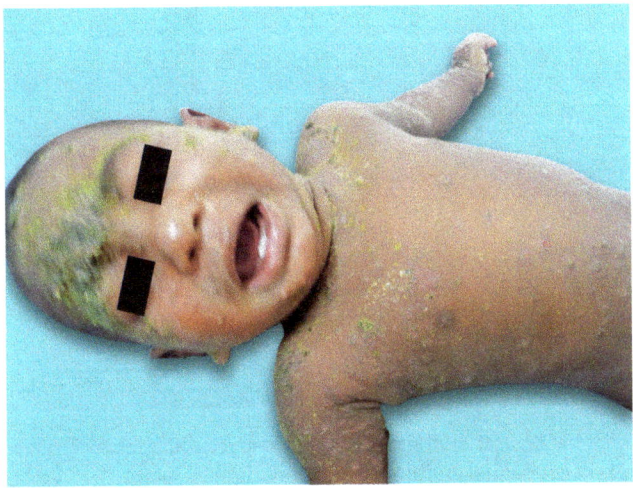

Fig. 46: Child with psoriasis evolved to erythroderma following irritation by local application.

CHAPTER 5 Pediatric Psoriasis

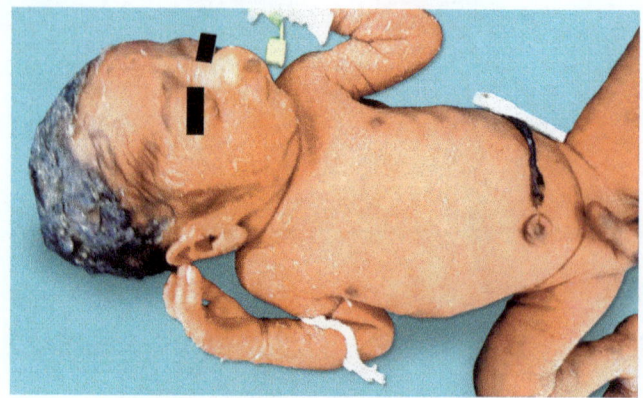

Fig. 47: Congenital erythrodermic psoriasis in a 5-day-old neonate.

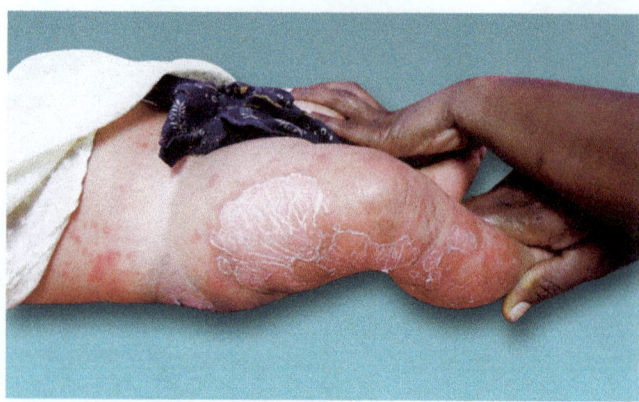

Fig. 50: Lower limbs of child shown in **Figure 49**.

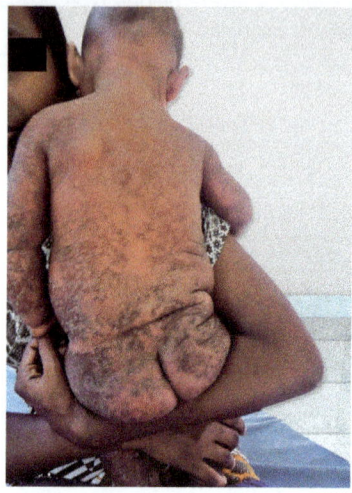

Fig. 48: Congenital erythrodermic psoriasis in an older infant.

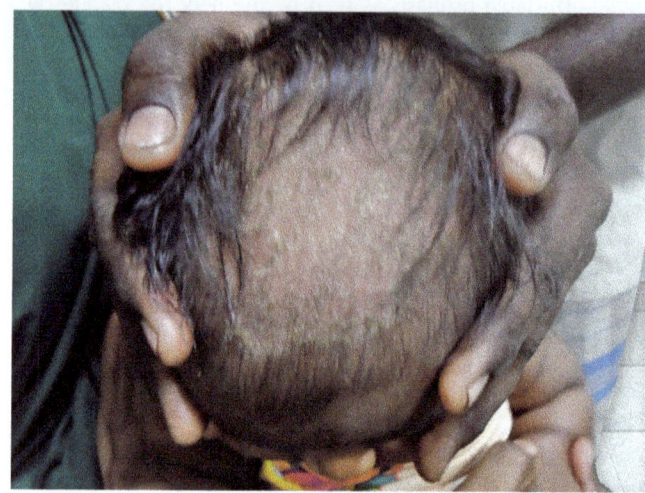

Fig. 51: Classical erythematous plaque over scalp with silvery scale in congenital erythrodermic psoriasis.

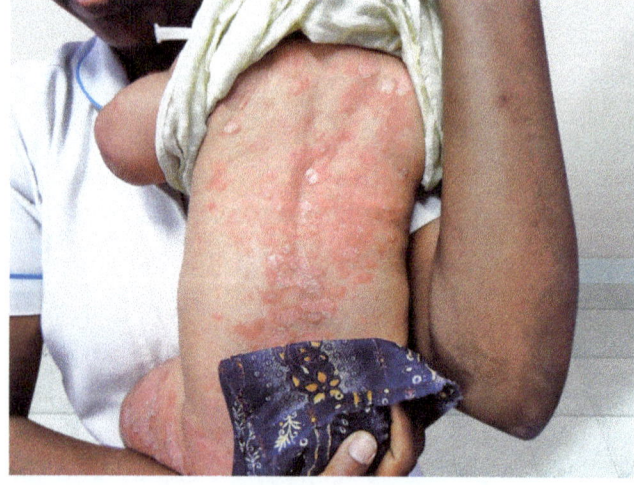

Fig. 49: Classical erythematous plaque over the back with silvery scale in congenital erythrodermic psoriasis in an infant.

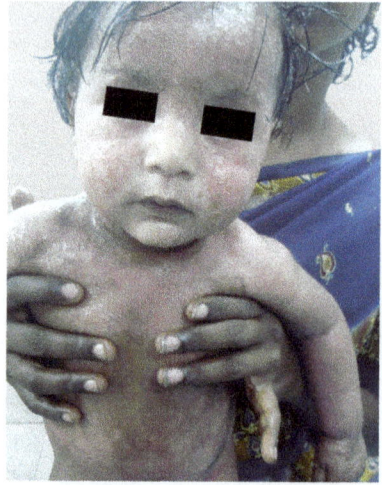

Fig. 52: Infant with erythroderma as presenting feature without history of plaque psoriasis.

CHAPTER 5 Pediatric Psoriasis

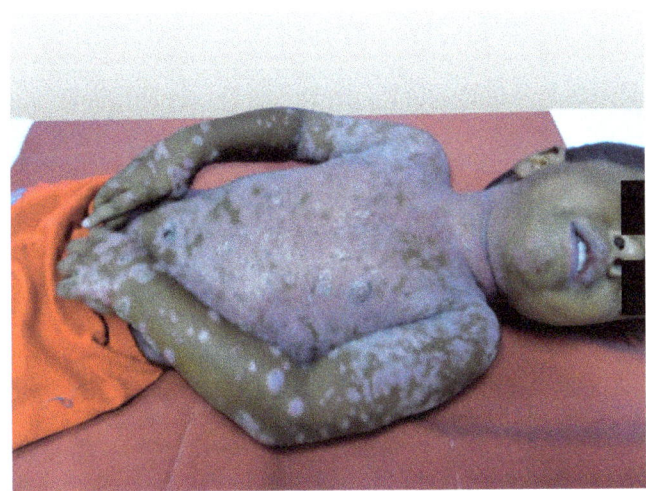

Fig. 53: Plaque psoriasis evolving into erythroderma in infant.

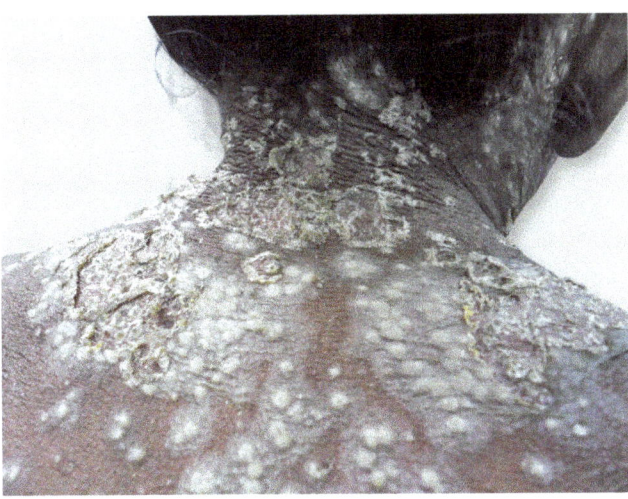

Fig. 56: Superficial pustules coalescing to form lake of pus in a known case of psoriasis after sudden withdrawal of systemic steroids.

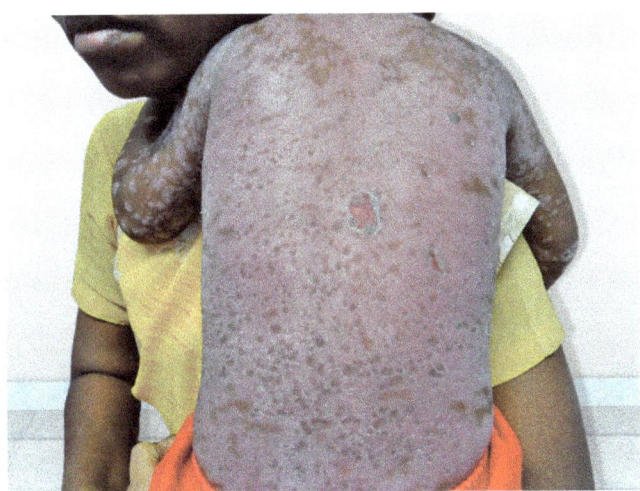

Fig. 54: Back of child seen in **Figure 53**.

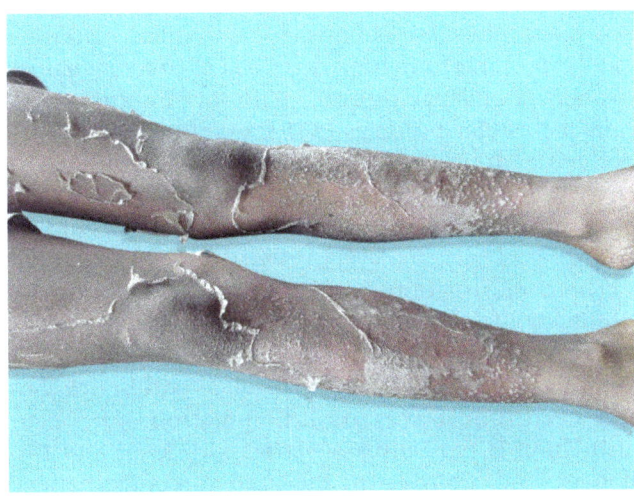

Fig. 57: Same child as in **Figure 56** showing resolution.

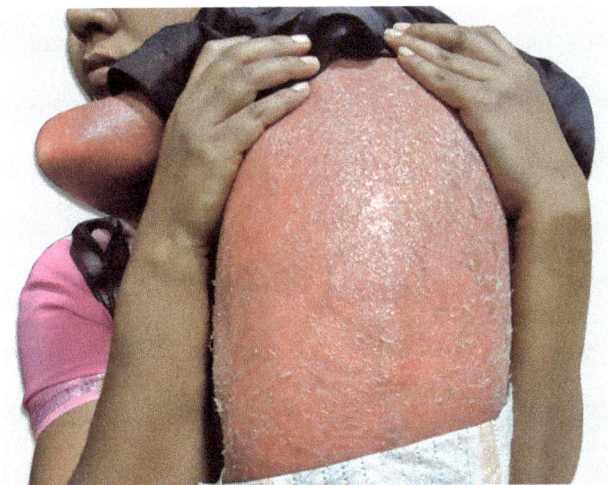

Fig. 55: Erythrodermic psoriasis in an infant.

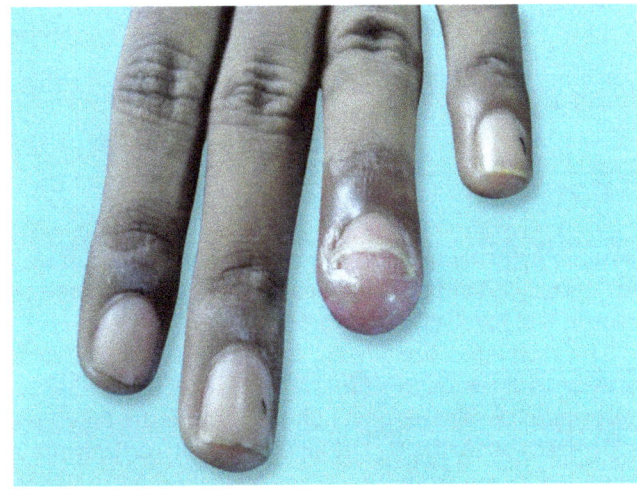

Fig. 58: Fingertip pustular lesion with nail change is an indicator of pustular psoriasis.

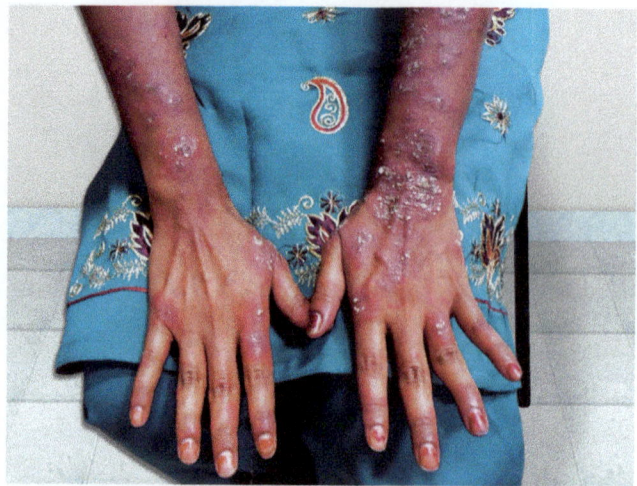

Fig. 59: Pustular psoriasis in an older girl.

A review of 1,262 cases of childhood psoriasis found a 0.6% rate of pustular variants.[29] Four clinical patterns of pustular psoriasis have been described in children: namely, generalized pustular psoriasis (GPP or von Zumbusch), annular pustular psoriasis (APP), exanthematic pustular psoriasis and localized pustular psoriasis. Annular form seems to be the most common presentation. They are not necessarily mutually exclusive and mixed variants are also possible.[58]

The clinical pattern of GPP (an acute, episodic, and potentially life-threatening form of psoriasis) classically presents as widespread sheets of sterile pustules on bright erythematous skin that resolves within 3-4 days, with recurrent waves of inflammation. The acute pustulation is typically associated with fever and toxic changes.[35,59,60] Considering the condition of the patients, GPP in children could be further classified as either the severe type or the mild type. Compared with the adult forms, the first manifestation of GPP in children is usually high fever accompanied by generalized pustules. Few of these cases converted to be psoriasis vulgaris.[61] The younger the age of onset, the more severe the patient's condition can be.[59]

Arthropathic Psoriasis

Psoriatic arthritis is relatively uncommon in children; it may occur with either plaque or guttate psoriasis and may precede skin involvement **(Fig. 60)**.

The estimated prevalence of psoriatic arthritis in all patients with psoriasis differs from 5 to 30%.[62,63] Eight to twenty percent of cases of childhood arthritis are diagnosed as psoriatic arthritis.[64] The age of onset of findings in childhood ranges from 9 to 12 years of age.[65] An incidence of < 2% was noted in studies conducted by Stefanaki, Al fouzan and Kumar.[9,31,32]

ASSOCIATIONS AND COMORBIDITIES

Psoriasis is commonly found to be associated with conditions like allergic contact dermatitis, eczema, vitiligo and alopecia areata.[41] It can also be easily mistaken for seborrheic dermatitis, avitaminosis with which it can coexist **(Figs. 61 to 64)**.

The association with AD commonly seen in adults is also seen in children with psoriasis.[66] Psoriatic children have a higher prevalence of obesity. It was also observed that overweight had different effects on childhood patients. Psoriasis in these children was more severe compared with psoriatic children of normal weight.[67] There is a strong association between psoriasis and obesity in children especially boys.[68] Increased incidence of hyperlipidemia, hypertension, and diabetes, has also reported to be associated with psoriasis in children/adolescents. It may be

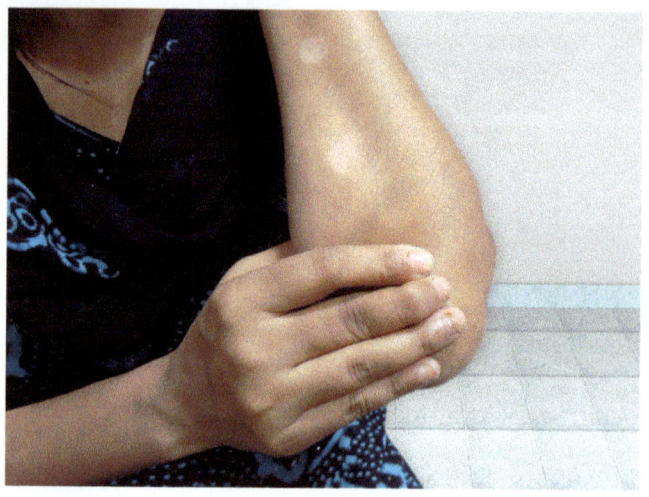

Fig. 60: Arthropathy of distal interphalangeal joints with lesion on the extensors in an adolescent girl with psoriasis.

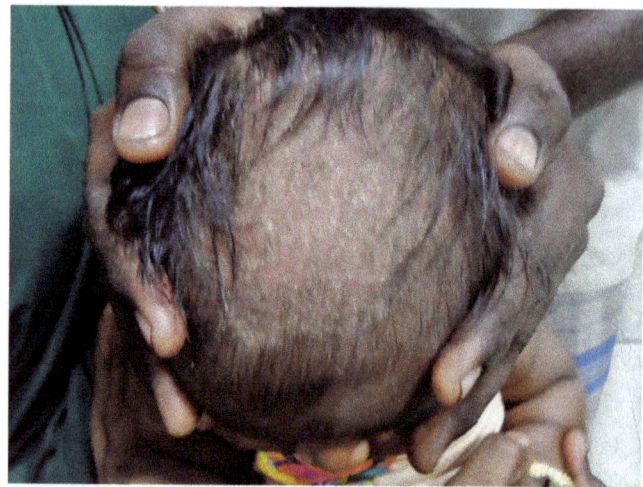

Fig. 61: Severe seborrheic dermatitis in an infant lasting longer than usual may be an indicator of psoriasis as is severe dandruff in an adult.

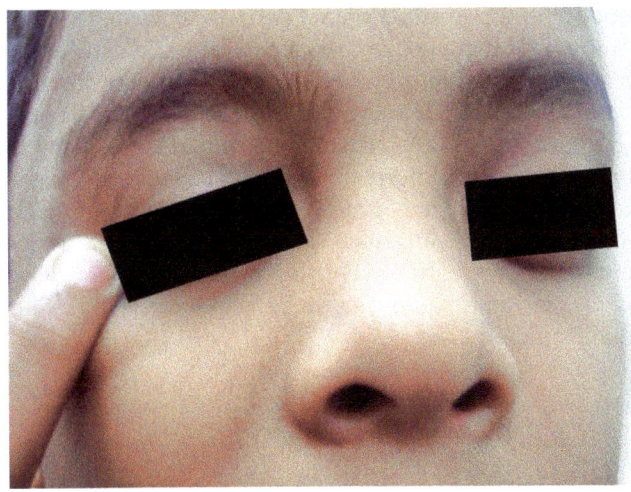

Fig. 62: Psoriasis in a boy mimicking seborrheic dermatitis.

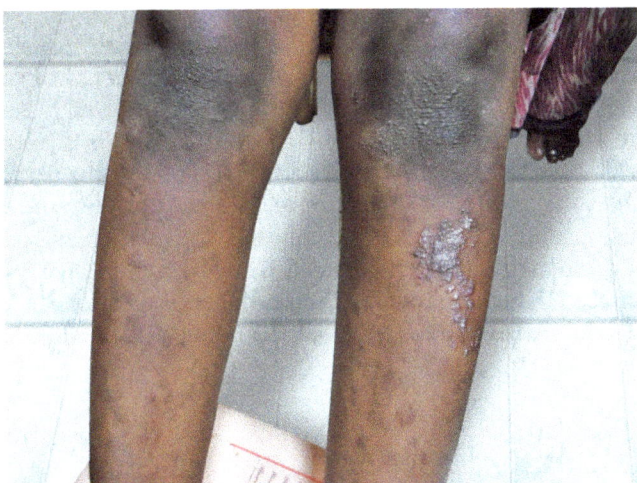

Fig. 63: Follicular psoriasis with phrynoderma.

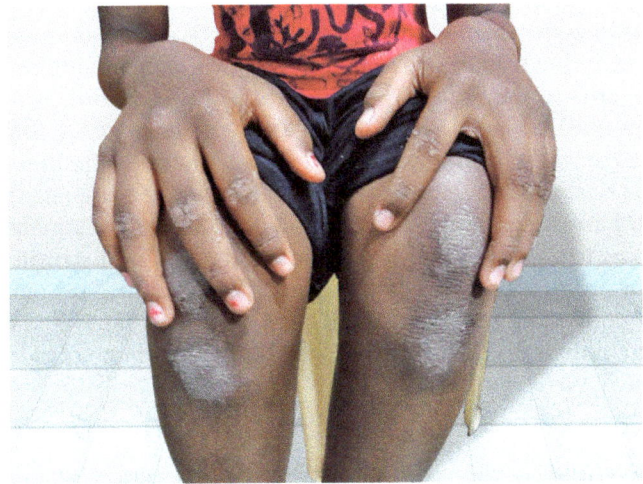

Fig. 64: Psoriasis in a boy with avitaminosis.

considered that in an obese child, disease severity can be a marker of cardiovascular risk. Prevalence of comorbidities in persons in the age range 0-20 years with psoriasis was found to be more than those without psoriasis. The following comorbidities were observed by Augustin et al.:[69] Crohn's disease, hyperlipidemia, diabetes mellitus, arterial hypertension, rheumatoid arthritis, obesity, ischemic heart disease and ulcerative colitis.[6]

TREATMENT

Childhood psoriasis is a cause for concern to the child, parent and the doctor alike. An effective therapy starts with counseling the patient and parent, explaining to them the nature of the disease, treatment options available, their pros and cons.[70]

This segment will review the treatment of childhood psoriasis under two headings:
1. The treatment options available
2. Treatment of different types of psoriasis.

Treating a child with psoriasis is a challenge. Success of the treatment partially lies on the compliance of the patient which means the safety and accessibility of treatment should be considered important.

Treatment options available can be symptomatic and specific. Antihistamines are given to alleviate itching. It would therefore, be preferable to give sedative antihistamines.

The available treatment options are broadly divided as:
- Topical therapy
- Phototherapy
- Systemic therapy
- Other modalities

Topical therapy is the mainstay for mild or localized disease with a PASI <10 or involvement of BSA of <20%.

Emollients, moisturizers, keratolytics, tar, anthralin, topical steroids, vitamin D analogs, calcineurin inhibitors, and retinoid are various topical preparations available.

The choice will depend upon the age of the child, type of psoriasis, PASI score, site of involvement, other comorbidities and associations, tolerance and affordability.

Emollients

Emollients are the most commonly used in management of childhood psoriasis. White soft paraffin reduces transepidermal water loss (TEWL), soothe and soften the skin and reduce scaling. They improve the barrier function and stratum corneum hydration, making the epidermis less amenable to trauma and stress, which is one of the trigger factors for the disease exacerbation. It is wise to start treatment with these agents and allow the disease to evolve before embarking to any stronger medications with side effects.

Keratolytics

Keratolytics, such as salicylic acid and urea, reduce scaling and enhance absorption of other drugs. Salicylic acid can be in lesions over the scalp, palms and soles in children older than 6 years. It is to be avoided in younger children because of the risk of percutaneous salicylate absorption leading to salicylism.[71] Topical salicylic acid reduces the efficacy of ultraviolet B (UVB) phototherapy because of a filtering effect.

Tar

Coal tar, which has antipruritic and anti-inflammatory effects, also suppresses deoxyribonucleic acid (DNA) synthesis and acts as antiproliferative agent.[72,73] It can be used alone or in combination with other agents such as corticosteroids, salicylic acid and ultraviolet therapy. However, it is not to be used on face and flexures, and in children below 12 years of age. Tar causes irritation, when combined with ultraviolet light in the Goeckerman regimen. Tar is also known to induce chromosomal aberrations in peripheral lymphocytes and bring on release of heat shock proteins.[74]

Dithranol

Dithranol, also known as anthralin, has anti-inflammatory and antiproliferative effects which are attributable to its ability to regulate keratinocyte differentiation and prevent T lymphocyte activation. The drug accumulates in keratinocyte mitochondria, dissipates mitochondrial membrane potential, and induces apoptosis through a pathway dependent on respiratory competent mitochondria.[75] "Short contact therapy" is the preferred method these days in which increasing concentrations of anthralin are applied for a short period (10–30 minutes) till a slight irritation develops, after which the dose and time are held constant till lesions clear.[76]

A significant remission in 81% of children was observed with 1% concentration.[77] It can be combined with UVB phototherapy, as in Ingram regimen, to improve the response. Anthralin 1% or dithranol are rarely used for localized areas and can cause localized irritation.[78] The usage of dithranol has been reducing with advent of new more cosmetically acceptable topical preparations.

Topical Steroids

Topical steroids are suitable for the treatment of childhood psoriasis among all age groups. They have anti-inflammatory, antiproliferative, immunosuppressive and vasoconstrictive effects.

Steroids low- to mid-potency corticosteroids, class 5–7, are chosen for facial and intertriginous lesions, while mid-potency class 2–4, are chosen for extremities and the scalp.[79] Topical clobetasol has been approved for use in children ages 12 and over in some formulations and can be quite effective for use in psoriatic lesions in adolescents.[80] Their inadvertent and long-term use can lead to local infections, skin atrophy, telangiectasia, striae distensae, acneiform eruption, and purpura. Contact dermatitis to the molecule or the vehicle is not uncommon. Rebound and tachyphylaxis are to be remembered while using topical steroids for a prolonged period. It is always advisable to follow the fingertip unit and adhere to the schedule. Systemic side effects are more common in children than adults because of a higher skin surface/body mass ratio. Ointments are to be avoided in flexural, facial, and genital skin. Lotions are preferred for hairy scalp. They can also be combined with other topicals such as calcipotriol and tazarotene to enhance efficacy and reduce irritation.

Topical Vitamin D Analogs

Topical vitamin D analogs have anti-inflammatory and antiproliferative actions. They also induce down regulation and correction of keratinocyte differentiation. Calcipotriol, calcitriol, maxacalcitol and tacalcitol are the various vitamin D analogs useful in the treatment of psoriasis. When combined with betamethasone the effect is better than either agent used alone. UVB phototherapy increases the efficacy of calcipotriol.[66,81] The most common adverse events are burning and stinging sensation, the drug is safe when the total dose does not exceed the recommended dose of not >75 g/week for children above 12 years and 50 g/week for children between 6 and 12 years. Over use can lead to hypercalcemia. Calcipotriene or calcitriol can be used for pediatric psoriasis, the latter being well tolerated for sensitive skin.[82,83]

Calcineurin Inhibitors

Topical calcineurin inhibitors act as nonsteroidal immunomodulatory drugs. They inhibit IL-2 production and subsequent T-cell activation and proliferation by blocking the enzyme calcineurin tacrolimus (0.03%, 0.1%) ointment and pimecrolimus (1%) cream are two drugs belonging to this class, which, although not food and drug administration (FDA) approved, have proven efficacy. This has recently been documented for treatment of childhood psoriasis.[84,85] They can be used as steroid sparing agents and are also useful for sequential and rotational regimens, so as to avoid long-term adverse effects of topical steroids. They are useful for sites such as face, flexures and anogenital region where topical steroids cannot be used safely.[86] Use in children under the age of 2 years is not recommended by the FDA.

Retinoids

Tazarotene is a third generation retinoid that acts on keratinocyte differentiation, diminishing hyperproliferation, and decreases expression of inflammatory markers. Skin irritation is the most common side effect and its use is thus usually restricted to thicker plaques in the nonintertriginous sites. Tazarotene 0.05% gel has been successfully used to treat nail psoriasis in a child in a single case report.[87]

Phototherapy

Ultraviolet radiation in the spectrum of ultraviolet A (UVA) and UVB act by inhibiting DNA synthesis and epidermal keratinocyte proliferation, inducing T-cell apoptosis. They also exhibit immunosuppressive and anti-inflammatory property. Broadband UVB (BB-UVB, 290–320 nm), narrow-band UVB (NB-UVB, 311 ± 2 nm) and UVA (320–400 nm) are the three spectra used in the treatment of psoriasis. Phototherapy is appropriate for carefully selected patients with refractory disease, diffuse (>15–20% BSA) involvement, or focal debilitating palmoplantar psoriasis. Guttate and thin plaque type lesions respond best to phototherapy. NB-UVB is the safest of the three and is used in children above six years of age. UVA or PUVA therapy is not advised in children below 12 years of age. In children, NB-UVB is more convenient and may be less carcinogenic, and given the independence of psoralens-related precautions and adverse effects, NB-UVB is now considered first-line phototherapy in pediatric age group for psoriasis. PUVA bath treatment should be preferred to oral PUVA in older children (>12 years) and adolescents in situations like recalcitrant hand and foot psoriasis because of avoidance of gastrointestinal side effects, lack of eye protection required, and shorter photosensitization time.[88] To limit the cumulative UVB dose and thereby the carcinogenic risk, combination with systemic therapy like acitretin or topical therapy like calcipotriol, tazarotene and anthralin has been found useful.[89] Ultraviolet treatment to children must be administered in an appropriate environment with constant supervision by parents and trained professional staff. One has to remember that any form of light therapy has to be commenced in children with enough considerations and thoughtfulness of the child being exposed to ultraviolet light-containing sunlight for many more years to come in their life time.

Systemic Therapies

Specific systemic therapy is rarely used in childhood psoriasis **(Figs. 65 to 71)**.

Systemic therapy including retinoid, methotrexate and cyclosporine, biologic is only used in severe forms of the disease such as erythrodermic, pustular and arthritic psoriasis. All these therapeutic options can be used as monotherapy or in various combinations.[90]

The indication for systemic therapy is one or more of the following:
- Involvement of BSA >20%
- Psoriasis area and severity index >10
- Erythrodermic psoriasis, with or without metabolic complication
- Generalized pustular psoriasis

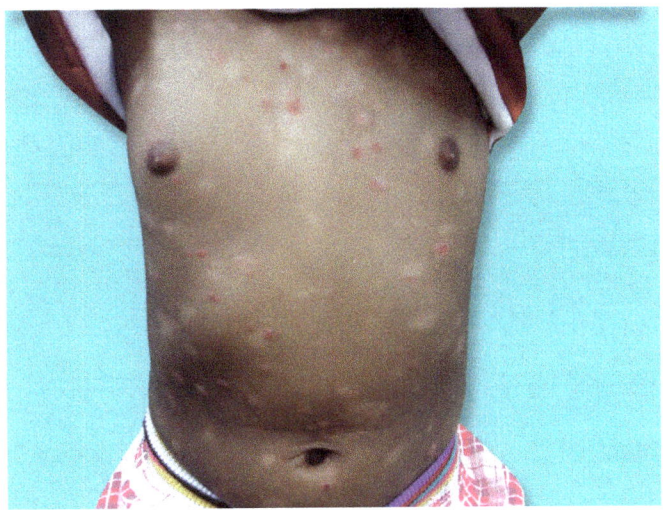

Fig. 65: Child 1 month after cyclosporine.

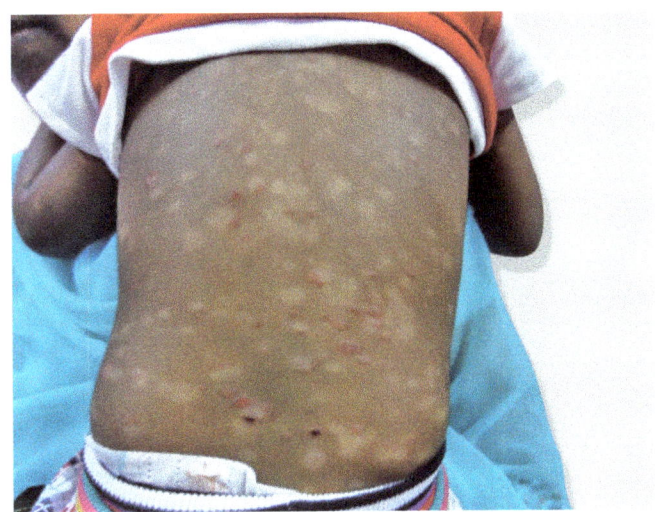

Fig. 66: Same child as in **Figure 65**.

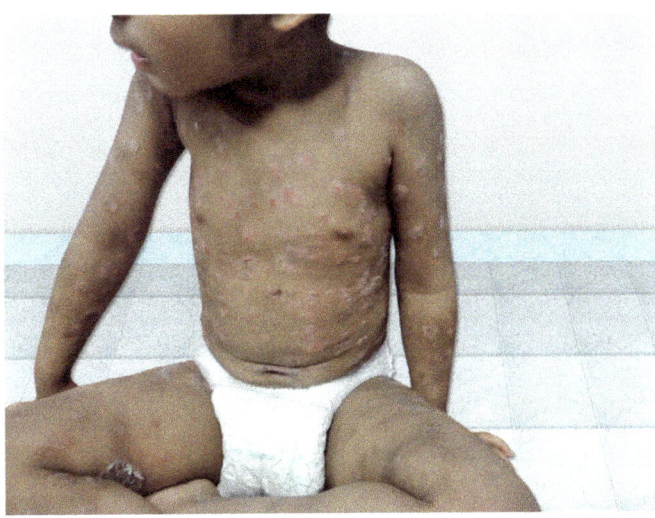

Fig. 67: Same child as in **Figure 65**—2 months after cyclosporine.

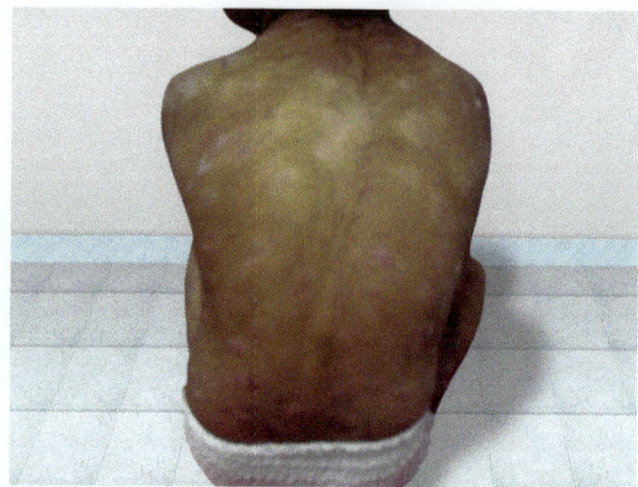

Fig. 68: Same child as in **Figure 66** after 2 months after cyclosporine.

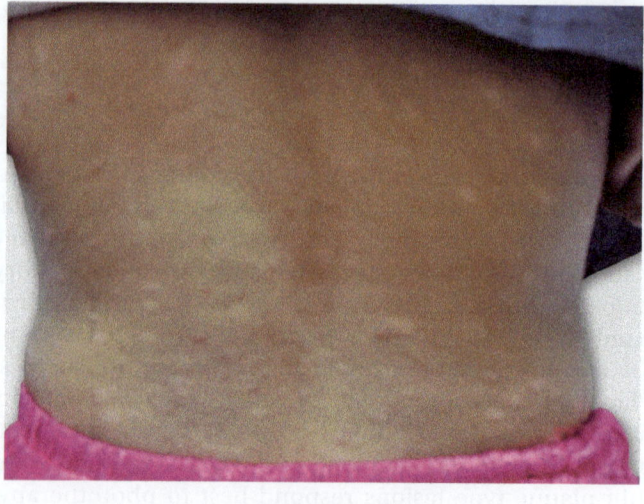

Fig. 71: Same child as in **Figure 70** showing the back.

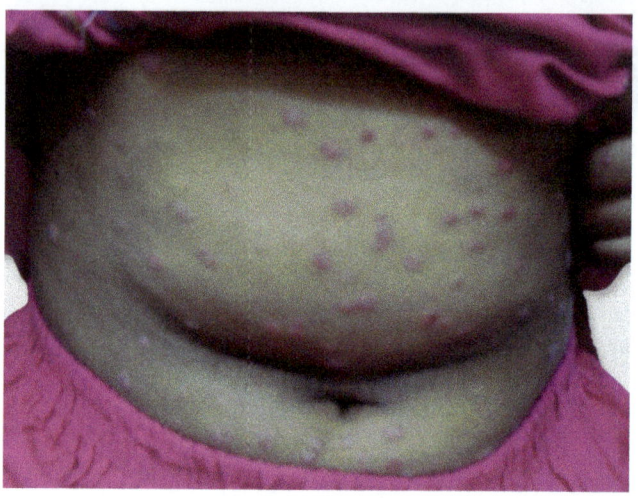

Fig. 69: Older child 1 month after methotrexate.

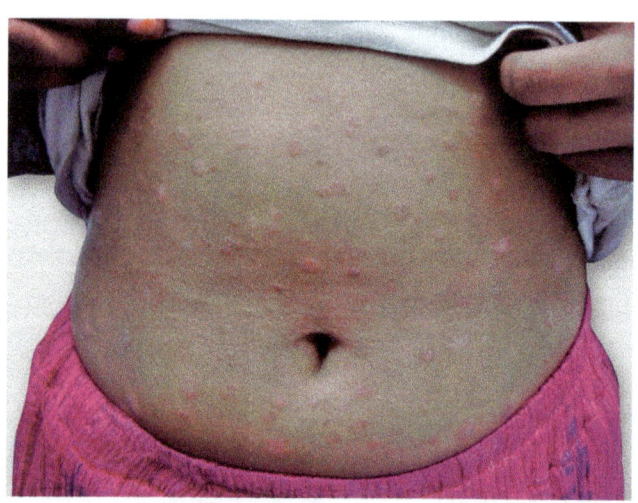

Fig. 70: Same child as in **Figure 69** after 2 months.

- Psoriatic arthropathy
- Localized disease not responding to topical therapy alone or with significant psychological morbidity.

Retinoids

Etretinate and acitretin, belonging to second generation retinoids, are the most commonly used systemic retinoids in children. The modes of action include modulation of the epidermal proliferation and differentiation, and anti-inflammatory activity. To begin with a low dose is started which can be increased up to 1 mg/kg/day and on improvement, tapered to 0.2 mg/kg body weight. The treatment continued for around 2–3 months postremission. Absorption is increased by milk or fatty foods and when dissolved in edible oils will enhance absorption.[91] The most common adverse effects are xerosis, cheilitis, epistaxis and reversible alteration in liver enzymes and serum lipids. Premature closure of epiphysis limits its use in children. Retinoids are best avoided while treating girls.

Methotrexate

It is an antimetabolite agent and one of the most commonly used systemic agent for the treatment of psoriasis, because of its efficacy, affordability and convenient dosing. It's usually given in a dosage of 0.2–0.4 mg/kg/week.[92] There are various studies documenting the successful use of methotrexate in various forms of juvenile psoriasis. Methotrexate is well-tolerated by children. It is effective as a single weekly oral dose of 3.75–25 mg. Most of the children tolerate the drug well-nausea; vomiting are the common side effects.[93] Serious adversities are a rare occurrence. When carefully monitored, methotrexate can be a safe and efficacious treatment option for severe forms of psoriasis in children. Obesity may be a relative contraindication, as associated nonalcoholic fatty liver disease is likely to increase hepatotoxicity.[94,95]

Relative Contraindications for Methotrexate Use

- Renal dysfunction (dosage adjustments needed)
- Significantly abnormal results on liver function tests

- Hepatitis
- Cirrhosis
- Significant pulmonary disease
- Blood dyscrasias (severe anemia, leukopenia, thrombocytopenia)
- Excessive alcohol consumption
- Active infectious disease (tuberculosis, pyelonephritis)

Cyclosporine

It is an immunosuppressive drug that primarily acts by inhibiting T-cell function and IL-2. Cyclosporin is an effective drug in the management of childhood psoriasis and is generally well tolerated.[96] It is used in a dose range of 3–5 mg/kg and is variably effective. In some patients, it is a true crisis buster. Nephrotoxicity, hypertension, immunosuppression are the major side effects and hence the drug is reserved only for severe cases.[97,98]

Biologics

The introduction of biologics in the armamentarium of antipsoriatic drugs is indeed a giant leap in the management of refractory pediatric psoriasis where other drugs like retinoids, methotrexate and cyclosporine cannot be used. Etanercept, an anti-TNF fusion protein, has been the one studied most extensively.[99-101] It has been found to be effective and well-tolerated in children and adolescents with moderate-to-severe plaque psoriasis. There are four case reports of the use infliximab in childhood psoriasis with good results.[102-105] When providing a child with biologics parents should be cautioned as to the side effects and potential life-threatening complications which can be associated. Being an immunosuppressive drug, the dosing of biologic agent is crucial ensuring that the child's immune system is not suppressed and allows for contacting infectious disease.

Administration of any of the above systemic drugs in a child should always be a team effort of dermatologist and pediatrician along with other specialist-like gastroenterologist as whenever necessary.

Other Modalities

Laser

A pilot study has reported 308 nm excimer lasers to be a safe and effective treatment for localized psoriasis in children as in adults.[106]

Oral antibiotics can be useful in treating psoriasis vulgaris, particularly in the setting of positive oral pharyngeal cultures, presence of perianal bacterial dermatitis, pustular psoriasis.[3,107]

Dietary Supplement

Fish oil, rich in omega-3 fatty acids is the best-known dietary supplement. Oral and intravenous supplementation of omega-3 and, less effectively, omega-6 fatty acids have been found effective in psoriatic adults, possibly through alterations in production and alterations in arachidonic acid (20:4 omega 6) and docosapentaenoic acid.[108]

Indigo naturalis, a traditional Chinese medicine, can be formulated into topical ointment with anecdotal reports of good results in childhood psoriasis when used for 8 weeks.[109]

Treatment According to Type of Psoriasis

Plaque Type Psoriasis

Treatments must be tailored to the age of the patient, quality of life issues, and surface area affected. Anthralin is an effective treatment of plaque psoriasis either with or without topical steroids. With the advent of newer drugs, the frequency of its use has come down. Topical steroids, calcipotriol, tazarotene are useful and safe if used properly. Salicylic acid can be used along with steroids in thick plaques. Systemic agents like methotrexate and phototherapy may be needed in moderate-to-severe recalcitrant disease.

Scalp Psoriasis

Topical steroid with or without salicylic acid as lotion applied at night followed by steroid/ketoconazole-based shampooing in the morning is helpful. For resistant plaques, tar based shampoos will help. A combination with NB-UVB/targeted phototherapy will give better results.

Guttate Psoriasis

Oral antibiotics are found to be useful in the treatment of guttate psoriasis. Systemic agents and phototherapy may be needed in moderate to severe disease. It should be remembered that guttate psoriasis can evolve into psoriasis vulgaris and hence the child should be followed up regularly.

Inverse Psoriasis

Nonsteroidal agents like-calcineurin inhibitor, low-potency topical corticosteroids are used with caution. Ointments should be avoided.

Nail Psoriasis

Psoriasis nail will frequently have super-added fungal infection after treatment of which, topical corticosteroids, tazarotene or calcipotriene can be applied to the paronychial skin. Intralesional triamcinolone can also be used in the same region to reduce the subungual inflammation. Calcipotriol or tazarotene under occlusion covering the nail folds, plate, and under the nail plate are useful.

Napkin Psoriasis

Mild topical corticosteroids with or without topical anticandidal agents can be helpful. Secondary infection if any should be attended to. Barrier therapy with zinc oxide pastes reduces secondary irritant reactions.

Pustular Psoriasis

Generalized pustular psoriasis responds well to methotrexate in children.[110] Maintenance of nutrition, fluid electrolyte balance prevention of organ failure should be stressed. Acitretin/isotretinoin (not for adolescent girls), and dapsone can be tried depending on the biochemical parameters. Oral steroids are used only to tide over the acute crisis. If the disease is localized, topical agents-like steroids will suffice.

Mucosal Psoriasis

No therapy is usually needed; however, topical medicaments in an oral base can be used when needed.

Congenital Erythrodermic Psoriasis

Regardless of underlying disease, the management of neonatal erythroderma includes fluid and electrolyte balance, correction of caloric and protein intake, and prevention and treatment of infections. Specific therapy is started once the diagnosis of underlying disease is established. The infant should be followed up. Topical calcipotriol is effective when emollients are not enough.[111]

Arthropathic Psoriasis

Methotrexate is the drug of choice in children with psoriatic arthropathy.

PSYCHOLOGICAL ASPECTS AND REHABILITATION

Psoriasis by itself is a disease that causes a lot of psychological stress and vice versa. Psoriasis was recently shown to have a great impact on quality of life in affected children **(Figs. 72 to 74)**.

Like AD, urticaria and acne, psoriasis in the pediatric age group can lead to a severe emotional burden to the extent of impairing the health-related quality of life. A study on children and adolescents aged between 5 and 16 years found that in children with psoriasis the values were as high

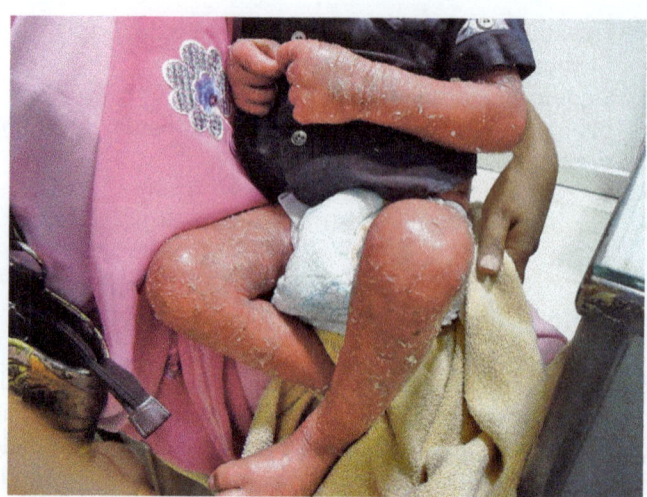

Fig. 72: Boy with erythrodermic psoriasis with severe psychological disturbance.

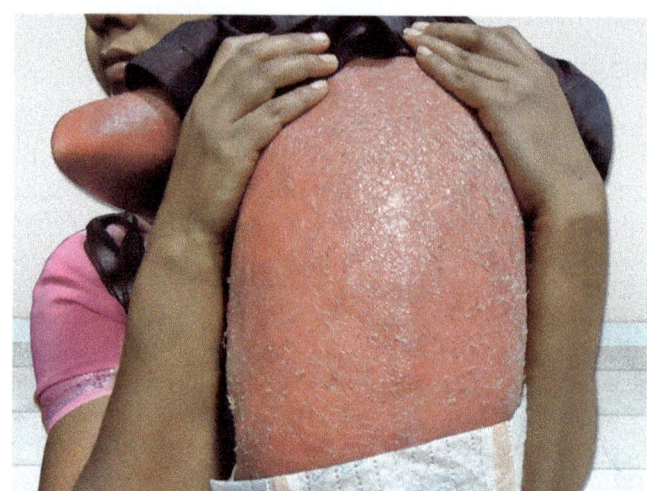

Fig. 73: Back of child seen in **Figure 72**.

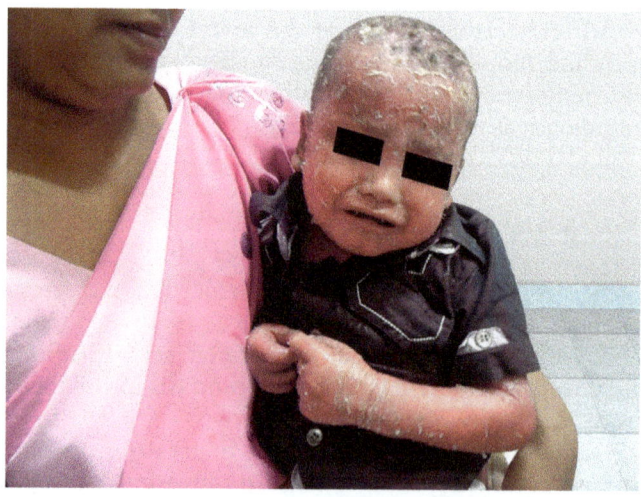

Fig. 74: Same boy as in **Figures 72 and 73** with note the facial expression.

as in children with AD, and higher than in children with urticaria or acne.[112]

The afflicted children must learn to cope with life and to adapt to their individual health situation. They must be counseled to choose a profession suitable to them in future. Rehabilitation of psoriatic children and adolescents can also supplement therapy of and prevent the disease.

Therapy goals of rehabilitation will include:
- Regular treatment of the skin under proper supervision clubbed with climate therapy, nutritional therapy and psychological interventions.
- Help in coping with the disease with respect to the psychosocial consequences of psoriasis.
- Help in finding an occupation.

SUMMARY

Childhood psoriasis signifies a special challenge. The varied etiopathological theories make the disease more diverse. The early onset of the disease and the congenital forms indicate a much stronger genetic background. Awareness of the characteristics of childhood psoriasis will aid clinicians in early diagnosis and management. Further work into the genetics and more research on pathology and controlled studies on therapy will throw more light on effective management protocol. It is essential to understand the impact of adiposity on childhood psoriasis. Besides proper treatment, counseling and supportive care is an important segment of effective management of childhood psoriasis. Although spontaneous remission is more frequent in pediatric-onset disease than in adult-onset patients, clearance is often followed by recurrence. Hence the parents, teachers and all the associates of the affected child should be adequately advised.

Early detection, appropriate management will avoid comorbidities that are likely to develop in adulthood due to chronic inflammation. Aggressive therapy should be considered in children with severe psoriasis in whom intermittent therapy has failed to control the disease.

REFERENCES

1. Kurd SK, Gelfand JM. The prevalence of previously diagnosed and undiagnosed psoriasis in US adults: results from NHANES 2003–2004. J Am Acad Dermatol. 2009;60(2):218-24.
2. Raychaudhuri SP, Gross J. A comparative study of pediatric onset psoriasis with adult onset psoriasis. Pediatr Dermatol. 2000;17(3):174-8.
3. Silverberg NB. Pediatric psoriasis: an update. Ther Clin Risk Manag. 2009;5:849-56.
4. Sharma V, Orchard D. Paediatric psoriasis. Paediatrics and Child Health. 2011;21(3):126-31.
5. Sticherling M, Augusti M, Boehncke W, et al. Therapy of psoriasis in childhood and adolescence–a German expert consensus. J Dtsch Dermatol Ges. 2011;9(10):815-23.
6. Augustin M, Glaeske G, Radtke MA, et al. Epidemiology and comorbidity of psoriasis in children. Br J Dermatol. 2010;162(3):633-6.
7. Swanbeck G, Inerot A, Martinsson T, et al. Age at onset and different types of psoriasis. Br J Dermatol. 1995;133(5):768-73.
8. Farber EM, Mullen RH, Jacobs AH, et al. Infantile psoriasis: a follow up study. Pediatr Dermatol. 1986;3(3):237-43.
9. Kumar B, Jain R, Sandhu K, et al. Epidemiology of childhood psoriasis: a study of 419 patients from northern India. Int J Dermatol. 2004;43(9):654-8.
10. Li Y, Begovich AB. Unraveling the genetics of complex diseases: Susceptibility genes for rheumatoid arthritis and psoriasis. Semin Immunol. 2009;21(6):318-27.
11. Lowes MA, Kikuchi T, Fuentes-Duculan J, et al, Psoriasis vulgaris lesions contain discrete populations of Th1 and Th17 T cells. J Invest Dermatol. 2008;128(5):1207-11.
12. Hüffmeier U, Lascorz J, Becker T, et al. Characterization of psoriasis susceptibility locus 6 (PSORS6) in patients with early onset psoriasis and evidence for interaction with PSORI. J Med Genet. 2009;46(11): 736-44.
13. Schäfer T. Epidemiology of psoriasis. Review and the German perspective. Dermatology. 2006;212(4):327-37.
14. Henseler T. The genetics of psoriasis. J Am Acad Dermatol. 1997;37(2 Pt 3):S1-11.
15. Benoit S, Hamm H. Childhood psoriasis. Clin Dermatol. 2007;25(6):555-62.
16. Takahashi H, Tsuji H, Takahashi I, et al. Plasma adiponectin and leptin levels in Japanese patients with psoriasis. Br J Dermatol. 2008;159(5):1207-8.
17. Takahashi H, Tsuji H, Takahashi I, et al. Prevalence of obesity/adiposity in Japanese psoriasis patients: adiposity is correlated with the severity of psoriasis. J Dermatol Sci. 2009;54(1):61-3.
18. Mobini N, Toussaint S, Kamino H, et al. In: Elder DE, Elenitsas R, Johnson BL, Murphy GF, Xu X (Eds). Lever's Histopathology of Skin, 10th edition. New York: Lippincott Williams & Wilkins Co; 2008. pp. 169-203.
19. Leclerc-Mercier S, Bodemer C, Bourdon-Lanoy E, et al. Early skin biopsy is helpful for the diagnosis and management of neonatal and infantile erythrodermas. J Cutan Pathol. 2010;37(2):249-55.
20. Walsh NM, Prokopetz R, Tron VA, et al. Histopathology in erythroderma: review of a series of cases by multiple observers. J Cutan Pathol. 1994;21(5):419-23.
21. Bitoun E, Micheloni A, Lamant L, et al. LEKTI proteolytic processing in human primary keratinocytes, tissue distribution, and defective expression in Netherton syndrome. Hum Mol Genet. 2003;12(9):2417-30.
22. Pruszkowski A, Bodemer C, Fraitag S, et al. Neonatal and infantile erythrodermas: a retrospective study of 51 patients. Arch Dermatol. 2000;136(7):875-80.
23. Beer WE, Smith AE, Kassab JY, et al. Concomitance of psoriasis and atopic dermatitis. Dermatology. 1992;184(4):265-70.

24. Guttman-Yassky E, Nograles KE, Krueger JG. Contrasting pathogenesis of atopic dermatitis and psoriasis- Part II: Immune cell subsets and therapeutic concepts. J Allergy Clin Immunol. 2011;127(6):1420-32.
25. Giustizieri ML, Mascia F, Frezzolini A, et al. Keratinocytes from patients with atopic dermatitis and psoriasis show a distinct chemokine production profile in response to T cell-derived cytokines. J Allergy Clin Immunol. 2001;107(5):871-7.
26. Cookson WO, Ubhi B, Lawrence R, et al. Genetic linkage of childhood atopic dermatitis to psoriasis susceptibility loci. Nat Genet. 2001;27(4):372-3.
27. Parimalam K, Thomas J. Congenital erythrodermic psoriasis with atopic dermatitis: An example of immunogenetic spinoff. Indian J Pathol Microbiol. 2013;56(1):72-3.
28. Seyhan M, Coşkun BK, Sağlam H, et al. Psoriasis in childhood and adolescence: evaluation of demographic and clinical features. Pediatr Int. 2006;48(6):525-30.
29. Morris A, Rogers M, Fischer G, et al. Childhood psoriasis: a clinical review of 1262 cases. Pediatr Dermatol. 2001;18(3):188-98.
30. Grjibovski AM, Olsen AO, Magnus P, et al. Psoriasis in Norwegian twins: contribution of genetic and environmental effects. J Eur Acad Dermatol Venereol. 2007;21(10):1337-43.
31. Stefanaki,C, Lagogianni E, Kontochristopoulos G, et al. Psoriasis in children: a retrospective analysis. J Eur Acad Dermatol Venereol. 2011;25(4):417-21.
32. Al-fouzan AS, Nanda A. A survey of childhood psoriasis in Kuwait. Pediatr Dermatol. 1994;11(2):116-9.
33. Altobelli E, Petrocelli R, Marziliano C, et al. Family history of psoriasis and age at disease onset in Italian patients with psoriasis. Br J Dermatol. 2007;156(6):1400-1.
34. Honig PJ. Guttate psoriasis associated with perianal streptococcal disease. J Pediatr. 1988;113(6):1037-9.
35. Cassandra M, Conte E, Cortez B. Childhood pustular psoriasis elicited by the streptococcal antigen: a case report and review of the literature. Pediatr Dermatol. 2003;20(6):506-10.
36. Lazar AP, Roenigk HH. Acquired immunodeficiency syndrome (AIDS) can exacerbate psoriasis. J Am Acad Dermatol. 1988;18(1 Pt 1):144.
37. Tsankov N, Angelova I, Kazandjieva J. Drug-induced psoriasis. Recognition and management. Am J Clin Dermatol. 2000;1(3):159-65.
38. Wolf R, Ruocco V. Triggered psoriasis. Adv Exp Med Biol. 1999;455:221-5.
39. O'Brien M, Koo J. The mechanism of lithium and beta-blocking agents in inducing and exacerbating psoriasis. J Drugs Dermatol. 2006;5(5):426-32.
40. Barisić-Drusko V, Rucević I. Psoriasis in childhood. Coll Antropol. 2004;28(1):211-85.
41. Wu Y, Lin Y, Liu HJ, et al. Childhood psoriasis: a study of 137 cases from central China. World J Pediatr. 2010;6(3):260-4.
42. Nanda A, Kaur S, Kaur I, et al. Childhood psoriasis: an epidemiological survey of 112 patients. Pediatr Dermatol. 1990;7(1):19-21.
43. Stern RS, Wu J. Psoriasis. In: Arndt KA, LeBoit PE, Robinson JK, Wintroub BU (Eds). Cutaneous Medicine and Surgery. Philadelphia: WB Saunders; 1996.
44. Gottlieb AB, Chaudhari U, Baker DG, et al. The natural psoriasis foundation score (NPF-PS) system versus the Psoriasis Area Severity Index (PASI) and Physicians Global Assessment. (PGA): a comparison. J Drugs Dermatol. 2003;2(3):260-6.
45. Dhar S, Banerjee R, Agrawal N, et al. Psoriasis in children: an insight. Indian J Dermatol. 2011;56(3):262-5.
46. Atherton DJ, Kahana M, Russell-Jones R. Naevoid psoriasis. Br J Dermatol. 1989;120(6):837-41.
47. Sarkar R, Garg VK. Erythroderma in children. Indian J Dermatol Venereol Leprol. 2010;76(4):341-7.
48. Dika E, Bardazzi F, Balestri R, et al. Environmental factors and psoriasis. Curr Probl Dermatol. 2007;35:118-35.
49. Fry L, Baker BS. Triggering psoriasis: the role of infections and medications. Clin Dermatol. 2007;25(6):606-15.
50. Naldi L, Gambini D. The clinical spectrum of psoriasis. Clin Dermatol. 2007;25(6):510-8.
51. Sarkar R. Neonatal and infantile erythroderma: "The Red Baby". Indian J Dermatol. 2006;51:178-82.
52. Salleras M, Sanchez-Regaña M, Umbert P. Congenital erythrodermic psoriasis: case report and literature review. Pediatr Dermatol. 1995;12(3):231-4.
53. Frost P, Van Scott EJ. Ichthyosiform dermatoses. Classification based on anatomic and biometric observation. Arch Dermatol. 1966;94(2):113-26.
54. Parimalam K, Thomas J. Congenital erythrodermic psoriasis: a case report. The Indian J Bio Research. 2012; 82:1-5.
55. Thomas J, Kumar P. Childhood psoriasis: a challenge to all. Ind J Pract Ped. 2011;13(1):98-100.
56. de Oliveira ST, Maragno L, Arnone M, et al. Generalized pustular psoriasis in childhood. Pediatr Dermatol. 2010; 27(4):349-54.
57. Burden AD. Management of psoriasis in childhood. Clin Exp Dermatol. 1999;24(5):341-5.
58. Liao PB, Rubinson R, Howard R, et al. Annular pustular psoriasis—most common form of pustular psoriasis in children: report of three cases and review of the literature. Pediatr Dermatol. 2002;19(1):19-25.
59. Zelickson BD, Muller SA. Generalized pustular psoriasis in childhood. Report of thirteen cases. J Am Acad Dermatol. 1990;24(2 PT 1):186-94.
60. Xiao T, Li B, He CD, et al. Juvenile generalized pustular psoriasis. J Dermatol. 2007;34(8):573-6.
61. Judge MR, Mcdonald A, Black MM. Pustular psoriasis in childhood. Clin Exp Dermatol. 1993;18(2):97-9.
62. Espinoza LR, Cuéllar ML, Silveira LH. Psoriatic arthritis. Curr Opin Rheumatol. 1992;4(4):470-8.
63. Zachariae H. Prevalence of joint disease in patients with psoriasis: implications for therapy. Am J Clin Dermatol. 2003; 4(7):441-7.
64. Southwood TR, Petty RE, Malleson PN, et al. Psoriatic arthritis in children. Arthritis Rheum. 1989;32(8):1007-13.
65. Shore A, Ansell BM. Juvenile psoriatic arthritis—an analysis of 60 cases. J Pediatr 1982;100(4):529-35.
66. Parimalam K, Thomas J, Kumar D. Histology of infantile erythrodermic psoriasis: a study of eight cases. E-Journal of Indian Society of Teledermatol. 2012;6(1):30-5.
67. Zhu KJ, He SM, Zhang C, et al. Relationship of the body mass index and childhood psoriasis in a Chinese Han population: a hospital-based study. J Dermatol. 2012;39(2):181-3.
68. Boccardi D, Menni S, La Vecchia C, et al. Overweight and childhood psoriasis. Br J Dermatol. 2009;161(2):484-6.
69. Augustin M, Reich K, Glaeske G, et al. Co-morbidity and age-related prevalence of psoriasis: analysis of health insurance data in Germany. Acta Derm Venereol. 2010;90(2):147-51.
70. Griffiths CE, Barker JN. Pathogenesis and clinical features of psoriasis. Lancet. 2007;370(9583):263-71.

71. Fluhr JW, Cavallotti C, Berardesca E. Emollients, moisturizers and keratolytic agents in psoriasis. Clin Dermatol. 2008;26(4):380-6.
72. Smith CH, Jackson K, Chinn S, et al. A double blind, randomized, controlled clinical trial to assess the efficacy of a new coal tar preparation (Exorex) in the treatment of chronic, plaque type psoriasis. Clin Exp Dermatol. 2000;25(8):580-3.
73. Thami G, Sarkar R. Coal tar: past, present and future. Clin Exp Dermatol. 2002;27(2):99-103.
74. Borska L, Andrys C, Krejsek J, et al. Genotoxic hazard and cellular stress in pediatric patients treated for psoriasis with the Goeckermann regimen. Pediatr Dermatol. 2009;26(1):23-7.
75. McGill A, Frank A, Emmett N, et al. The anti-psoriatic drug anthralin accumulates in keratinocyte mitochondria, dissipates mitochondrial membrane potential, and induces apoptosis through a pathway dependent on respiratory competent mitochondria. FASEB J. 2005;19(8):1012-4.
76. Lebwohl M, Ali S. Treatment of psoriasis. Part 1. Topical therapy and phototherapy. J Am Acad Dermatol. 2001;45(4):487-98.
77. Zvulunov A, Anisfeld A, Metzker A. Efficacy of short-contact therapy with dithranol in childhood psoriasis. Int J Dermatol. 1994;33(11):808-10.
78. Farber EM, Nall L. Childhood psoriasis. Cutis. 1999;64(5):309-14.
79. Kiken DA, Silverberg NB. Atopic dermatitis in children, part 2: treatment options. Cutis. 2006;78(6):401-6.
80. Kimball AB, Gold MH, Zib B, et al. Clobetasol Propionate Emulsion Formulation Foam Phase III Clinical Study Group. Clobetasol propionate emulsion formulation foam 0.05%: review of phase II open-label and phase III randomized controlled trials in steroid-responsive dermatoses in adults and adolescents. J Am Acad Dermatol. 2008;59(3):448-54.
81. Rim JH, Choe YB, Youn JI. Positive effect of using calcipotriol ointment with narrow-band ultraviolet B phototherapy in psoriatic patients. Photodermatol Photoimmunol Photomed. 2002;18(3):131-4.
82. Oranje AP, Marcoux D, Svensson A, et al. Topical calcipotriol in childhood psoriasis. J Am Acad Dermatol. 1997;36(2 Pt 1):203-8.
83. Liao YH, Chiu HC, Tseng YS, et al. Comparison of cutaneous tolerance and efficacy of calcitriol 3 µg/g^{-1} ointment and tacrolimus 0.3 mg/g^{-1} ointment in chronic plaque psoriasis involving facial or genitofemoral areas: a double-blind, randomized controlled trial. Br J Dermatol. 2007;157(5):1005-12.
84. Brune A, Miller DW, Lin P, et al. Tacrolimus ointment is effective for psoriasis on the face and intertriginous areas in pediatric patients. Pediatr Dermatol. 2007;24(1):76-80.
85. Mansouri P, Farshi S. Pimecrolimus 1 percent cream in the treatment of psoriasis in a child. Dermatol Online J. 2006;12(2):7.
86. Jain VK, Aggarwal K, Jain K, et al. Narrow-band UV-B phototherapy in childhood psoriasis. Int J Dermatol. 2007;46(3):320-2.
87. Diluvio L, Campione E, Paternò EJ, et al. Childhood nail psoriasis: a useful treatment with tazarotene 0.05%. Pediatr Dermatol. 2007;24(3):332-3.
88. Holme SA, Anstey AV. Phototherapy and PUVA photochemotherapy in children. Photodermatol Photoimmunol Photomed. 2004;20(2):69-75.
89. Pasić A, Ceović R, Lipozenćić J, et al. Phototherapy in pediatric patients. Pediatr Dermatol. 2003;20(1):71-7.
90. Ceović R, Pasić A, Lipozenćić J, et al. Treatment of childhood psoriasis. Acta Dermatovenereol Croat. 2006;14(4):261-4.
91. Pang ML, Murase JE, Koo J. An updated review of acitretin: a systemic retinoid for the treatment of psoriasis. Expert Opin Drug Metab Toxicol. 2008;4(7):953-64.
92. Cordoro KM. Topical therapy for the management of childhood psoriasis: part I. Skin Therapy Lett. 2008;13(3):1-3.
93. Kumar B, Dhar S, Handa S, et al. Methotrexate in childhood psoriasis. Pediatr Dermatol. 1994;11(3):271-3.
94. Collin B, Vani A, Ogboli M, et al. Methotrexate treatment in 13 children with severe plaque psoriasis. Clin Exp Dermatol. 2009;34(3):295-8.
95. Kalb RE, Strober B, Weinstein G, et al. Methotrexate and psoriasis: 2009 National Psoriasis Foundation Consensus Conference. J Am Acad Dermatol. 2009;60(5):824-37.
96. Perrett CM, Ilchyshyn A, Berth-Jones J. Cyclosporin in childhood psoriasis. J Dermatol Treat. 2003;14(2):113-8.
97. Alli N, Gónger E, Karakayali G, et al. The use of cyclosporin in a child with generalized pustular psoriasis. Br J Dermatol. 1998;139(4):754-5.
98. Pereira TM, Vieira AP, Fernandes JC, et al. Cyclosporin A treatment in severe childhood psoriasis. Eur Acad Dermatol Venereol. 2006;20(6):651-6.
99. Paller AS, Siegfried EC, Langley RG, et al. Etanercept treatment for children and adolescents with plaque psoriasis. N Engl J Med. 2008;358(3):241-51.
100. Trueb RM. Therapies for childhood psoriasis. Curr Probl Dermatol. 2009;38:137-59.
101. Kress DW. Etanercept therapy improves symptoms and allows tapering of other medications in children and adolescents with moderate to severe psoriasis. J Am Acad Dermatol. 2006;54(3 Suppl 2):S126-8.
102. Pereira TM, Vieira AP, Fernandes JC, et al. Anti-TNF-alpha therapy in childhood pustular psoriasis. Dermatology. 2006;213(4):350-2.
103. Farnsworth NN, George SJ, Hsu S. Successful use of infliximab following a failed course of etanercept in a pediatric patient. Dermatol Online J. 2005;11(3):11.
104. Menter MA, Cush JM. Successful treatment of pediatric psoriasis with infliximab. Pediatr Dermatol. 2004;21(1):87-8. 44.
105. Weishaupt C, Metze D, Luger TA, et al. Treatment of pustular psoriasis with infliximab. J Dtsch Dermatol Ges. 2007;5(5):397-9.
106. Pahlajani N, Katz BJ, Lozano AM, et al. Comparison of the efficacy and safety of the 308 nm excimer laser for the treatment of localized psoriasis in adults and in children: a pilot study. Pediatr Dermatol. 2005;22(2):161-5.
107. Pacifico L, Renzi AM, Chiesa C. Acute guttate psoriasis after streptococcal scarlet fever. Pediatr Dermatol. 1993;10(4):388-9.
108. Grattan C, Burton JL, Manku M, et al. Essential-fatty-acid metabolites in plasma phospholipids in patients with ichthyosis vulgaris, acne vulgaris and psoriasis. Clin Exp Dermatol. 1990;15(3):174-6.
109. Lin YK, Yen HR, Wong WR, et al. Successful treatment of pediatric psoriasis with Indigo naturalis composite ointment. Pediatr Dermatol. 2006;23(5):507-10.
110. Kumar P, Nithya P, Saratha KP, et al. Effect of methotrexate in juvenile generalised pustular psoriasis. J Applied Med Surg. 2012;1(3):28-31.
111. Parimalam K, Thomas J. Infantile erythrodermic psoriasis: successful treatment with topical Calcipotriol. E-Journal of the Indian Society of Teledermatology. 2011;5:9-14.
112. Beattie PE, Lewis-Jones MS. A comparative study of impairment of quality of life in children with skin disease and children with other chronic diseases. Br J Dermatol. 2006;155(1):145-51.

Psoriasis and Pregnancy

INTRODUCTION

It is well established that psoriasis fluctuates during pregnancy, likely due to the hormonal changes in estrogen and progesterone resulting in a state of altered immune surveillance **(Fig. 1)**.

The majority of women usually experience an improvement in their cutaneous disease during pregnancy. According to a study by Murase et al., 55% of the patients reported improvement during pregnancy, 21% no change, and 23% reported worsening.[1] However, only 9% of patients reported improvement, 26% no change, and 65% reported worsening postpartum. In patients with 10% or greater body surface area involvement who reported improvement, lesions decreased by 83.8% during pregnancy. Similar data were obtained by Raychaudhuri et al.[2] Of the 91 pregnant women involved in the study, 51 (56%) improved, 24 (26.4%) worsened, and 16 (17.6%) had no change during pregnancy. Relapse during the early postpartum period was common. The mechanism by which psoriasis tends to improve during pregnancy is not well understood. However, there is now data to suggest that the upregulation of Th2 cytokines during pregnancy counteracts the effects of proinflammatory Th1 cytokines which are key players in the pathogenesis of psoriasis.

Women with psoriasis generally progress through conception, pregnancy and birth just like anyone else.

Rates of pregnancy and spontaneous abortion were found to be similar in both in pregnant women with inflammatory skin diseases and women without inflammatory skin diseases. However, studies have shown that women with severe psoriasis (defined as those who had received photochemotherapy or systemic therapy within 2 years before delivery) had a higher risk for the delivery of low birth weight infants compared with mothers without psoriasis.

But it was noted that receiving systemic therapy during pregnancy did not appear to contribute to the increased risk of low birth weight; rates of low birth infants were similar among mothers who received systemic medications during pregnancy and those who did not. Indicating that psoriasis by itself due to the chronic inflammatory process increases the risk of low birth weight babies which was also proved in a retrospective cohort study which identified psoriasis as an independent risk factor for spontaneous abortions, induced abortions, premature rupture of membranes and infant macrosomia.[3]

SAFETY OF DRUGS IN PREGNANCY WHILE TREATING PSORIASIS

The appropriate treatment for psoriasis in a woman who is pregnant, or who plans pregnancy, will depend on the extent and severity of the skin condition.

Topical therapy can be used with confidence, but using large quantities of salicylic acid, calcipotriol, topical steroids and calcineurin inhibitors for long periods of time should be avoided.

Ultraviolet light B (UVB) phototherapy is safe for pregnant women with more severe psoriasis. Cyclosporin can be prescribed when systemic therapy is essential, providing blood pressure and kidney function are very carefully monitored.

There is little research on the impact of psoriasis and psoriatic arthritis treatments on pregnant and nursing

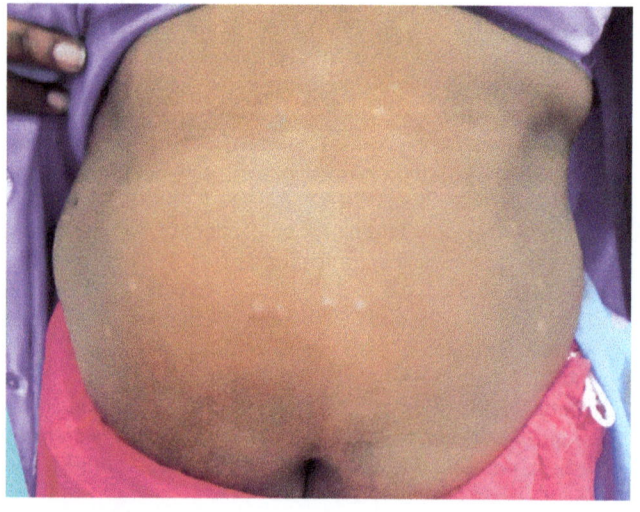

Fig. 1: Mild psoriasis in pregnancy, topical therapy will suffice.

women. The National Psoriasis Foundation released guidelines in 2012 for treating psoriasis in pregnant or breastfeeding women. Topical treatments are the first choice of treatment, particularly moisturizers and emollients, such as petroleum jelly. Limited use of low-to-moderate dose topical steroids appears safe, but women should use caution when applying topical steroids to the breasts to avoid passing the medication to the baby while nursing. Read more about using topical treatments during pregnancy or nursing.

Narrow-band ultraviolet light B (NBUVB) phototherapy should be the second-line treatment. If NBUVB is not available, then broadband UVB may be used. Nursing women should avoid psoralen and UVA because psoralen enters breastmilk and could cause light sensitivity to infants.

For a better understanding of drug therapy in psoriasis, it is advisable that a clear knowledge of drug categories used in psoriasis is agreed.

Australian Drug Evaluation Committee Pregnancy Categories

- **A** Drugs which have been taken by a large number of pregnant women and women of childbearing age without an increase in the frequency of malformations or other direct or indirect harmful effects on the fetus have been observed.
- **B1** Drugs which have been taken by only a limited number of pregnant women and women of childbearing age, without an increase in the frequency of malformation or other direct or indirect harmful effects on the human fetus having been observed. Studies in animals have not shown evidence of an increased occurrence of fetal damage.
- **B2** Drugs which have been taken by only a limited number of pregnant women and women of childbearing age, without an increase in the frequency of malformation or other direct or indirect harmful effects on the human fetus having been observed. Studies in animals are inadequate or may be lacking, but available data show no evidence of an increased occurrence of fetal damage.
- **B3** Drugs which have been taken by only a limited number of pregnant women and women of childbearing age, without an increase in the frequency of malformation or other direct or indirect harmful effects on the human fetus having been observed. Studies in animals have shown evidence of an increased occurrence of fetal damage, the significance of which is considered uncertain in humans.
- **C** Drugs which, owing to their pharmaceutical effects, have caused or may be suspected of causing, harmful effects on the human fetus or neonate without causing malformations. These effects may be reversible.
- **D** Drugs which have caused are suspected to have caused or may be expected to cause, an increased incidence of human fetal malformations or irreversible damage. These drugs may also have adverse pharmacological effects.
- **X** Drugs that have such a high risk of causing permanent damage to the fetus that they should not be used in pregnancy or when there is a possibility of pregnancy.

TREATMENT OF PSORIASIS IN PREGNANCY

Psoriasis is known to be associated with metabolic syndrome. Comorbidities such as diabetes, obesity or hypertension in pregnancy may worsen psoriasis and vice versa. Therefore, the management of psoriasis in such patients means medical, dermatological and obstetric challenge which has to be born in mind while treating a pregnant woman with psoriasis. It is also possible that some women experience spontaneous improvement of psoriasis during pregnancy.

Topical Therapies for Psoriasis in Pregnancy and Lactation

Simple emollients appear safe to use in pregnancy.

Salicylic acid is absorbed through the skin (10–25%). It is proved that oral salicylates are associated with bleeding and are harmful to the baby it is better to avoid topical salicylic acid over large areas of the body for prolonged periods.

Coal tar products are considered safe, if used for short periods or on localized areas such as the scalp. Though the risk of coal tar and injury to the baby is unknown, it is better to avoid their use over large areas of the body for prolonged periods as they contain potentially hazardous polycyclic aromatic hydrocarbons.

Since Dithranol/anthralin is not absorbed through skin, the risk in pregnancy is unknown but the drug is not frequently advised due to its irritant nature.

Topical corticosteroids appear to be safe during pregnancy if used judiciously. Mild-to-moderate potency topical corticosteroids should be preferred to more potent corticosteroids during pregnancy. Potent to very potent topical corticosteroids should be used only as second-line therapy for as short a time as possible. They are better avoided over high-absorption areas like the eyelids, genitals and flexures. Whether the newer potent lipophilic topical corticosteroids (e.g., mometasone, fluticasone and methylprednisolone) are associated with less risk to fetus is not fully determined.

Mild, moderate and potent topical corticosteroids are also considered safe to use when breastfeeding. Patient should be instructed to wash-off any steroid cream applied to breasts, before feeding. It is advisable that, very potent topical corticosteroids are not recommended to use over the chest while breastfeeding.

Calcipotriol, a category B drug, with 6% systemic absorption, should be used with caution though the risk in pregnancy is unknown. Dose should not exceed 100 g/week, and should not be applied over the chest area, if the mother is breastfeeding.

Calcineurin inhibitors tacrolimus, pimecrolimus belong to category C and their risk in pregnancy is unknown.

Tazarotene, although topical, is a category X medication therefore, is to be strictly avoided in pregnancy.

Phototherapy for Psoriasis in Pregnancy and Lactation

Phototherapy with broadband UVB and NBUVB appears as safe in pregnancy as at other times. The risk of topical psoralen ultraviolet light A (PUVA) in pregnancy is considered very low, but oral PUVA should be avoided during pregnancy.

Systemic Therapies for Psoriasis in Pregnancy and Lactation

It is always better to avoid systemic therapy in pregnancy. Most of the systemic drugs used in the treatment of psoriasis are unsafe in pregnancy and lactation (Box 1). Cyclosporine and biologics are the only drugs relatively safe in pregnancy come under category C.

Though cyclosporine belongs to category C drug, it may cause high blood pressure and kidney damage, which might harm the baby. If treatment is essential, it must be monitored carefully. It is best not to breastfeed during treatment as cyclosporine passes into the milk.

Biologics, the category C drugs are better avoided during pregnancy and breastfeeding as little information is available about their safety in pregnancy and lactation.

The appropriate treatment for psoriasis in a woman who is pregnant, or who plans pregnancy, will depend on the extent and severity of the skin condition.

Topical therapy can be used with confidence, but large quantities of salicylic acid, calcipotriol, topical steroids and calcineurin inhibitors should be avoided for long periods of time.

Ultraviolet light B phototherapy is safe for pregnant women with more severe psoriasis. If there is a need to prescribe cyclosporine, blood pressure and kidney function should be monitored very prudently.

BOX 1: Systemic drugs in pregnancy.

- *Methotrexate*: Category D
- *Acitretin*: Category X
- *Cyclosporine*: Category C
- *Hydroxyurea*: Category D
- *Mycophenolate mofetil*: Category D
- *Biologics*: Category C

IMPETIGO HERPETIFORMIS OR GESTATIONAL PUSTULAR PSORIASIS

Impetigo herpetiformis (IH) was first described by Hebra and an endocrine cause was suspected. The claims that IH stands as an entity separate from gestational pustular psoriasis (GPP) have been restated. IH or GPP is a rare form of pustular psoriasis related to pregnancy which normally occurs during the 3rd trimester. However, there are reports of cases occurring earlier, and has been recorded in the 1st month of pregnancy and in the 1st day of the puerperium. The disease tends to persist until the child is born, and occasionally long afterwards. Familial occurrence has been reported.

Pathogenesis

Primiparous women are at the highest risk, though severity increases in subsequent pregnancies. The worsening of pustular psoriasis just before menstruation is well recognized and challenge with progesterone or clomifene has produced pustular exacerbations in such patients. Maternal hypocalcemia, stress and infection are considered as triggering factors.

Clinical Features

It presents superficial pustules with a tendency for grouping in a herpetiform distribution. The pustular eruption typically starts symmetrically over the inguinogenital region and other the flexural skin of axillae, groin, inframammary and the periumbilical area. Pustules are sometimes seen over the abdominal striae. The lesions start as minute pustules arising on an acutely inflamed area of skin which extend centrifugally, drying in the center, or form plaques in which eroded greenish-yellow pustules become fetid. Crusted or vegetating condyloma like lesions may form in the flexures. The eruption soon spreads to become generalized with desquamation. The pustules heal, leaving behind reddish brown pigmentation. The tongue, buccal mucosa and even the esophagus may be involved, with circinate or erosive lesions following short-lived pustules.

Constitutional disturbance is characteristically severe with fever, and death may occur, attributable to cardiac or renal failure. Delirium, diarrhea, vomiting and tetany have been described.

Differentiation between acute generalized exanthematous pustulosis (AGEP) and pustular psoriasis is very difficult during the first episode in the absence of history or evidence of psoriasis. The duration of pustules is shorter lived in AGEP as against IH. Histology will be the most important diagnostic tool under such situations, where in AGEP, there is eosinophilic exocytosis and necrotic keratinocytes in the epidermis with marked dermal edema and evidence of vasculitis. Whereas, IH will show acanthosis and papillomatosis with neutrophilic pustules.

Course and Prognosis

Impetigo herpetiformis is a medical emergency involving the mother as well as the fetus. Apart from the complications of hypocalcemia, the other complications include fluid and electrolyte imbalance and maternal secondary infection and sepsis. The more severe and long-standing the disease, the greater are the risks of placental insufficiency leading to stillbirth, neonatal death or fetal abnormalities **(Figs. 2 and 3)**.

In many cases, there is derangement of liver enzymes. Even when the disease is controlled in the mother and an increased stillbirth risk and fetal abnormalities are noted.

Lesions are expected to regress after delivery but invariably recur at times of stress and at an earlier gestational age in further pregnancies, as a characteristic eruption of erythemato-squamous plaques with or without pustules. Characteristically, the disease recurs in subsequent pregnancies and on subsequent use of oral contraceptives. There is one report where the disease continued unabated despite termination of the pregnancy.

Investigations

Blood investigations should be carried out to look for, leukocytosis elevated erythrocyte sedimentation rate (ESR), hypocalcemia, electrolyte imbalance, low vitamin D levels, altered liver and renal functions. Biopsy should be performed to confirm diagnosis in patients who present with IH for the first time in the absence of a history of psoriasis.

Treatment

Impetigo herpetiformis can be successfully treated with topical and systemic corticosteroids. Antibiotics may be indicated for secondary bacterial infection. Fluid and electrolytes especially calcium should be monitored and normalized. Unresponsive cases can be given cyclosporine, NBUVB, PUVA, clofazimine or induction of early delivery. During the postpartum period, oral retinoid can be given. Treatment is imperative due to the life-threatening nature of the disease. The treatment of choice in pregnancy is prednisone 15–30 mg/day. Cyclosporine is used only if the potential benefits justify the potential risk to the fetus. As the fetal mortality is high, even when the disease appears well controlled with corticosteroids, fetal well-being should be monitored using biophysical profile and umbilical artery Doppler studies. If fetal or maternal conditions deteriorate, pregnancy should be terminated by induction of labor or Cesarean section, as indicated. Though maternal mortality is less with the advent of treatment options available, stillbirth and intrauterine growth retardation may occur even when the disease appears to be controlled with corticosteroids. Low-dose methotrexate can be substituted in the postpartum period to prevent rebound of rashes, but is contraindicated in pregnancy and lactation. The disease remits after delivery but may recur in successive pregnancies.

SUMMARY

Psoriasis in pregnancy does affect both the mother's health and the fetal outcome. Which is more so when the disease is severe.

The disease fortunately does not affect the reproductive system. However, there is higher incidence of infertility in psoriatics than the normal females **(Figs. 4 and 5)**.

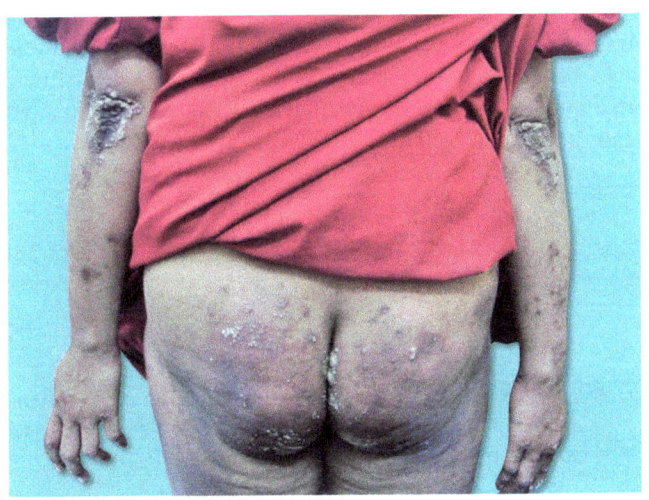

Fig. 2: Impetigo herpetiformis in a pregnant woman.

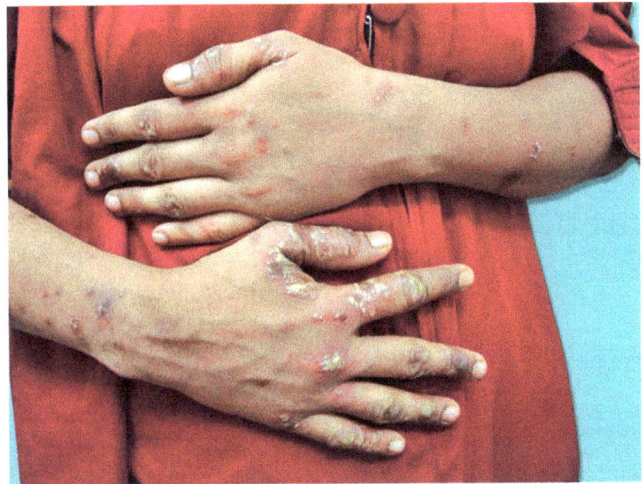

Fig. 3: Same patient as in **Figure 2**, pustules persisting after termination of pregnancy, Impetigo herpetiformis resulted in fetal loss.

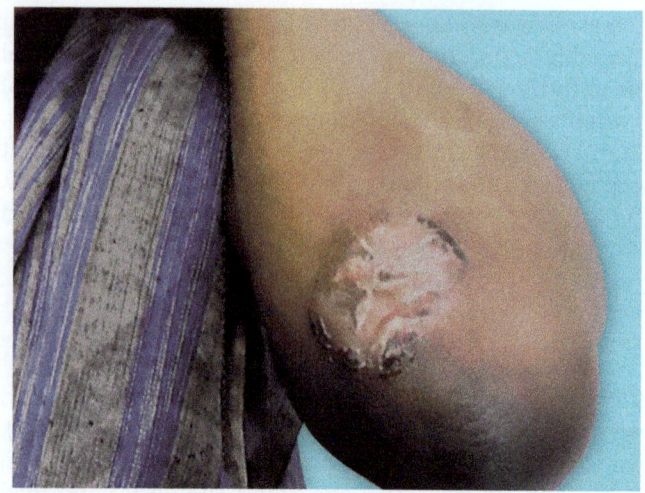

Fig. 4: Woman on treatment for primary infertility.

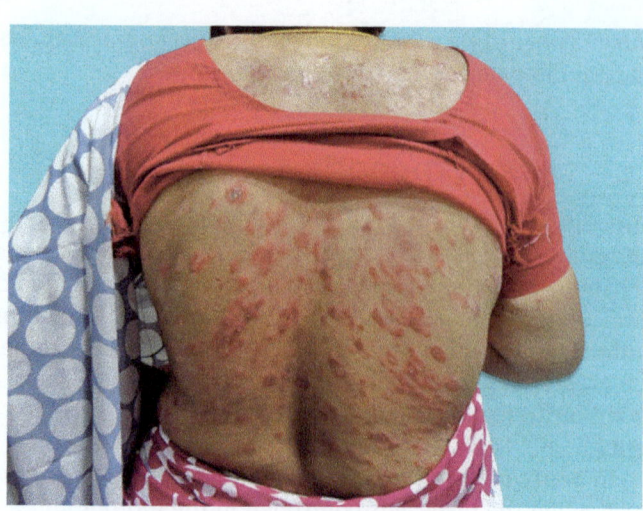

Fig. 5: Woman with psoriasis since childhood with infertility.

Therapy of pregnant woman with psoriasis when administered judiciously does not harm the mother or fetus. Drugs which are contraindicated during pregnancy should be avoided.

Impetigo herpetiformis is a medical emergency requiring multidisciplinary approach. Even if the disease is controlled in the mother, there can still be an adverse effect on the fetus which should be born in mid while following up the patient.

Impetigo herpetiformis is known to recur during subsequent pregnancy about which the patient and the family should be kept aware of.

REFERENCES

1. Murasse JE, Chan KK, Garite TJ, et al. Hormonal effect on psoriasis in pregnancy and postpartum. Arch Dermatol. 2005;141(5):601-6.
2. Raychaudhuri SP, Navare T, Gross J, et al. Clinical course of psoriasis during pregnancy. Int J Dermatol. 2003;42(7):518-20.
3. Cohen-Barak E, Nachum Z, Rozenman D, et al. Pregnancy outcomes in women with moderate-to-severe psoriasis. J Eur Acad Dermatol Venereol. 2011;25(9):1041-7.

Psoriasis in HIV

INTRODUCTION

Unlike some dermatoses that have a higher frequency in patients infected with human immunodeficiency virus (HIV), psoriasis presents a similar prevalence in these patients to that in the general population. Psoriasis in these patients, however, presents certain clinical and therapeutic characteristics **(Figs. 1 to 7)**.

The main features of HIV-associated psoriasis are shown in **Box 1**.

Sudden exacerbation of extensive and severe inflammatory psoriasis should indicate suspected HIV inspection

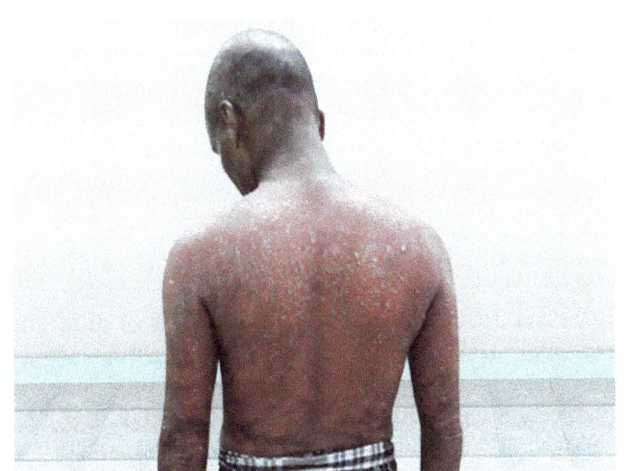

Fig. 1: Human immunodeficiency virus (HIV)-positive man with sudden onset of psoriasis.

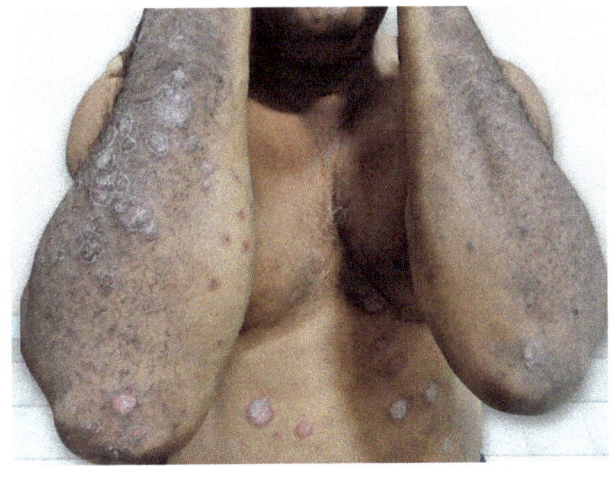

Fig. 3: Patient on zidovudine showing improvement with acitretin.

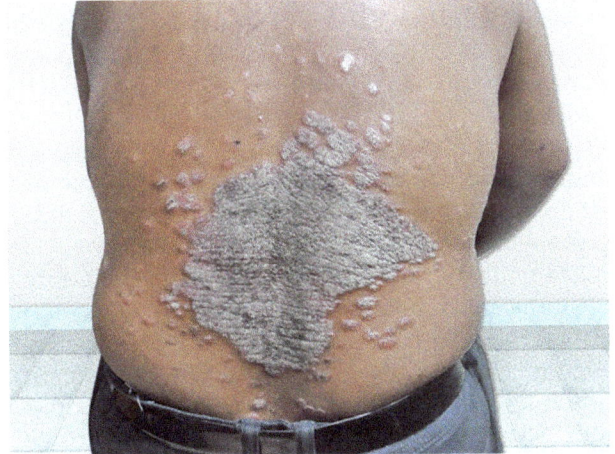

Fig. 2: Severe form of psoriasis in human immunodeficiency virus (HIV)-positive man resistant to treatment.

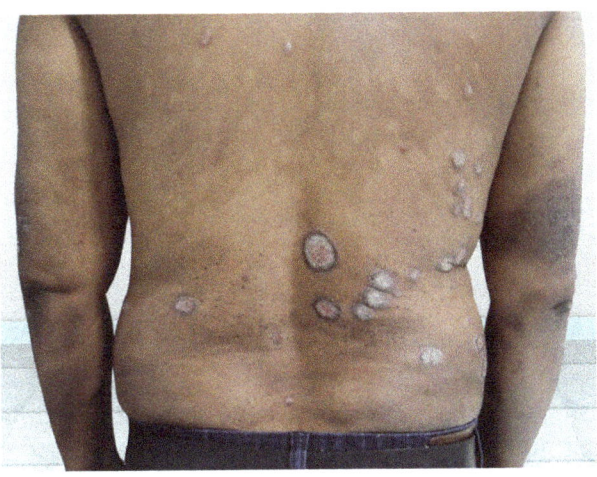

Fig. 4: Same as in **Figure 3** on zidovudine.

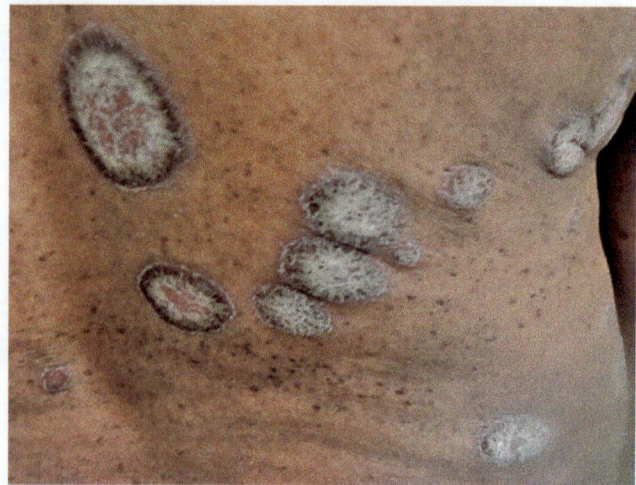

Fig. 5: Same as in **Figure 4** on zidovudine close-up view.

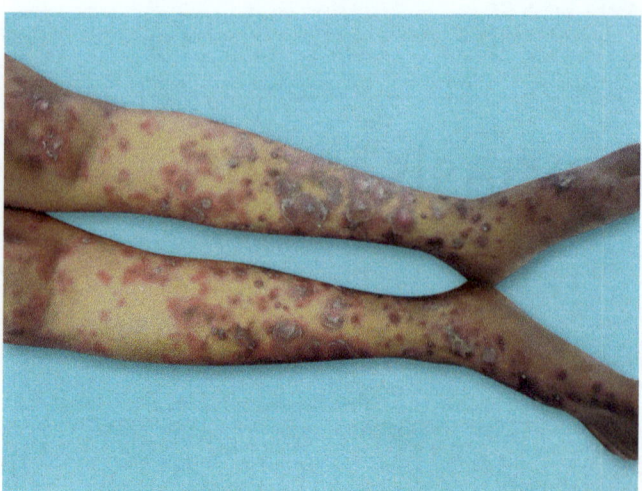

Fig. 7: Pustular lesions in human immunodeficiency virus (HIV)-positive psoriasis patient.

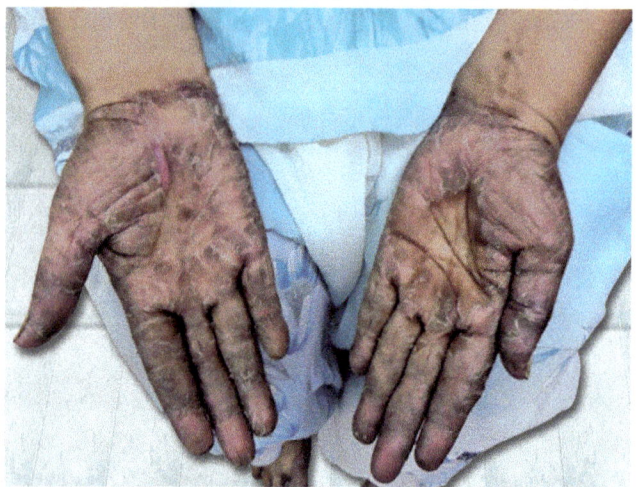

Fig. 6: Severe involvement of palm as keratoderma in human immunodeficiency virus (HIV)-positive woman.

> **BOX 1: Features of human immunodeficiency virus (HIV)-associated psoriasis.**
>
> - Sudden onset
> - Palmoplantar keratoderma
> - Severe nail dystrophy
> - Involvement of skin folds
> - Pustular forms
> - High frequency of arthritis

and requires a serological analysis. In patients already diagnosed with HIV, the considerable efficacy of the new antiretroviral drugs has meant that the classical clinical forms predominate due to the improved immune status of these patients. HIV-positive patients present different types of spondyloarthropathy in which severe joint involvement is observed, with joint destruction; they also present nail involvement and associated palmoplantar lesions. Joint involvement in patients with psoriasis and HIV infection is aggressive and is more prevalent and clinically more florid than in HIV-negative patients. Unlike in Reiter's disease, sacroiliac involvement is rare in these patients. The prevalence of Reiter's disease is therefore higher in HIV-positive patients than in the general population.[1]

REITER'S DISEASE

Reiter's syndrome illustrates the difficulty of differential diagnosis in HIV-positive patients, due to the severe joint involvement and the varied morphology of the lesions that may develop in patients with psoriasis **(Figs. 8 to 10)**.

Diagnosis of Reiter's disease is indicated by the characteristic triad of polyarthritis, urethritis, and conjunctivitis, together with the typical psoriasis form skin lesions.

The disease is most frequent among young men and the association with HLA-B27 is a characteristic finding, which is present in between approximately 80 and 90% of patients. Patients with this association typically have more serious disease.

Typical of the disease are episodes of vesicular-pustular lesions on the palms and soles; over the course of the episode, the lesions coalesce, progressing to scabs and hyperkeratosis.

Also typical are genital involvement in the form of circinate balanitis and involvement of the nails. The extensor surface of the limbs and the scalp may also be affected, though to a lesser extent. Due to the clinical similarity to psoriasis lesions, however, diagnosis requires the presence of more elements of the triad. There seems to be an intimate link between "psoriatic arthritis" and "Reiter's syndrome".[2] The association with HIV is higher than those with psoriasis.

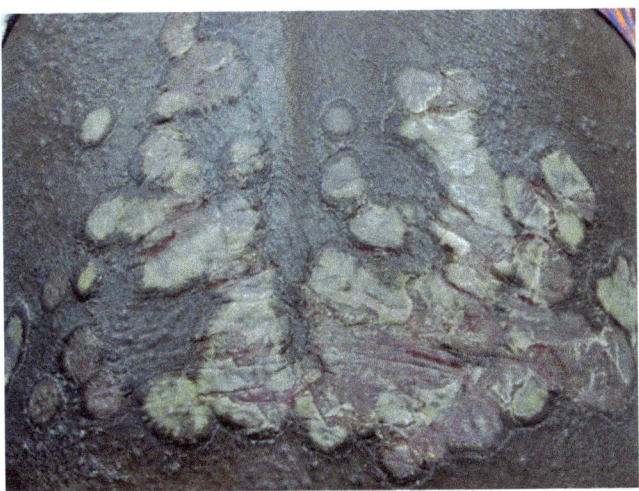

Fig. 8: Skin lesions of patient with Reiter's syndrome.

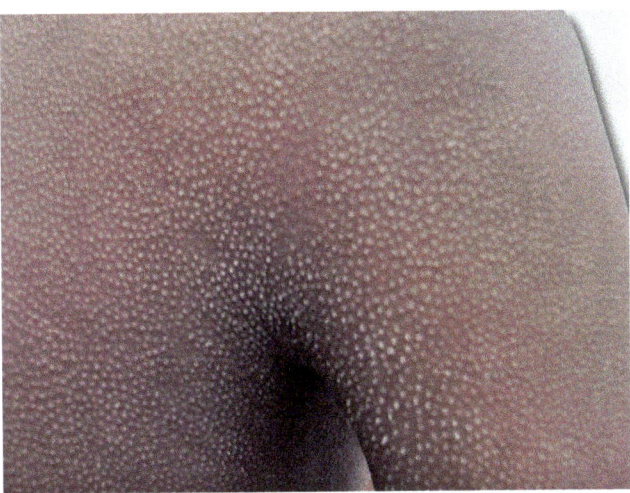

Fig. 11: Classical grouped follicular papules of pityriasis rubra pilaris (PRP).

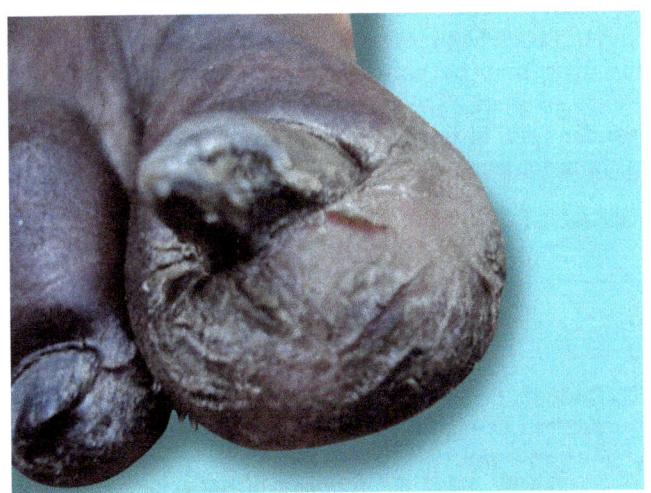

Fig. 9: Human immunodeficiency virus (HIV)-positive patient with Reiter's syndrome having nail change.

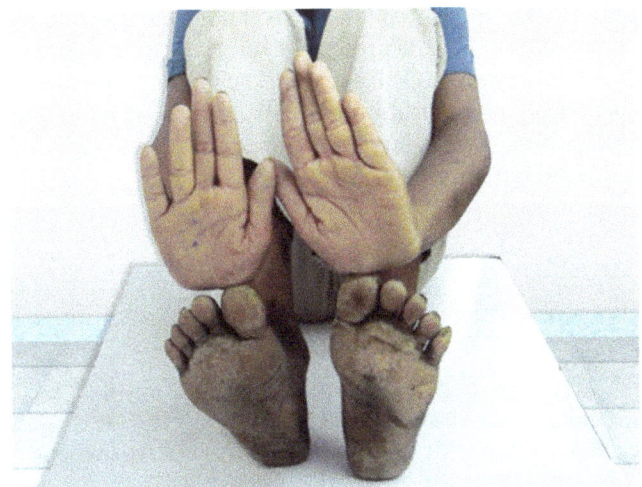

Fig. 12: Palmoplantar keratoderma of pityriasis rubra pilaris (PRP). This child was seronegative.

PITYRIASIS RUBRA PILARIS

Pityriasis rubra pilaris (PRP), also called follicular psoriasis, is a rare disease that is clinically characterized by the appearance of follicular hyperkeratotic papules on an erythematous base. The lesions show a marked tendency to coalesce, extending in a caudal direction and leaving islands of sparing. Involvement of the palms and soles also often occurs in the form of reddish-orange keratoderma with a waxy appearance. Development of varying degrees of erythroderma is characteristic of the disease. Most cases of PRP are acquired, though occasional familial cases occur. Different environmental factors have been suggested as triggers, including infections—particularly HIV. Pityriasis rubra pilaris is divided into five categories—depending on age, duration, and type of skin involvement. A sixth category has been proposed for the form of PRP-associated with HIV infection **(Figs. 11 and 12)**.

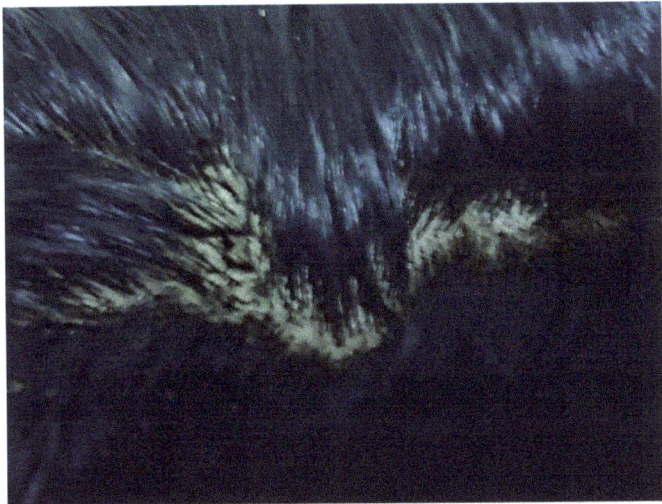

Fig. 10: Thick scales on the scalp in Reiter's syndrome in a patient on zidovudine.

TREATMENT OF PSORIASIS IN HIV-AFFECTED PATIENTS

Psoriasis occurs with at least undiminished frequency in HIV-infected individuals. The behavior of psoriasis in HIV disease is of interest, in terms of pathogenesis and therapy because of the background of profound immunodysregulation. It is paradoxical that, while drugs that target T-lymphocytes are effective in psoriasis, the condition should be exacerbated by HIV infection.

Intravenous (IV)-associated psoriasis is often refractory to traditional treatments. Treatment is challenging and requires careful consideration and should be tailored to patients based on disease severity and the input from an infectious disease specialist. Close monitoring for potential adverse events is necessary.[3]

Psoriasis in the setting of HIV disease may be mild, moderate, or severe. Standard therapies and zidovudine are effective in management. Survival does not seem to be adversely affected by the presence of psoriasis or its therapy. Zidovudine therapy, at a dosage of 1,200 mg/day, appears to be beneficial in the treatment of HIV-associated psoriasis, although long-term relapses occurred and the associated arthritis did not improve.[4]

Oral gold was found to be safe and useful in a woman in the treatment of disabling psoriatic arthritis with HIV infection, in whom CD4 count during oral gold therapy showed a significant, sustained increase in CD4 cells.[5]

SUMMARY

Mild-to-moderate disease: Topical therapy is the first-line recommended treatment.

UVB can be considered as second-line therapy.

Moderate-to-severe disease: Phototherapy is the recommended first-line therapeutic choice. Oral retinoids may be used as second-line treatment.

Refractory, severe disease: Cyclosporine, methotrexate, hydroxyurea and tumor necrosis factor-α inhibitors may be considered and used with extreme caution. Since skin lesions of patients with therapy-resistant AIDS-associated psoriasis have been reported to clear with oral zidovudine, this drug may be considered retinoid-resistant AIDS-associated psoriasis, where, methotrexate, cyclosporine and psoralen (oral or topical) photochemotherapy (PUVA) may be contraindicated.

REFERENCES

1. Leal L, Ribera M, Daudénb E. Psoriasis and HIV infection. Actas Dermosifiliogr. 2008;99:753-63.
2. Wright V, Reed WB. The link between Reiter's syndrome and psoriatic arthritis. Ann Rheum Dis. 1964;23:12-21.
3. Menon K, Van Voorhees AS, Bebo BF, et al. Psoriasis in patients with HIV infection: from the medical board of the National Psoriasis Foundation. J Am Acad Dermatol. 2010;62:291-9.
4. Duvic M, Crane MM, Conant M, et al. Zidovudine improves psoriasis in human immunodeficiency virus-positive males. Arch Dermatol. 1994;130:447-51.
5. Shapiro DL, Masci JR. Treatment of HIV associated psoriatic arthritis with oral gold. J Rheumatol. 1996;23:1818-20.

Psoriasis as a Systemic Disease

INTRODUCTION

Psoriasis is now classified as an immune-mediated inflammatory disease (IMID) of the skin. Patients with various IMIDs are at higher risk of developing "systemic" comorbidities. IMIDs may impact these comorbid conditions through shared genetic, environmental factors, or common inflammatory pathways that are coexpressed in IMIDs and target organs **(Fig. 1)**.

Psoriasis patients are frequently obese, unknowingly at greater risk than general population for myocardial infarction (MI), metabolic syndrome and other comorbidities. There is strong evidence to suggest that psoriasis is an independent risk factor for the development of metabolic and CV comorbidities. Having observed these findings consistently by many authors, the questions that arise are:
- Is psoriasis a cutaneous disease or systemic disease?
- Is psoriasis a marker of underlying systemic disease?
- Is psoriasis a risk factor for systemic disease?
- What are the potential mechanistic "links" between psoriasis and systemic comorbid conditions?

With the advancing research that is going on, it is proved beyond doubt that psoriasis can now be considered as a systemic disease. Psoriasis by itself predisposes an individual to other systemic diseases and therefore is viewed as a marker of such systemic disorders. There is strong evidence to suggest that psoriasis is an independent risk factor for the development of metabolic and cardiovascular comorbidities. Probably the connecting link is the persistent inflammation that triggers off, and perpetuates the comorbid manifestations.

Mediators of inflammation produced in the skin are released into the systemic circulation and thus may contribute to the increased risk of inflammation in additional organs or tissues **(Fig. 2)**. Psoriasis, being an immune-mediated inflammatory disease, is capable of injuring the other organ system through a cascade of events. Insulin resistance and endothelial damage lead to organ dysfunction either directly or indirectly. There seems to exist a common pathway driven by many of the proinflammatory cytokines such as tumor necrosis factor alpha (TNF-α), Th1 and IL-6 in the pathogenesis of psoriasis and its comorbidities.[1]

The systemic disease that are more common in psoriatics **(Fig. 3)** are, arthropathy/arthritis, psychological disorders, hypertension, cardiovascular disease, chronic obstructive pulmonary disease (COPD), metabolic syndrome, insulin resistance/diabetes, celiac disease, autoimmune and collagen vascular diseases and malignancy **(Box 1)**.

PSORIATIC ARTHROPATHY AND ARTHRITIS

When genetically primed individual is exposed to a bacterial, stress, or entheseal-related peptide, the innate immune response, gets activated resulting in CD8 infiltration and chemokine/cytokine release. The process is amplified with angiogenesis and cellular infiltration of involved tissues. Human leukocyte antigen (HLA) and other genes expressed may determine the exact pattern of tissue involvement. In as many as 15–20% of patients, arthritis appears before the psoriasis.[2] 40–57% have deforming arthritis. Nearly one-fifth of them have more than five joints involved. Spine is involved in as high as 40%. Psoriatic arthritis leads to disability in nearly one-fifth of the affected individuals. The mortality is increased than the general population. The morbidity

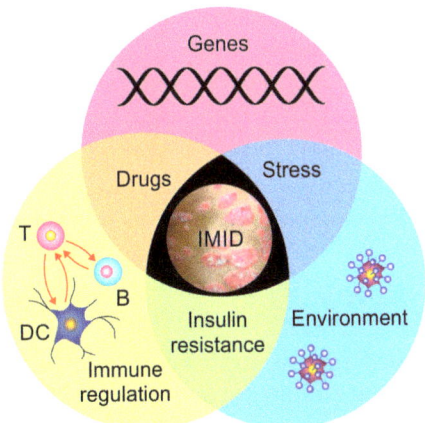

Fig. 1: Psoriasis—a systemic disease—the missing link.

CHAPTER 8: Psoriasis as a Systemic Disease

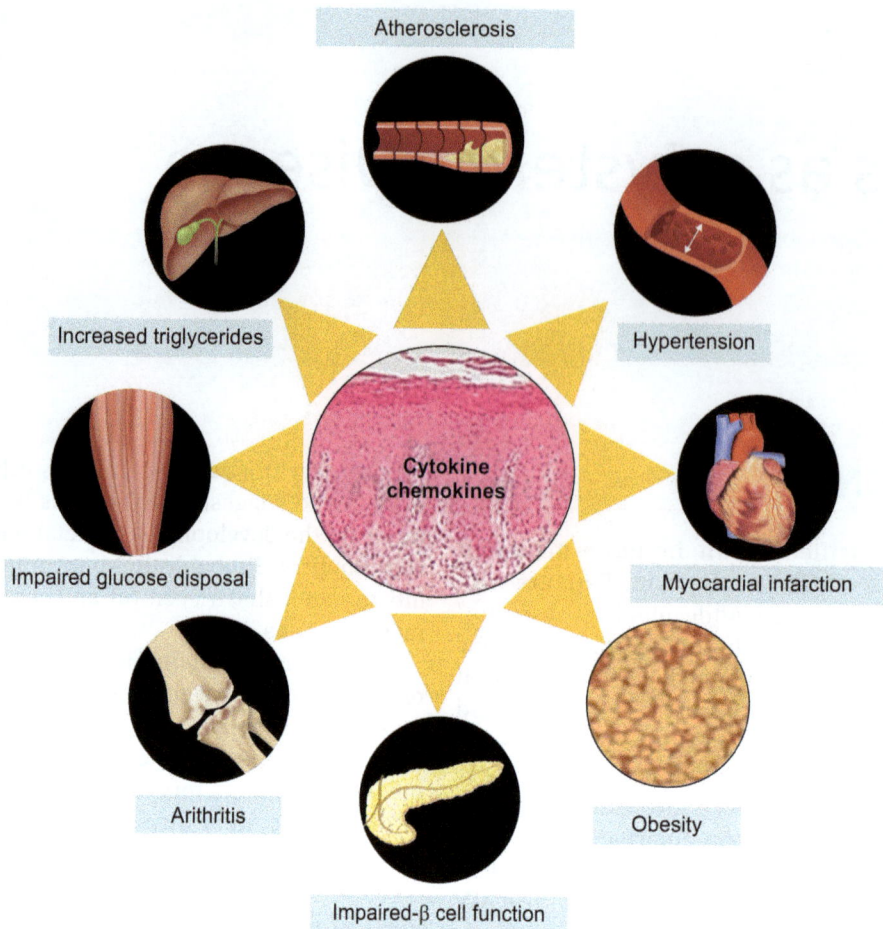

Fig. 2: Inflammatory mediators of psoriasis leading to systemic damage.

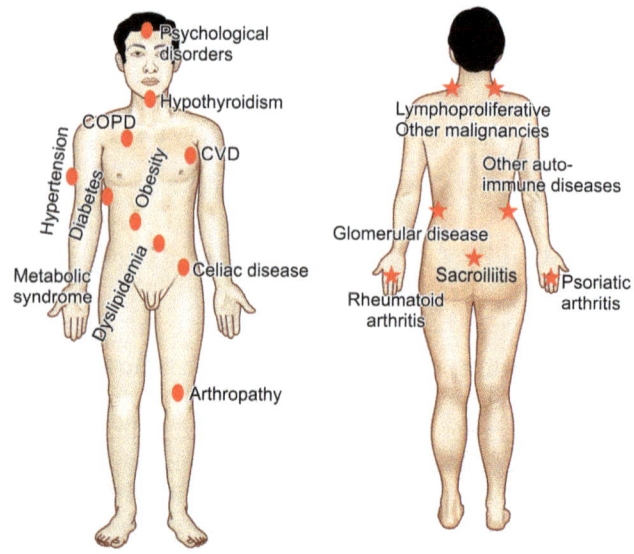

Fig. 3: Systemic diseases in psoriasis.

BOX 1: Systemic disease associated with psoriasis.

- Arthropathy/arthritis
- Psychological disorders
- Hypertension
- Cardiovascular disease
- Metabolic syndrome
- Diabetes
- Chronic obstructive pulmonary disease
- Celiac disease
- Autoimmune and collagen vascular diseases
- Renal disease
- Multiorgan failure
- Malignancy

and mortality can be reduced if the inflammation can be controlled at an early stage (Chapter 4).

"Psychological aspects" of psoriasis have been discussed separately in Chapter 12.

HYPERTENSION

There are many reports supporting the fact that patients with psoriasis are more prone to develop hypertension **(Figs. 4 to 6)**.

Drugs like beta-blockers used in the management of hypertension can precipitate, sustain or perpetuate psoriasis. In a large study with multivariate analysis, hypertension was associated with psoriasis after controlling for age, sex, smoking status, obesity, diabetes, nonsteroidal anti-inflammatory drugs (NSAIDs) and use of COX-2 inhibitors supporting the previously noted association between psoriasis and hypertension.[3] Association between psoriasis and hypertension may be attributed to angiotensin II, a product of angiotensin-converting enzyme (ACE) that regulates vascular tone and stimulates the release of proinflammatory cytokines. Elevated plasma renin activity and endothelin-1 seen both sera and lesional skin of patients with psoriasis may contribute to hypertension in psoriasis patients. Endothelial damage due to oxidative stress present in patients with psoriasis, may further add to the development of hypertension by destructive effects of reactive oxygen species, damaging endothelium-dependent vasodilatation. NSAID and COX-2 inhibitors used for psoriatic arthritis could also contribute to increased blood pressure. Similarly, beta-blockers used for control of hypertension can further worsen psoriasis thus inducing a vicious cycle. When adjusted for age and sex, the association between psoriasis and hypertension appears to be significant only above the age of 40 years. Therefore, it is mandatory that all psoriatics above 40 years of age are screened for hypertension.

PSORIASIS AND CARDIOVASCULAR DISEASE/ATHEROTHROMBOTIC DISEASES

Of emerging significance is the relationship between cardiovascular disease and severe psoriasis, as this may explain the increased mortality of the latter.[4] Psoriasis and psoriatic arthritis are associated with increased atherothrombotic diseases, including MI, deep venous thrombosis and reduced lifespan **(Figs. 7 and 8)**.

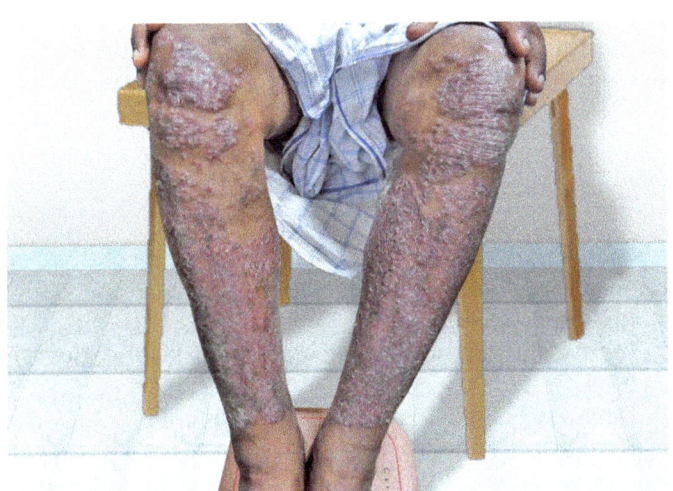

Fig. 4: Patient with psoriasis detected to have systemic hypertension on screening.

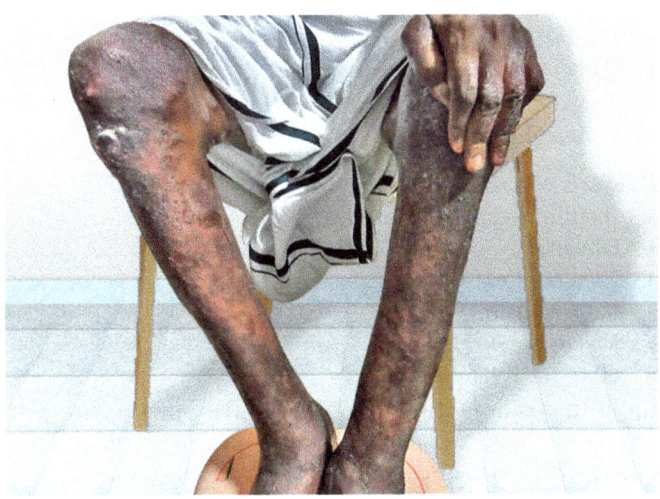

Fig. 6: Patient with systemic hypertension on long-term beta blockers.

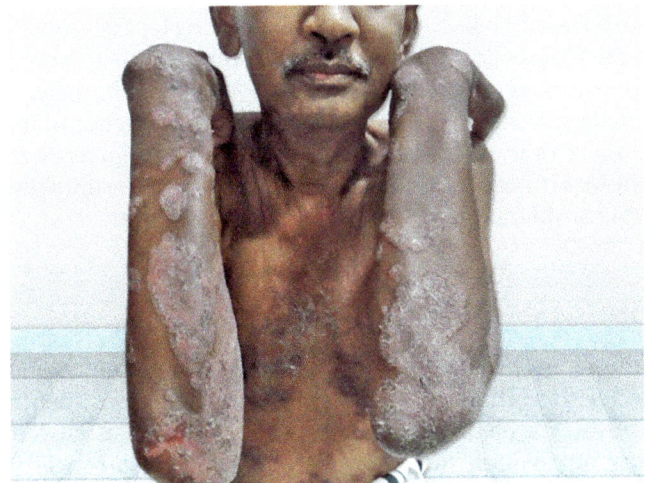

Fig. 5: Patient with hypertension.

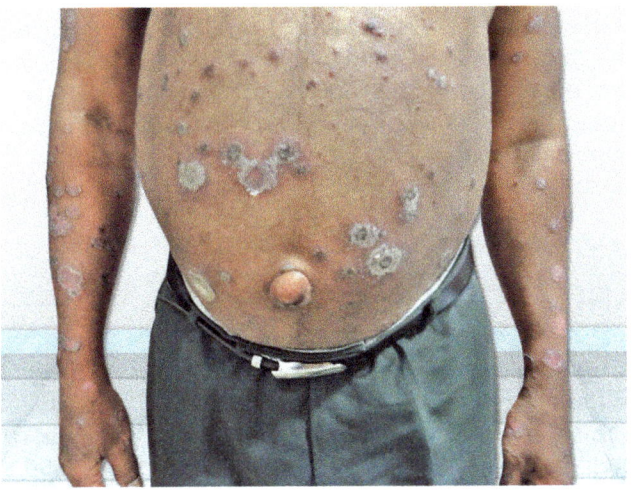

Fig. 7: Man developed myocardial infarction (MI) who was having psoriasis for 5 years before the infarct.

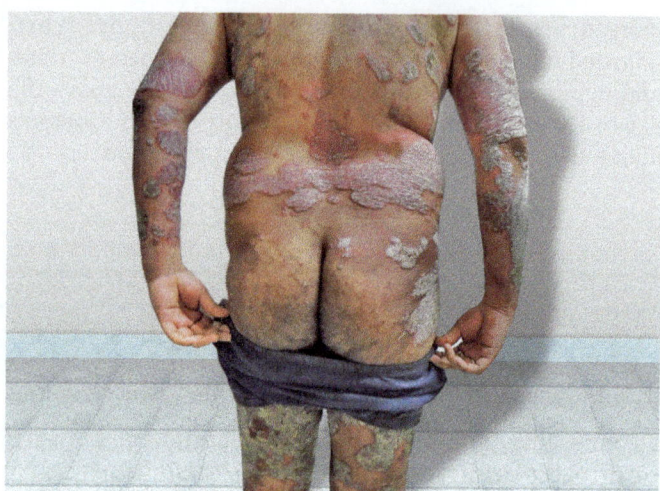

Fig. 8: Patient had myocardial infarction 1 year after the onset of psoriasis.

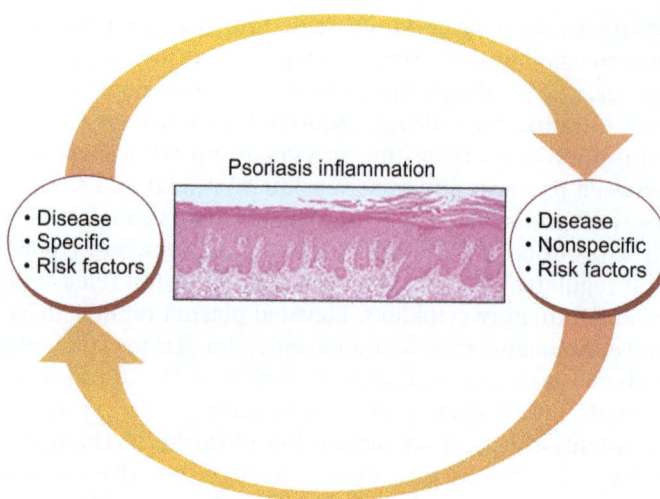

Fig. 9: Risk factors involved in perpetuation of cardiac disease.

Disease-specific risk factors are those that are a direct consequence of psoriasis inflammation:
- Hyperhomocysteinemia
- Elevated C-reactive protein (CRP)
- Elevated blood inflammatory cytokines
- Platelet hyperactivity.

Psoriasis nondisease-specific risk factors:
- Insulin resistance/diabetes
- Obesity
- Dyslipidemia
- Hypertension
- Metabolic syndrome
- Habitual tobacco smoking.

Both disease-specific and nondisease-specific risk factors are likely to fuel one another in deleterious vicious circles **(Fig. 9)**. Patients with psoriasis should be treated effectively and encouraged to aggressively correct their modifiable cardiovascular risk factors.

Cytokine-activated leukocytes in the skin enter circulation after rolling on inflamed endothelial cells in psoriatic plaques. The inflammatory chemokines released into the systemic circulation, like TNF, IL-1, or IL-6, may alter the function of hepatocytes, vascular cells, leukocyte physiology and increase cardiovascular risk factors or overt pathological pathways.

MYOCARDIAL INFARCTION AND PSORIASIS

There is an age-dependent increase in MI among psoriatic patients compared with control population. Young patients with severe disease have the greatest risks, which is still worse in females. Psoriasis was found to be an independent risk factor for MI, after adjustment for other confounding conditions for cardiovascular disease, such as hypertension, diabetes, history of MI, hyperlipidemia, age, sex, smoking and body mass index (BMI). According to Gelfand JM, psoriasis may confer an independent risk of MI. The relative risk was greatest in young patients with severe psoriasis.[5]

METABOLIC SYNDROME

Metabolic syndrome is defined as the presence of three or more of the following components:
1. Abdominal obesity
2. Increased insulin resistance/elevated fasting glucose level
3. Decreased high-density lipoprotein cholesterol
4. Hypertriglyceridemia
5. Hypertension.

The factors defining metabolic syndrome go hand in hand with an increased risk for diabetes and atherosclerotic cardiovascular disease. Emerging data clearly indicate that psoriasis might be an independent risk factor for cardiovascular disease even after correcting for components of the metabolic syndrome. The incidence of one or more of the components of metabolic syndrome is much higher in female patients over 40 years of age.[6] The incidence of one or more of the components in females is as high as 88.5% whereas it ranges from 52 to 56% if both genders are taken into consideration.

Obesity and Psoriasis

Adipocytes produce CRP and proinflammatory cytokines under the influence of inflammatory mediators such as TNF-α, suggesting that an interplay may exist between adipocytes and the inflammation that drives psoriasis. There is distinct interaction between adipokines and Th17 cytokines is involved in the pathogenesis of psoriasis.

As systemic inflammation drives the development of disease, adiponectin is downregulated while leptin and resistin are simultaneously upregulated. Leptin plays a key role in metabolism and enhances macrophage activity, upregulating TNF-α and IL-6, the latter of which promotes CRP production. Resistin being a secretory factor linked to inflammation that drives insulin resistance favors the development of atherosclerosis. Overall, compared with the general population, psoriasis patients have higher prevalence and incidence of obesity. Patients with severe psoriasis have greater odds of obesity than those with mild psoriasis.[7]

Whether obesity is a contributing factor to or a manifestation of psoriasis is still under debate. Recent data suggest that obesity is a risk factor for the development of psoriasis **(Figs. 10 to 13)**.

Those data which indicate that BMI increased in patients after psoriasis diagnosis, suggest that obesity is secondary to psoriasis. Irrespective of whether obesity is cause or consequence of psoriasis, it has been noted that increased BMI coincides with a greater degree of psoriasis disease severity.

Insulin Resistance/Diabetes and Psoriasis

There is significant association between psoriasis, diabetes and insulin resistance. Several measurements indicative of insulin resistance were found to be significantly correlated with the psoriasis area and severity index (PASI) score. The concept of insulin resistance as a consequence of chronic inflammation and possible pathogenetic cause for comorbidities known to be associated with psoriasis is supported by these data **(Fig. 14)**.[8]

Systemic inflammation causing insulin resistance, in turn triggers endothelial cell dysfunction, subsequently leading to atherosclerosis and finally MI or stroke. Obesity being a known risk factor for psoriasis may induce the phenotype

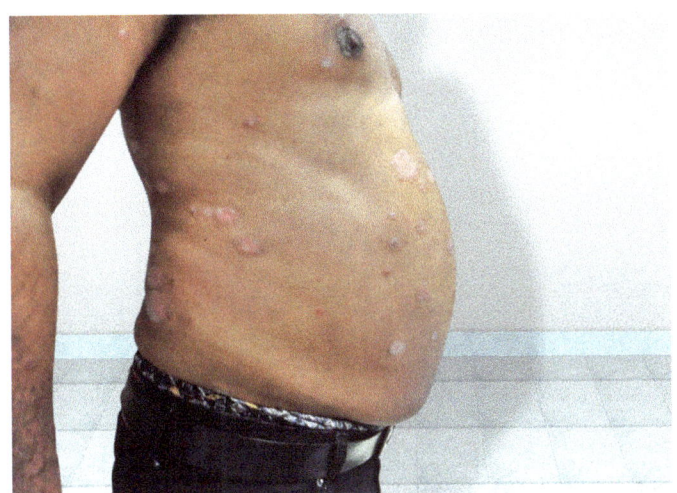

Fig. 10: Psoriasis and obesity a potential risk factor.

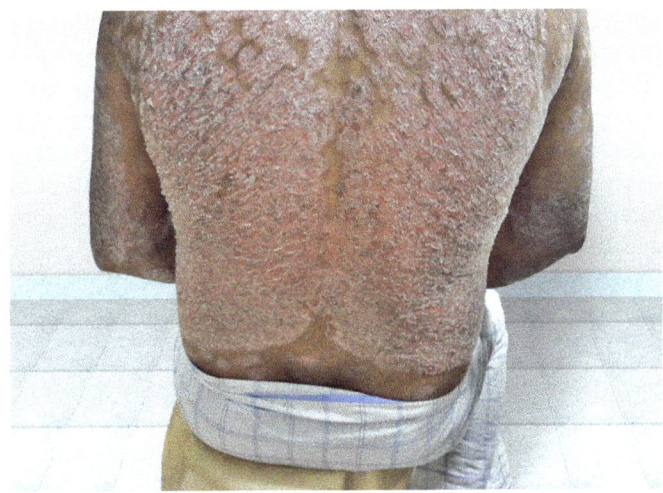

Fig. 12: Patient on statin for dyslipidemia needs strict control of both skin disease and lipid profile.

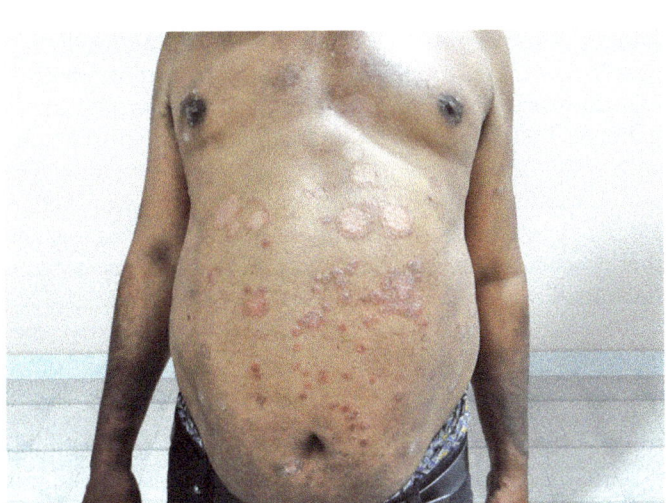

Fig. 11: Same patient as in **Figure 10**.

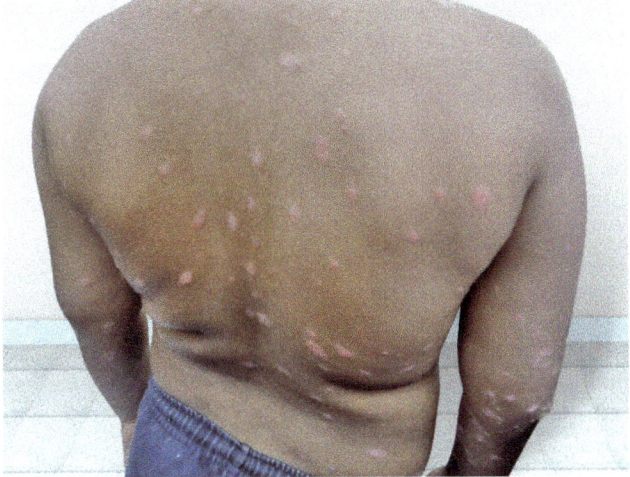

Fig. 13: Same patient as in **Figure 12**.

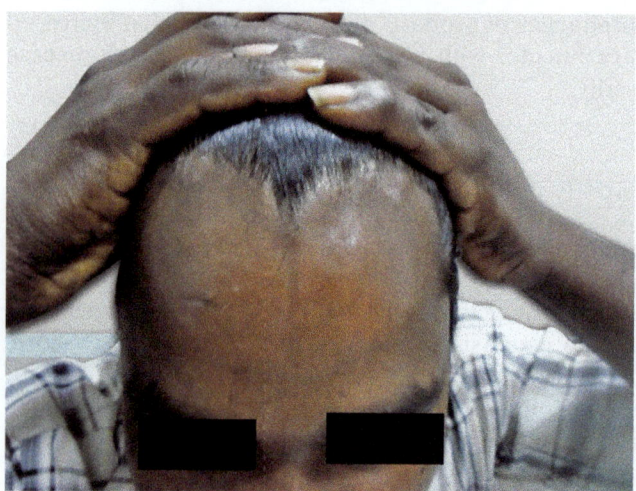

Fig. 14: Obese man with patterned hair loss, obesity, dyslipidemia whose father a known case of psoriasis died of myocardial infarction.

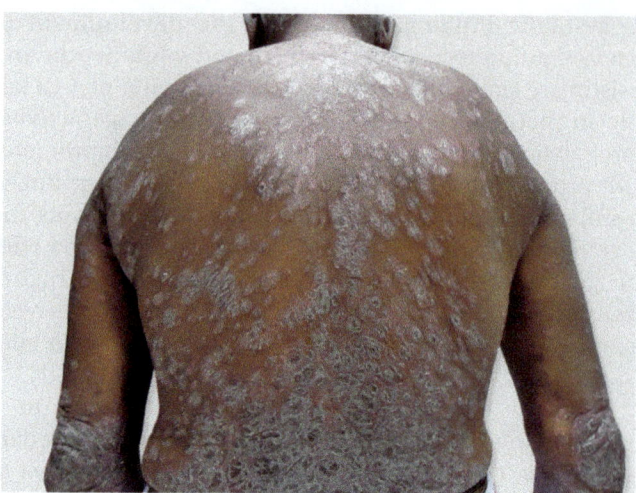

Fig. 15: This man with psoriasis developed chronic obstructive pulmonary disease (COPD).

through systemic inflammation further leading to insulin resistance which increases keratinocyte proliferation and reduce differentiation further perpetuating the skin disease thus keeping the vicious cycle on. There increased prevalence and incidence of diabetes in psoriatics, the association being strongest among patients with severe psoriasis. According to a research data, those with severe psoriasis, were 46% more likely to get a diabetes than people without the condition, after weight and other health measures were taken into account.

Pulmonary Disease and Psoriasis

The lung condition COPD, which is mainly caused by smoking, is significantly more common among psoriasis patients than the general population, researchers have found **(Figs. 15 and 16)**.[9]

Up to 5.7% of psoriasis patients had been diagnosed with COPD compared with just 3.6% of those without the skin condition. Even though the difference is small, this has to be born in mind while treating patients with psoriasis. Methotrexate and other immune suppressive agents, biologics may lead to development of tuberculosis. Lung fibrosis can be precipitated by long-term methotrexate. Increased incidence of malignancy has also been noted. The triad of stress-smoking—worsening of disease—should be broken lest may further lead to more severe consequences.

Gastrointestinal System and Psoriasis

It has been documented that there is a decrease in the small bowel surface area in patients with severe psoriasis. Smoothing of the intestinal wall in the jejunal area of the bowel was demonstrated as a feature of severe psoriasis. There is an increased prevalence of psoriasis in Crohn's disease and ulcerative colitis and their first degree relatives

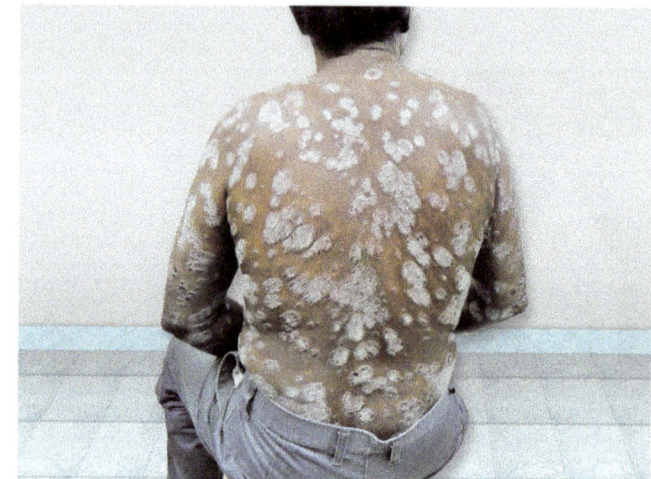

Fig. 16: Man with psoriasis who is on treatment for chronic obstructive pulmonary disease (COPD).

than control.[10] There is an increase in mast cells, eosinophils, duodenal intraepithelial lymphocytes, IgA antibodies to gliadin, serum eosinophil cationic protein and numbers of EG2 positive eosinophils in the duodenal mucosa of psoriasis patients. There are reports quoting that in psoriatic patients with celiac disease having gluten sensitivity avoidance of gluten induces remission of psoriasis and re-introduction led to active skin disease. There are enough studies to show that psoriasis is associated with alcoholic liver disease and hepatitis C virus (HCV) infection **(Figs. 17 and 18)**.

Autoimmune Diseases and Psoriasis

Psoriasis was positively associated with many autoimmune diseases, which are statistically significant. The strongest association was with rheumatoid arthritis. Patients with psoriasis are >50% more likely than patients without

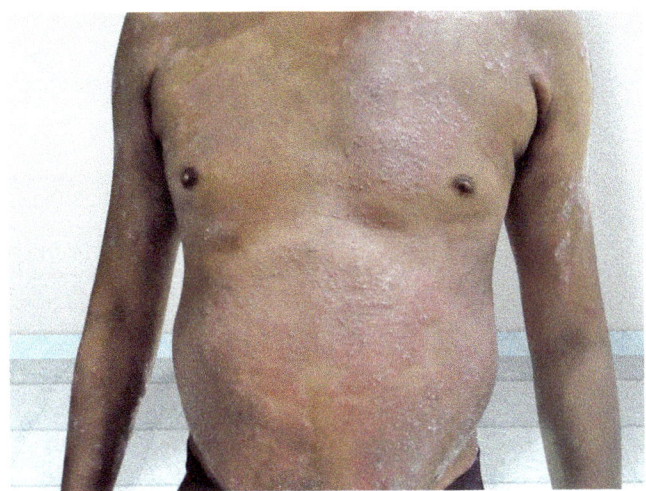

Fig. 17: Man with alcoholic liver disease.

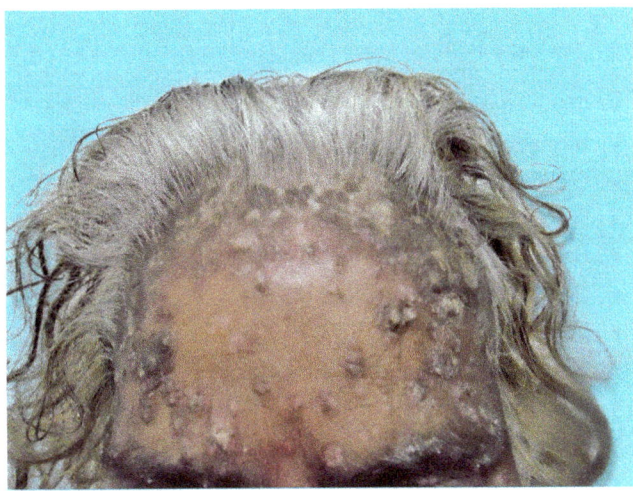

Fig. 19: Lady with severe psoriasis having hypothyroid, dyslipidemia.

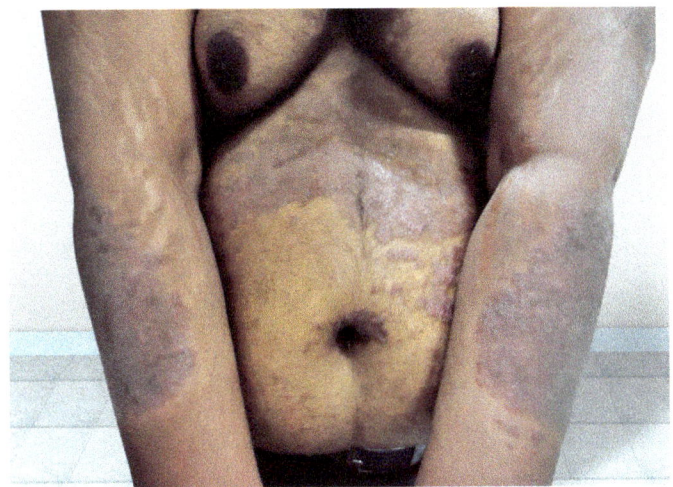

Fig. 18: Patient with hepatitis C virus (HCV) infection.

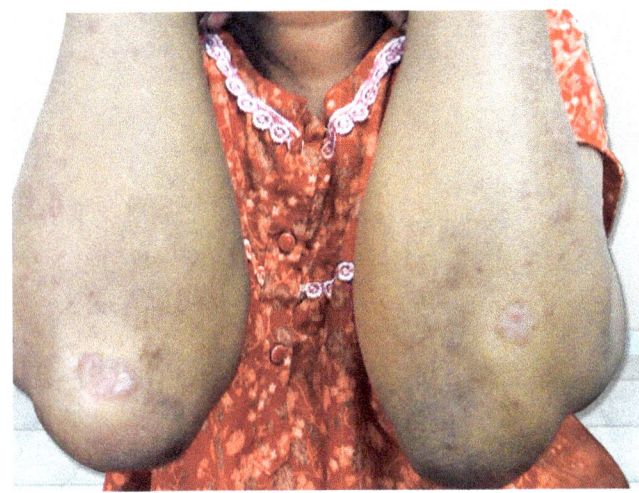

Fig. 20: Psoriasis and hypothyroidism in a woman.

psoriasis to have at least one other autoimmune disease and are nearly twice as likely to have at least two other autoimmune diseases.[11] The autoimmune diseases known to be associated with psoriasis are given in **Box 2 (Figs. 19 and 20)**.

Renal Disease and Psoriasis

While the existence of a "psoriatic nephropathy" having been proposed based on case reports of glomerulonephritides in patients with psoriasis, the association between psoriasis and kidney disease are now studied more widely. Studies found a fourfold increase in death from nephritic or nonhypertensive kidney disease among those with severe psoriasis. Multiple cross-sectional studies have also observed greater prevalence of microalbuminuria, a sign of subclinical glomerular dysfunction, in patients with psoriasis. Though some studies have detected no association between psoriasis and renal disease.

It is now hypothesized that patients with psoriasis, especially if it is severe, have an increased risk of moderate to advanced (Stage 3–5) chronic kidney disease (CKD) compared with patients without psoriasis **(Fig. 21)**.

Moderate-to-severe psoriasis is associated with moderate to advanced CKD independent of traditional risk factors. Closer monitoring for renal insufficiency, such as routine screening urinalysis for microalbuminuria and serum creatinine and blood urea nitrogen testing, should be considered for patients with psoriasis affecting 3% or more of the body surface area. Increased screening efforts will allow for earlier detection and intervention to reduce the substantial morbidity and mortality associated with CKD. Additionally, the risk versus benefit of potentially nephrotoxic drugs in patients with moderate-to-severe psoriasis should be carefully considered. Moderate-to-severe psoriasis is associated with an increased risk of CKD independent of traditional risk factors, such as diabetes and heart disease indicates the most recent study.[12]

BOX 2: Autoimmune disease in psoriasis.

- Crohn's disease
- Ulcerative colitis
- Celiac disease
- Type 1 diabetes mellitus (T1DM)
- Hemolytic anemia
- Giant cell arteritis
- Multiple sclerosis
- Systemic lupus erythematosus (SLE)
- Graves' disease
- Hashimoto's disease
- Chronic glomerulonephritis
- Pulmonary fibrosis
- Sjögren's syndrome
- Addison's disease
- Immune thrombocytopenia
- Primary biliary cirrhosis
- Alopecia areata
- Vitiligo
- Chronic urticaria

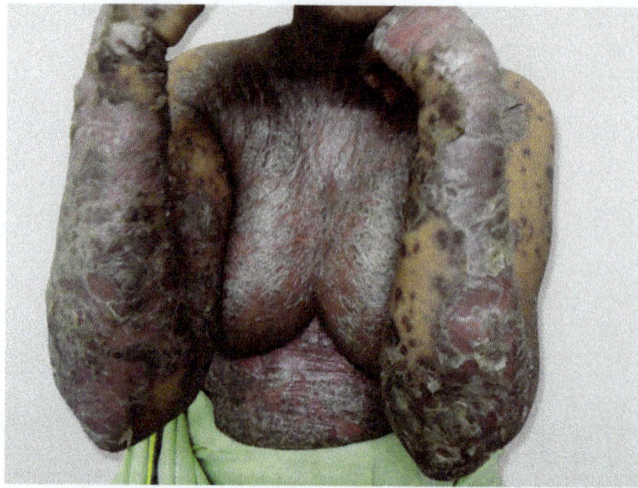

Fig. 22: Lady with severe psoriasis, diabetes mellitus, hypertension, hypothyroid, dyslipidemia with multiorgan failure.

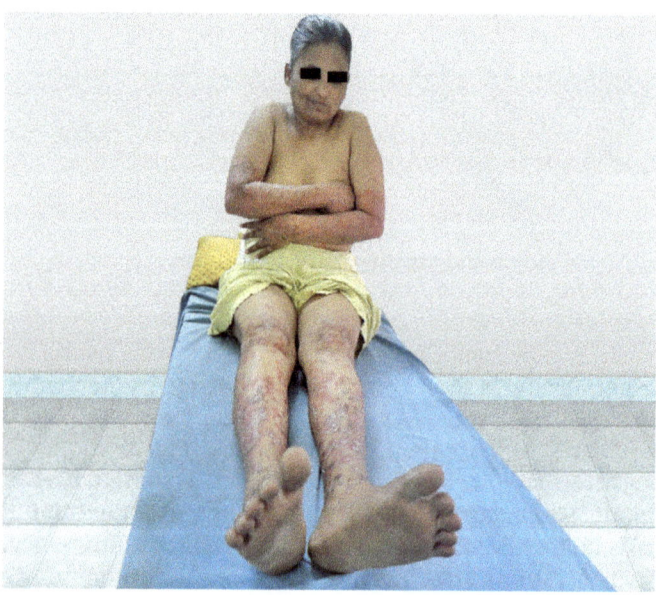

Fig. 21: Pustular psoriasis in a lady with chronic kidney disease.

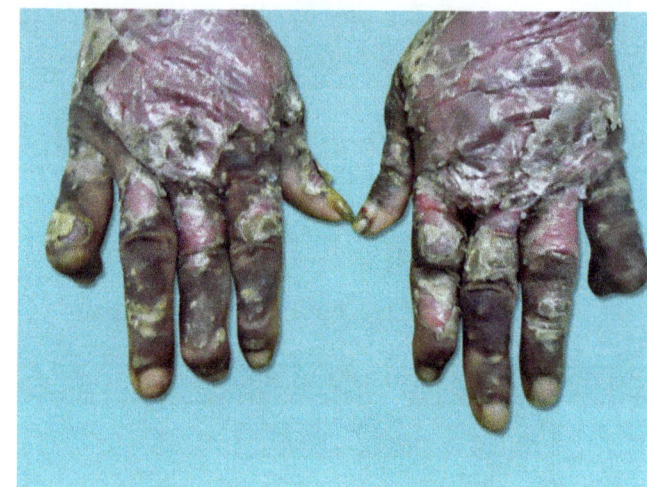

Fig. 23: Severe psoriasis in a patient with multiorgan failure.

Multiorgan Failure due to Psoriasis

Multiorgan failure (multisystem organ failure) has been reported by people with coronary artery bypass, blood pressure management, high blood pressure and rheumatoid arthritis.

Now there are reports staining occurrence of multiorgan failure in patients with psoriasis **(Figs. 22 and 23)**.

In a study where 57,508 people with psoriasis are studied, 64 people (0.11%) were found to have multiorgan failure with a female male ratio of 32.10:67.90%. The top most coexisting conditions for these people was found to be psoriasis which was found in all 64 patients amounting to 100.00%.[13] In another report, a woman developed multiorgan failure as a result of erythrodermic psoriasis and shortly thereafter developed bronchial pneumonia. There are reports where generalized pustular psoriasis appearing in patients after organ transplantation subsequently leading to multiorgan failure, while the European guidelines for renal transplantation reported by the European Best Practices Guidelines (EBPG) Expert Group in 2000 do not include psoriasis in the exclusion criteria. With only two cases reported so far, whether psoriasis or a history of psoriasis in patients with chronic renal failure is a contraindication for transplantation or not is a question that remains unanswered.[14]

MALIGNANCY AND PSORIASIS

Patients with psoriasis are at an increased risk of developing malignancy, particularly nonmelanoma skin cancer and lymphoproliferative cancers **(Fig. 24)**.

The fact that risk is greatest for those with severe disease, may probably be a reflection of treatment with systemic agents and phototherapy. The risk of psoriatic patients developing lymphoid malignancies may be attributable to the abnormal immune activation that has been demonstrated in them.

In addition to lymphoma, psoriatic patients have an increased risk for other malignancies, including those of the head and neck, solid organs (liver, pancreas, lung, breast and kidney) and genitals.[15]

Psoriatic patients with diabetes are prone to develop digestive organ cancers. Chronic inflammation acts as the driving force that enhances the risk of malignancy in psoriatic. Prevalent cancers in the population should be carefully monitored in the psoriatic over 40 years of age especially for those with concomitant diabetes. There is increased risk of mortality for these psoriasis patients, when compared with the general population.

COMORBIDITY IN CHILDHOOD PSORIASIS

Psoriatic children have a higher prevalence of obesity. It was also observed that overweight had different effects on childhood patients. Psoriasis in these children was more severe compared with psoriatic children of normal weight. There is a strong association between psoriasis and obesity in children especially boys.[16] Increased incidence of hyperlipidemia, hypertension and diabetes, has also reported to be associated with psoriasis in children/adolescents. It may be considered that in an obese child, disease severity can be a marker of cardiovascular risk. Prevalence of comorbidities in persons in the age range 0-20 years with psoriasis was found to be more than those without psoriasis. Crohn's disease, hyperlipidemia, diabetes mellitus, arterial hypertension, rheumatoid arthritis, obesity, ischemic heart disease, ulcerative colitis were the comorbidities observed in childhood psoriasis.

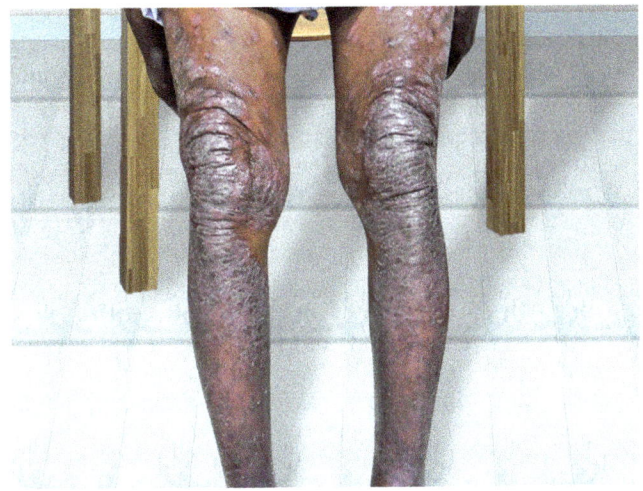

Fig. 24: Man developed lymphoma who was on immunosuppressive drugs for psoriasis for 5 years.

SUMMARY

Psoriasis is a debilitating chronic inflammatory disease that predisposes patients both young and old to serious comorbidities. Pediatricians and primary care physicians should be aware of potential cardiometabolic conditions and risk factors when treating patients with psoriasis. Certain predictive factors can help detect patients who will be at risk of developing comorbidities. In such patients, early therapeutic intervention will help prevent the onset of these comorbidities?

- Young females with severe psoriasis suffer cardiovascular event five times more than their counterpart.[17]
- Antecedents of skin disorders and skin infection within the last year predisposes to development of comorbidities.[18]
- Smoking was found to be an independent risk factor for psoriasis.
- Obesity is a definite risk factor in psoriasis in the induction of comorbid conditions, no matter whether it is a cause or consequence, whether it is a child or adult.

REFERENCES

1. Reich K. The concept of psoriasis as a systemic inflammation: implications for disease management. J Eur Acad Dermatol Venereol. 2012;26:3-11.
2. Hammadi A, Badsha H. (2013). Psoriatic arthritis. [online] Available from Medscap http://emedicine.medscape.com/article/331037-overview. [Accessed November, 2013].
3. Cohen AD, Weitzman D, Dreiher J. Psoriasis and hypertension: a case-control study. Acta Derm Venereol. 2010;90:23-6.
4. Gelfand JM, Troxel AB, Lewis JD, et al. The risk of mortality in patients with psoriasis: results from a population-based study. Arch Dermatol. 2007;143:1493-9.
5. Gelfand JM, Neimann AL, Shin DB, et al. Risk of myocardial infarction in patients with psoriasis. JAMA. 2006;296:1735-41.
6. Kumar P, Thomas J. Comorbid conditions in psoriasis—higher frequency in females: a prospective study. Indian Dermatol Online J. 2012;3(2):105-8.

7. Armstrong AW, Harskamp CT, Armstrong EJ. The association between psoriasis and obesity: a systematic review and meta-analysis of observational studies. Nutr Diabetes. 2012;2:e54.
8. Boehncke S, Thaci D, Beschmann H, et al. Psoriasis patients show signs of insulin resistance. Br J Dermatol. 2007;157:1249-51.
9. Cowen M. Lung disease common in psoriasis patients. Br J Dermatol. 2008: Advance online publication. [online] Available from the URL http://www.medwirenews.com/52/76543/Consumer_Health/Lung_disease_common_in_psoriasis_patients.htm [Accessed November, 2013].
10. Yates MV, Watkinson G, Kelman A. Further evidence for an association between psoriasis, Crohn's disease and ulcerative colitis. Br J Dermatol. 1982;106:323-30.
11. Kelly JC. (2013). Psoriasis linked to autoimmune diseases. [online] Available from Medscape http://www.medscape.com/viewarticle/773015 [Accessed November, 2013].
12. Wan J, Wang S, Haynes K, et al. Risk of moderate to advanced kidney disease in patients with psoriasis: population based cohort study. BMJ. 2013;347:f5961.
13. eHealthMe. (2013). Review: Psoriasis and Multi-organ failure. [online] Available from http://www.ehealthme.com/cs/psoriasis/multi-organ+failure. [Accessed November, 2013].
14. Vougas V, Dedemadi G, Noutsis K, et al. Generalised Pustular Psoriasis (von Zumbusch type) following renal transplantation. Report of a case and review of the literature. Hospital Chronicles. 2007;2(2):89-93.
15. Gottlieb AB, Dann F. Comorbidities in Patients with Psoriasis. Am J Med. 2009;122:1150.e1-1150.e9.
16. Boccardi D, Menni S, La Vecchia C, et al. Overweight and childhood psoriasis. Br J Dermatol. 2009;161:484-6.
17. Gelfand JM, Troxel AB, Lewis JD, et al. The risk of mortality in patients with psoriasis. Arch Dermatol. 2007;143(12):1493-9.
18. Huerta C, Rivero E, García Rodríguez LA. Incidence and risk factors for psoriasis in the general population. Arch Dermatol. 2008;143:1559-65.

9

Investigations

INTRODUCTION

Diagnosis of psoriasis is essentially clinical except in variants like erythrodermic psoriasis, pustular psoriasis when they present for the first time. Linear psoriasis and persistent plaque psoriasis are common diagnostic challenges, if the classical features of psoriasis are lost. Under such situations, to establish the diagnosis and to rule out the differential diagnosis, biopsy is warranted.[1] By and large, investigations *per se* in psoriasis are needed only under the following circumstances:
- To rule out infection as a cause of psoriasis
- To assess the disease activity
- To assess extent and type of damage as in psoriatic arthritis (PA)
- To screen for comorbidity and systemic involvement
- To assess the patient's general condition during the acute presentation like erythrodermic psoriasis, pustular psoriasis
- To assess the patient for specific therapy
- Evaluation of drug therapy
- To assess the prognosis.

Baseline investigations to be done in all patients with psoriasis above the age of 40 years will include:
- All patients should have their blood pressure and body mass index (BMI) read and recorded:
  - Complete blood count including total count (TC), differential count (DC), erythrocyte sedimentation rate (ESR), hemoglobin (Hb), total red blood cells (RBC) and platelets
  - Blood sugar fasting and postprandial
  - Lipid profile
  - Liver function test (LFT)
  - Uric acid
  - Rheumatoid (RA) factor
  - Antinuclear antibody (ANA)
  - Renal function test including urine analysis.

TO RULE OUT INFECTION AS A CAUSE OF PSORIASIS

Throat swab culture, ESR and antistreptolysin O (ASO) titer will help in children with guttate psoriasis.

TO ASSESS THE DISEASE ACTIVITY[2-4]

- *Markers of neutrophil activation*: Elastase, lactoferrin and lipid peroxidation.
- *Markers of endogenous antioxidant*: Total plasma antioxidant capacity (TAC), transferrin, ceruloplasmin, alpha-1-antitrypsin and alpha 2-macroglobulin.
- *Markers of inflammation*: Antiprotease systems, and fibrinogen, erythrocyte sedimentation rate, C-reactive protein (CRP), haptoglobin, C3 and C4 complement.

These markers show a raised value in active psoriasis when compared to inactive psoriasis. Most of these are essentially done for research purpose.

TO ASSESS EXTENT AND TYPE OF DAMAGE IN PSORIATIC ARTHRITIS[5-11]

X-ray of the affected joint, computerized tomogram (CT) scan and magnetic resonance imaging (MRI), ultrasonography (USG), nuclear imaging studies are required in assessing the type and extent of involvement.

In particular, CT scanning is useful in identifying inflammatory lesions, even when pre-existing degenerative disease is present; in demonstrating the articular surfaces of bone in an exact fashion; and, in some cases of sacroiliitis, in clearly demonstrating erosive changes that can appear equivocal or negative with radiography.

TABLE 1: Distinguishing features between psoriatic arthritis (PA) and rheumatoid arthritis (RA).

Findings	PA	RA
Subcutaneous nodules	–	+
RA factor	–	+
Bony ankylosis	+	–
Periarticular bony proliferation	+	–
Osteopenia	–	+
Bone mineralization and has periosteal reaction and new-bone formation	Maintained	Lost
Sausage digit and spontaneous joint fusion	Common	Rare

Findings on MRI are the most sensitive and specific for sacroiliitis and for other changes in the axial skeleton and in the hands and feet. With MRI, it is possible to identify the early inflammatory phase of enthesitis before the development of erosion, as seen on radiographs. MRI can depict early cortical erosion, inflammatory granulation tissue and bone marrow edema.

Ultrasonography is useful for assessing the extent of disease, but it is not the method of choice for monitoring bone involvement in psoriatic arthritis (PA). Whole-body scintigraphy shows the distribution of active joint disease. Abnormal radiotracer uptake precedes findings on plain radiographs.

The radiographic appearance of PA can be similar to that of RA. The distinguishing features of PA are enlisted in **Table 1**.

TO SCREEN FOR COMORBIDITY AND SYSTEMIC INVOLVEMENT

All patients should have their blood pressure and BMI read and recorded. The following investigations must be carried out in all patients with psoriasis, wherever possible which will detect the systemic involvement early.
- Complete blood count including TC, DC, ESR, Hb, total RBC and platelets
- Blood sugar fasting and postprandial
- Lipid profile
- Liver function test
- Uric acid
- RA Factor
- ANA
- Renal function test including urine analysis.

INVESTIGATIONS DURING ACUTE STAGES

Tests to be done in erythroderma patients:
- *Complete hemogram*: Hb, TC, DC, ESR
- Peripheral smear
- Motion for occult blood
- X-ray chest, electrocardiogram (ECG)
- Ultrasonography abdomen
- Serum electrolytes, creatinine
- Lactate dehydrogenase (LDH)
- Liver function test including bilirubin and protein level
- Blood glucose
- Gamma globulin, immunoglobulin E (IgE)
- Lymph node biopsy should be considered in long standing or recurrent cases of erythroderma
- *Laboratory findings*: Gastrointestinal pathogen panel (GPP)
- Culture of the pus does not yield organisms
- There may be an absolute lymphopenia at the onset
- Quickly followed by polymorphonuclear leukocytosis
- The ESR is usually raised
- Plasma albumin, zinc and calcium may be abnormally low
- Liver enzymes may be elevated.

TO ASSESS THE PATIENT FOR SPECIFIC THERAPY

It is mandatory to exclude tuberculosis and other infections before initiating any immunosuppressive drugs including biologics.
- Complete blood count for all patients to be started on immunosuppressant drug
- Renal function test (RFT) and LFT for methotrexate
- Renal function test for cyclosporine along with maintenance of blood pressure
- Lipid profile and LFT in case of retinoid therapy.

EVALUATION OF DRUG THERAPY

While the patient is started on a drug like methotrexate or biological agent, there are certain protocols to be followed while investigating the patients. These have to be meticulously adhered to and the results interpreted appropriately.

Methotrexate

Premethotrexate evaluation:
- Complete blood count with differential and platelet count
- Blood urea nitrogen and serum creatinine
- Urinalysis
- Liver function tests including serum bilirubin
- Chest X-ray (if not taken in the last 6 months)
- Repeat every 2 weeks till 6 weeks thereafter every 2 months. X-ray repeated once a year
- Liver biopsy
- Pretreatment liver biopsy in alcoholics suggested.

During treatment liver biopsy is suggested, if there is persistent elevation of aspartate transaminase (AST) and elevation of peptide of type III procollagen (PIIINP) above 10 mcg/L in three samples in 1 year, or after a cumulative dose of 1.5 g of methotrexate.

Biological Agents

Screening tests recommended prior to starting etanercept usually include full blood count, liver enzymes, serum creatinine, urine analysis, pregnancy test, if relevant (urine or serum), hepatitis B virus (HBV)/hepatitis C virus (HCV) and human immunodeficiency virus (HIV).

Tuberculosis screening includes chest X-ray and Mantoux intradermal test or QuantiFERON-TB gold blood test. The following protocol can be followed for monitoring patients on biological therapies:

- *Annual screening for tuberculosis*: Mantoux test, X-ray chest alternatives include the QuantiFERON-TB gold blood test
- CD4+ T-lymphocyte count every 2 weeks for alefacept
- Complete metabolic panel with LFTs for each infliximab infusion and with any sign of hepatic injury
- Complete blood count and metabolic panel every 3–6 months on all biological therapies
- Hepatitis screen and HIV testing when risk factors present on all biological therapies
- Avoid all live and live-attenuated vaccines

Evaluation of CD4 lymphocyte count may be indicated in the event of development of opportunistic infection while on any immunosuppressant drug.

TO ASSESS THE PROGNOSIS

With the advancement in the field of genetics, there are many human leukocyte antigen (HLA) and non-HLA genes found to be associated with certain disease outcome and treatment response.

The following are some of the documented associations. Detection of these will help to manage the patient in a better way:

- HLA B27 in congenital erythrodermic psoriasis, where the etiology of erythroderma is not established. HLA-B27—spinal involvement
- HLA-B38, B39—peripheral polyarthritis
- HLA-B39, HLA-B27 in the presence of HLA-DR7 and HLA-DQw3—increased risk for disease progression
- HLA-B22—protective for disease progression
- HLA-Cw6 and HLA-DRB1*07 together—less severe course of arthritis
- MHC class I chain-related antigen A (MICA)-A9 variant positive—60% chance of developing PA
- MICA-A9 variant negative—70% chance of not developing PA.

SUMMARY

Psoriasis is invariably diagnosed clinically needing biopsy only on certain clinical presentations where the close mimickers need to be excluded. Investigations are by and large done in order to exclude associations, complications and for planning treatment and follow-up.

REFERENCES

1. Kim WB, Jerome D, Yeung J. Diagnosis and management of psoriasis. Can Fam Physician. 2017;63(4):278-85.
2. Dowlatshahi EA, van der Voort EA, Arends LR, Nijsten T. Markers of systemic inflammation in psoriasis: a systematic review and meta-analysis. Br J Dermatol. 2013;169(2):266-82.
3. Punzi L, Podswiadek M, Oliviero F, Lonigro A, Modesti V, Ramonda R, et al. Laboratory findings in psoriatic arthritis. Reumatismo. 2007;59(Suppl 1):52-5.
4. Farshchian M, Ansar A, Sobhan M, Hoseinpoor V. C-reactive protein serum level in patients with psoriasis before and after treatment with narrow-band ultraviolet B. An Bras Dermatol. 2016;91(5):580-3.
5. Poggenborg RP, Østergaard M, Terslev L. Imaging in Psoriatic Arthritis. Rheum Dis Clin North Am. 2015;41(4):593-613.
6. Fassio A, Matzneller P, Idolazzi L. Recent Advances in Imaging for Diagnosis, Monitoring, and Prognosis of Psoriatic Arthritis. Front Med (Lausanne). 2020;29;7:551684.
7. McQueen F, Lassere M, Østergaard M. Magnetic resonance imaging in psoriatic arthritis: a review of the literature. Arthritis Res Ther. 2006;8(2):207.
8. Maldonado-Ficco H, Sheane BJ, Thavaneswaran A, Chandran V, Gladman DD. Magnetic Resonance Imaging in Psoriatic Arthritis: A Descriptive Study of Indications, Features and Effect on Treatment Change. J Clin Rheumatol. 2017;23(5): 243-5.
9. Naranje P, Prakash M, Sharma A, Dogra S, Khandelwal N. Ultrasound Findings in Hand Joints Involvement in Patients with Psoriatic Arthritis and Its Correlation with Clinical DAS28 Score. Radiol Res Pract. 2015;2015:353657.
10. Kumar P. Usefulness of ultrasonography in the early detection of psoriatic arthritis at: https://doi.org/10.1016/j.jaad.2017.04.1077.
11. K Parimalam, R Subha, M Ananthi, V Suganthi, B Karpagam. Clinico radiological correlation of psoriatic arthropathy: A prospective study. International Journal of Recent Trends in Science and Technology, ISSN 2277-2812 E-ISSN 2249-8109, Volume 18, Issue 1, 2016. Available at https://statperson.com/Journal/ScienceAndTechnology/Article/Volume18Issue1/18_1_21.pdf

Treatment

INTRODUCTION

Psoriasis is a cause for concern to the patient, parent, and the doctor alike. An effective therapy starts with counseling the patient and the parents. Whether the patient is a child, adolescent or an adult, treatment options available, pros and cons of medication suggested, and the outcome should be explained. Above all the recurring nature of the disease must be described. This segment will review the treatment under the following headings:
- Symptomatic
- Topical
- Phototherapy
- Systemic therapy
- Biologics and other agents
- Treatment according to site/type
- Erythroderma
- Arthropathy
- Treatment of psoriasis in special populations
- Childhood psoriasis

SYMPTOMATIC TREATMENT

Itching being the most common symptom, a histamine to suit the patient's age, job nature and other factors like associated systemic conditions should be taken into consideration.

In case of arthropathy, pain is the most difficult symptom to treat which is dealt separately.

Patients with guttate, erythrodermic, or pustular psoriasis may present to the emergency department. In each of these cases, restoration of the barrier function of the skin is of prime concern. The simplest treatment of psoriasis is daily sun exposure, sea bathing, topical moisturizers, and relaxation. Moisturizers, such as petrolatum jelly, are helpful. Daily application of moisturizing cream to the affected area is inexpensive and successful adjunct to psoriasis treatment. Application immediately after a bath or shower helps to minimize itching and tenderness.

TOPICAL THERAPY

Therapeutic focus trivializes seriousness and extent of psoriasis so that it cannot be a factor for stressful life and improves patient's well-being. For most patients, the initial decision point around therapy will be between topical and systemic therapy. However, even patients on systemic therapy will likely continue to need some topical agents. Topical therapy may provide symptomatic relief, minimize required doses of systemic medications, and may even be psychologically cathartic for some patients.

Topical therapy is the mainstay for mild or localized disease with a psoriasis area and severity index (PASI) < 10 or involvement of body surface area (BSA) of <20%. Topical therapy easily manages mild to moderate psoriasis. For people suffering with psoriasis involving <10% BSA can be easily managed with topical therapy.
- Topical treatment is mainly concentrated on areas such as flexures, face, and genitals (delicate areas).
- It is also used as supportive therapy.
- Along with systemic medication impacting >10% BSA.
- Refractory palmoplantar or scalp psoriasis
- The important topical therapies are emollients, corticosteroids, coal tar, dithranol, retinoids, and vitamin D and its analogs.
- New developments include the topical Janus kinase inhibitors although not yet permitted.

Emollients and Keratolytics

- Emollients are not so expensive, secure, and mobile but not strong topical treatment for psoriatic patients as these can act only by hydrating and softening the hyperkeratotic areas of the plaques.[1]

But, these are useful in decreasing the itching, scaling, redness, and spread of the disease.

The side effects are minimal and they are contact dermatitis and folliculitis.
- Oil-based like petrolatum and aquaphor cream are used less commonly as they are sticky.

They contain keratolytic agents as salicylic acid which is needed for conversion of scaly fissured plaques into smoother one's.
- 2-10% salicylic acid used as adjuvant with corticosteroids or coal tar so that the drug penetration is improved.[2]
- A randomized control study of 408 psoriasis patients demonstrated that salicylic acid 5% and mometasone furoate 0.1% was more worthwhile compared to topical corticosteroid given alone after 22 days of treatment.
- Harmful effects of salicylate include tinnitus, dizziness, and gastrointestinal disturbance.
- Salicylic acid desquamates the corneocytes by reducing intercellular adhesions of the horny cells by breaking down the intercellular cement.[2]
- PH of horny layer decreases and in turn improves the hydration and smoothness.
- Emollients and keratolytics are avoided around sensitive areas such as eyes, genitals, and mucous membranes.
- Application of salicylic acid in the upper part of the body at night and lower parts of body in morning on affected areas can be done in case of involvement of larger surface areas.
- Salicylic acid inactivates calcipotriol.
- Apply it after phototherapy as it restricts the ultraviolet (UV) light.
- For localized psoriasis in pregnancy, these agents can be applied but restricted in pediatric age groups.

Topical Corticosteroids[3,4]

- Effective therapies for outpatient use are the potent topical corticosteroids and these are also recommended by the National Institute for Health and Care Excellence. These are efficient, user friendly, and economical.
- At areas which contain hard skin such as palms and soles superpotent corticosteroids are being used.
- Regulation of gene transcription which codes for proinflammatory cytokines can be done by binding to intracellular corticosteroid receptors.
- Thickness of stratum corneum plays a role in determining the penetration capacity which is inversely proportional.
- In case of treating plaque psoriasis, clobetasol and halobetasol works wonder when used applied twice a day for 2 weeks and can be continued with an intermittent can be continued with an intermittent dosing regimen. In case of plaque psoriasis, fluticasone propionate found to be effective.
- Lotions, foams, and solutions are available as treatment regimens.
- Psoriasis involving the nail bed and nail matrix can be treated with 8% clobetasol propionate. Prolonged use of topical corticosteroids has a tendency to lead to tachyphylaxis.
- Secondary infection, skin atrophic changes, striae distensae, and telangiectasia are common side effects seen with prolonged usage of corticosteroids.
- Cushing's syndrome, increase in calcium levels, and HPA axis repression have also been noticed with topical corticosteroids usage.
- And when corticosteroids are suddenly withdrawn or patients suddenly stop using corticosteroids then it leads to rebound phenomenon and higher dosages lead to flaring up of psoriasis in the form of pustular psoriasis can be seen.
- In infants and young children, the use of corticosteroids is limited as increased value of skin surface area to body mass ratio. In case of prolonged use of topical therapy in children with corticosteroids, suppression of HPA axis and growth suppression have been noted.
- To lessen the side effects of these corticosteroids we introduce intermittent pulse dosing therapy. We treat patients with a topical steroid two times a day for 2-3 weeks. Tips for safe usage of topical corticosteroids are given in **Box 1**.
- Clobetasol propionate unit cream 0.05%, diflorasone diacetate ointment 0.05% comes under superpotent corticosteroids.
- As these are superpotent, avoid using on groin, face, axilla, and area with active infection.
- Betamethasone dipropionate ointment, betamethasone dipropionate cream, betamethasone valerate ointment (0.1%), triamcinolone acetonide ointment (0.1%) come under high potent category of corticosteroids.
- Low potential corticosteroids include betamethasone valerate lotion (0.05%) and hydrocortisone acetate cream (1%). These are safe to use in children.

Lotions: Liquid preparations in which there is suspended active medication that contains the most water, good for oily skin and people living in warm areas.

Powder: Pulverized form of creams.

Creams: Mixture of water and oil-thicker because they have less water that is good for dry itchy skin.

Ointments: Semisolid medication that can be spread over the skin, greasy, and useful for cracked dry-chapped areas.

Face: Low and medium potency—creams.

Intertriginous areas: Low and medium potency—creams.

Trunk and extremities: Moderate to potent—ointment.

Palms and soles: Potent to superpotent—ointment.

Scalp: Moderate to high—solution, lotion, and shampoo.

> **BOX 1: Safe usage of topical corticosteroids.**
>
> - Topical steroids + topical agents (combination treatment)
> - Following recommendations
> - Being alert while using in vulnerable areas
> - Careful monitoring while using in infants and children
> - Treatment regimens that reduce side effects

Vitamin D Analogs[5-8]

- Treatment of chromic plaque psoriasis and nail psoriasis can be easily managed with topical vitamin D analogs.
- Helpful in treating the areas which are hard to treat like face or intertriginous areas that are prone to atrophy induced by steroids.
- Synthetic analogs of vitamin D have been developed to improve the antipsoriatic effect of Vitamin D and decrease hypercalcemic role.
- Regulation of genes coding for inflammation, keratinization, and epidermal proliferation are regulated by binding of vitamin D analogs to intracellular receptors pf vitamin D and therefore, they exhibit the action by shifting the Th1 cytokine profile of plaques toward Th2 by acting on immunocytes [Vitamin D receptor (VDR) mediated genomic mechanism].
- Preparations include naturally occurring active metabolite of vitamin Da, 1,25-dihydroxyvitamin Da (calcitriol) and synthetic analog that is calcipotriol and 1,24-dihydroxyvitamin Da (tacalcitol).
- Calcipotriene available as 0.005% that is 5 mg/g cream, scalp lotion, and ointment. The effect on calcium metabolism is very minimal.
- Late onset of action is seen with calcipotriene but has longer disease-free time period.
- Combination of calcipotriene and topical corticosteroids has proven higher level effect to either agent used alone.
- Calcipotriol (50 ug/g) cream, reported to be at least as effective as 0.1% betamethasone valerate ointment. It is widely used.
- It acts by inhibiting human β-defensin and proinflammatory cytokines which can be easily found elevated in psoriasis.
- In children with psoriasis using 50 μg/g calcipotriol shown to be safe.
- Local irritation mainly when applied on face is common adverse effect associated with calcipotriol.
- Disturbance in systemic calcium homeostasis with hypercalciuria and hypercalcemia is seen with vitamin D analogs.
- When dose regimen exceeds the normal range, we should be carefully monitoring the serum and urinary calcium levels.
- Potent topical corticosteroid cream applied in the night with a calcipotriol cream applied in the morning for 2 weeks shown better results than using either of the cream alone in treatment of psoriasis.
- Calcipotriene has lesser effects on calcium metabolism when compared to calcipotriol.
- Also, a study showed that prolonged continuation with halobetasol ointment two times a day on weekends and calcipotriene two times a day on weekdays was more beneficial to weekend treatment with halobetasol and placebo during the week.
- The common side effect is the irritant contact dermatitis mostly involved areas are face and intertriginous areas.
- Studies shown the association among psoriasis, obesity, and vitamin D deficiency. Reports shown correlation between increased C-reative protein (CRP) levels and PASI score and psoriasis and waist circumference.
- Due to hyperproliferation and desquamation of the epidermal layer of skin leads to increased loss of nutrients in specific of vitamin D, psoriasis has been associated with nutritional deficiencies.
- To prevent the comorbidity associated with psoriasis, supplements needed to be provided in patients of psoriasis with nutritional deficiencies to prevent metabolic syndrome and hypertension.
- Food sources of vitamin D include cod liver oil, tuna fish, liver, beef, egg, and cheese.
- Vitamin D analogs are nearly equivalent to corticosteroids in efficacy, these can be utilized as adjuncts of long-term treatment modalities.
- Maxacalcitol, paricalcitol, and becocalcidiol are the newer vitamin D analogs which are in consideration in treating plaque psoriasis.
- Vitamin D analogs can be prescribed during pregnancy. The use of calcipotriene in children is productive and dosage should not be >50 g/week.

Coal Tar[9,10]

- It was described by the Greek philosopher. It is affordable with less side effects and safe to use on large BSAs. Also used as portion of daily dressing regimen.
- It is antibacterial and antipruritic anti-inflammatory, and photosensitizing effect that hampers deregulated epidermal proliferation and dermal infiltrates without affecting the normal skin, and also inhibits DNA synthesis.
- Coal tar (5% liquor carbonic detergents suspension) shown to be more reliable than emollient following 4 weeks of therapy by improving 47% in disease prognosis. But, some studies shown that calcipotriol is superior to coal tar after 5 weeks of treatment.
- Exorex (1% coal tar) is a new coal tar-based preparation, it has an esterified essential fatty acid that is similar to component of banana skin which is beneficial in treating inflammatory skin conditions.
- Dosage is one or two times a day applied with massaging and then leave it for 3 hours.
- The major concern is that it has unpleasant odor and it stains clothing. It can also cause irritation of skin which leads to acneiform eruptions and folliculitis and formation of keratoacanthoma.
- As of now for treating scalp psoriasis shampoos consisting of tar preparations used and also as a sensitizing regimen before to phototherapy in Goeckerman therapy.
- Restricted use in xeroderma pigmentosum, basal cell nevus syndrome, folliculitis and acne in the area of psoriasis and acute inflammatory psoriasis may trigger erythroderma.

- Psoralen with ultraviolet A (PUVA) therapy increases the risk of skin cancer by treating with coal tar. So, it is not used along with PUVA.
- Coal tar belongs to category C so it might be used in treating psoriasis in pregnancy.
- This should be used carefully in the pediatric age group.
- *New regimen coal tar from 1 to 15%* has been unfolded declaring to be nonstained nonodorous and can be spread easily. Efficacy has also been improved to compare to old coal tar preparations.

Anthralin (Dithranol) (1,8-dihydroxy-9-anthrone)[11-14]

- Stable plaque psoriasis can be topically treated effectively with anthralin.
- Plaque psoriasis which has not been resolved with other therapies can be treated with short duration of anthralin.
- It decreases keratinocyte proliferation and anthralin accumulation in the mitochondria reducing the energy to the cells leading to mitochondrial dysfunction and inhibits T cell activation and replaces cell differentiation through free radical oxidation.
- It also acts on DNA and impairs its replication decreases the cell dividing capacity that usually seen in plaque psoriasis.
- Attempts are done to include anthralin with different drug delivery systems in order to get control of their limitations.
- For example, a formulation containing microcrystalline monoglyceride-based micro-encapsulated anthralin is evolved in the modern era and resulted in very mild irritation and nonstaining of clothes.
- Other examples involving drug incorporation into vesicular carriers nanoemulsion, phospholipid microemulsion, and nanocapsules, e.g., liposomes and niosomes.
- The vesicles showed greater permeation by mouse abdominal skin in comparison with creams, polypropylene mine dendrimers have been incorporated into in vitro anthralin.
- The dendrimer-loaded drug shown increased permeation rate constant and very mild to moderate irritation of skin. Anthralin that is loaded into lipid-core nanocapsules have greater strength when compared to UVA light-induced degradation.
- Ethosomes are recently discovered vesicular carriers containing largely of ethanol phospholipids and H_2O.
- The fascinating quality of these ethosomes are because of its elevated ethanol that ease the penetration through stratum corneum and it also aims at deeper skin surface areas.
- This is far better compared with liposomes which has been restricted penetration through skin and restricted to the upper layer of the skin that is stratum corneum.
- In comparison with liposomes, ethosomes have higher retention of methotrexate into the skin for a prolonged duration of given time, resulting into a superior therapeutic net result.
- The PASI score that is observed showed that ethosomes were much more superior and efficient in comparison to liposomes. Taken altogether, outcome showed the advantage of the advanced anthralin ethosomal gel as a superior and safe therapy in patients with psoriasis.
- It is used as SCAT of which greater concentrated application of anthralin 1% applied for 20 minutes to 1 hour prior removal. In other method, it is applied in a 1% preparation for 5 minutes on the first day. Everyday application keeps up with increasing 5 minutes every alternate day till patient notices mild to moderate irritation. Then it is maintained until clearing.

Topical Immunomodulators[15]

Calcineurin Inhibitors

- These are the mainstay of treatment in atopic dermatitis but the therapeutic use of these calcineurin inhibitors in psoriasis is off label.
- They act by inhibiting the activity of the calcineurin phosphatase and suppress the making of inflammatory substances.
- Topical preparations include tacrolimus ointment (0.03% and 0.1%) and pimecrolimus cream (1%).
- Topical application of the calcineurin inhibitors is limited due to their large molecular size and lack of ability to pass through thicker plaques of psoriasis.

However, the penetration always be improved by occlusion or by combining these calcineurin inhibitors with salicylic acid.

However, they are less potent than 0.1% betamethasone valerate or 0.005% calcipotriol.

Latest vehicle of topically applied tacrolimus a 0.3% gel and 0.5% creams has been introduced to enhance its penetration into thicker plaques of psoriasis. The above agents do not cause skin atrophy, these topical agents can be applied on face, intertriginous areas.

Side effects include stinging sensation which is normally short-term irritation that is moderately common with tacrolimus in comparison to pimecrolimus.

Increased risk of cancer can be seen with prolonged use of topical calcineurin inhibitors and a caution is put on to the labels of this medication as a outcome the Food and Drug Administration (FDA) recommends that topical preparations of immunomodulators should not be used as prolonged therapy over larger surface areas or in pediatric age group <2 years of age.

Both the widely used topical calcineurin inhibitors comes under category C and these are not known to cause any teratogenic effects because of their little systemic absorption and topical calcineurin inhibitors can be found in human milk and these are not approved for application in lactating mothers.

We know that topical calcineurin inhibitors can be given to patients as youngest as 3 years of age suffering from atopic dermatitis and to use them for psoriasis in young children is not recommended and approved by the FDA.

But recently, studies have shown that tacrolimus when applied topically proven to be effective on the face and intertriginous areas with limited side effects.

Sirolimus is a recently developed topical preparation of calcineurin inhibitor which is under consideration for treating persistent that is >6 weeks plaque psoriasis.

Topical Retinoids[16]

- Tazarotene ethyl 6-[2-(4,4-dimethylthiochroman-6-yl)-ethynyl] nicotinate
- Vitamin A derivative which is the earliest synthetically developed retinoid used for treating psoriasis topically.
- It is obtainable as creams and gels at concentration of 0.1% and 0.05% indicated for fixed plaque psoriasis that is given along with a topical corticosteroid and calcipotriene (vitamin D analogue). The combination therapy of above agents has been effective for patients with psoriasis.
- In nail psoriasis, this compound selectively binds to beta and gamma retinoic acid on the cell membrane of keratinocytes and is later transported to the nucleus altering transcription of gene in keratinocytes, this results in decreased epidermal hyperproliferation normalizing carotenoid differentiation decreasing inflammation.
- Recent studies have shown that tazarotene is as effective as fluocinonide with very mild irritation and 0.01% topical application of tazarotene is as good as in comparing with clobetasol propionate in treating palmoplantar psoriasis.
- Combination of topical steroid like mometasone with tazarotene has showed great results in comparison to treatment with topical steroid alone.
- Applying 0.1% tazarotene for 12–23 weeks has been effective in treating psoriasis involving nails includes hyperkeratosis, distal separation of nail plate from nail bed, pitting and oil drop pigmentation.
- Side effect is localized irritating effect of these topical retinoids at the site of application.
- To minimize the side effects, we can use them at low concentrations, day-by-day application and minimal exposure period with the topical agent.
- Topical application in sensitive areas such as faceand genitals is not recommended.
- The FDA given a warning in concern of using of this and exposure to sunlight, and strictly recommended to use sunscreen regularly while applying tazarotene. The dosage needs to be monitored when combined with phototherapy to avoid burning of skin.
- Tazarotene is used as off-label therapy for children as topical retinoids are well tolerated by them. But, these are not recommended in pregnancy belonging to category X, as they are prone to be teratogenic nature of retinoids.
- Recent advances in topical retinoids include bexarotene 1% gel.
- Mechanism of action of bexarotene is binding to the nuclear retinoid X receptor.
- They are studied as an effective therapy for psoriatic patients and used as a combination therapy with narrowband ultraviolet B (UVB) therapy.

Recent Advances in Topical Treatment[17-23]

- Halobetasol propionate-tazarotene lotion 0.01%/0.045% (Duobrii)
- FDA approved this topical treatment in 2019 for effectively treating plaque psoriasis. It is a combination of topical corticosteroid and topical retinoid.
- Corticosteroids act by anti-inflammatory property which clears the plaques, while topical retinoid which is a derivative of vitamin A acts by inhibiting the excess growth of skin cells.
- Side effects include inflammation of the hair follicles, excoriation, and rashes at the site of application.
- Halobetasol propionate foam, 0.05% (Lexette)
- FDA approved in 2018 for treating plaque psoriasis in adults. Common adverse effects include pain and headache.
- TAPINAROF (Vtama) cream 1% is a new steroid free topical treatment that is an aryl hydrocarbon receptor agonist.
- Applied once daily and can be used in sensitive areas of skin and is also safe for prolonged use. Approved for mild, moderate, and severe psoriasis with no restrictions on duration of use and can be used on sensitive areas of skin.[22,23]
- Dermavant sciences, a bio-pharmaceutical company announced the US FDA has approved VTAMA a steroid free cream for treating psoriasis.
- Common side effects include folliculitis, nasopharyngitis, and contact dermatitis.
- New treatment for children includes calcipotriene foam 0.005% (sorilux) used in children from 4 years of age. It helps in slowing down the process of abnormal cell growth. applied two times a day for 7 weeks.
- Calcipotriene-betamethasone dipropionate foam, 0.005%/0.064% (Enstilar).
- Approved by FDA for adolescents between 12 and 17 years of age. Former decreases the rate of cell growth and latter acts by reducing inflammation.

PHOTOTHERAPY

It is well known that psoriasis improves during the summer months and ultraviolet (UV) irradiation has long been recognized as beneficial for the control of psoriatic skin lesions. UV radiation has antiproliferative effect thereby slowing keratinization. Due to its anti-inflammatory effects, there induces apoptosis of pathogenic T-cells in psoriatic plaques. In choosing UV therapy, consideration must be given to the potential for UV radiation to accelerate photodamage and increase the risk of cutaneous malignancy. This must be particularly remembered while suggesting phototherapy for children. Phototherapy can be administered with UV radiation or LASER, both as an office procedure or home unit delivery. Whatever be the modality, the dermatologists should meticulously calculate the dose and monitor the patient for both clinical improvement and side effect.

The common modalities of light therapy used include:
- UVB
  - Broadband
  - Narrowband
- Photochemotherapy with UVA: Psoralen with UVA
- Combined therapy
- LASER

Ultraviolet B

Phototherapy with UVB spectrum light (290–320 nm) has been used to treat psoriasis for at least the past 70 years. Phototherapy induces immunosuppression that involves induction of apoptosis in both T lymphocytes and keratinocytes, leading to decreased inflammation and epidermal hyperplasia. Exposure to UVB, alone or in combination with emollients or tar preparation is an effective therapy in the treatment of psoriasis. Successful clearance of psoriasis using UVB, with or without petrolatum, typically occurs within 6 weeks of treatment and weekly regimens range from 3 to 5 exposures per week, take an average of 25 doses to achieve clearance

- Broad band ultraviolet B (UVB) radiation (290–320 nm). This treatment is used in patients with extensive disease, alone or in combination with topical tar. The mechanism of action of UVB is likely through its immunomodulatory effects. Patients receive near-erythema-inducing doses of UVB at least three times weekly until remission is achieved, after which a maintenance regimen for 2 months is usually recommended to prolong the remission.
- Narrow-band (NB) UVB phototherapy consists of a subset of the UVB spectrum, with a peak at 311 nm. This is an alternative to standard (broadband: 290–320 nm) UVB in the treatment of psoriasis. Apoptosis of T cells is also more common with 311 nm than with broadband UVB. The advantage being maximum clinical response with minimum erythema that is faster and more complete.

- *Home phototherapy*: An alternative to office-based phototherapy is the use of a home UVB phototherapy unit prescribed by the treating clinician. This option may be preferred by patients who are not in close proximity to an office-based phototherapy center, whose schedules do not permit frequent office visits, or for whom the costs of in-office treatment exceed those of a home phototherapy unit. When used with adequate safety measures, they are as good as office unit, reducing time and travel.

Photochemotherapy

Photochemotherapy (PUVA) involves treatment with either oral or bath psoralen followed by UVA radiation (320–400 nm) under strict medical supervision. UVA penetrates deeper into the dermis than UVB and does not have the latter's potential for burning the skin.

This can be oral PUVA, Bath PUVA or Topical PUVA.

In oral PUVA, 8-methoxypsoralen is ingested at a dose 0.6 mg/kg/2 h before irradiation, followed within 2 hours by exposure to UVA; this sequence is performed three times weekly the dose is increased by increments of 0.5–1.5 J/cm^2 according to response until remission, then twice or once weekly as a maintenance dose. Higher clearance UVA doses (13–14 J/cm^2), higher cumulative doses (up to 200 J) and 10–12 weeks may be needed in selected cases.

With bath/topical PUVA, the psoralen capsules are dissolved in water, and affected skin (hands, feet, or total body) is soaked for 15–30 minutes prior to UVA exposure.

Pre- and posttreatment photoprotection (e.g., hat, sunscreen, and sun-protective goggles) are critical in preventing serious burn injury to the skin and eyes from being outside.

PUVA is advisable for patients over 55 years of involving >20% of the body surface, not controlled by conventional topical therapy. Treatment is given two to four times weekly. UVA dosage is increased by increments of 0.5–1.5 J/cm^2 according to response.

Contraindications to PUVA therapy are given in **(Box 2)**.

> **BOX 2: Contraindications to PUVA therapy.**
>
> - Exposure to inorganic arsenic
> - Radiotherapy
> - Cutaneous malignancy
> - Hepatic disorders
> - Photosensitive disorders
> - Xeroderma pigmentosum
> - Lupus erythematosus
> - Pregnancy
> - Lactation
> - Children under 18 years
> - PUVA should not be suggested for hairy scalp

Of all the clinical types, psoriasis vulgaris responds best to PUVA therapy with a clearance rate as high as up to 90%. PUVA is also of value in generalized pustular psoriasis, erythrodermic psoriasis, palmoplantar pustulosis and nail psoriasis, but success rates are much lower in these atypical patterns of disease. It would be advisable to give maintenance treatment for 2 months and stop PUVA if remission is maintained.

Pretreatment emollients have long been thought to improve results with UVB. However, while thin oils do not impede UV penetration, emollient creams can actually inhibit the penetration of the UV and should not be applied before treatment. Gentle removal of plaques by bathing does help prior to UV exposure.

Since PUVA is associated with potential systemic side effects (erythema, pruritus, nausea, ocular damage, and increased risk of skin cancer) as well as death from accidental overexposure, it is generally not recommended as an option for home phototherapy.[19]

Combination Therapy

The following combinations are used with success in the management of psoriasis that does not respond to conventional therapy.
- Etretinate or acitretin and PUVA
- Dithranol and PUVA
- Methotrexate in combination with PUVA as in erythrodermic or pustular psoriasis
- Topical corticosteroids and PUVA
- Calcipotriol combined with PUVA
- Carcinogenicity is a risk while combining PUVA with cytotoxic drugs like methotrexate.
- Hepatotoxicity should also be borne in mind before combining PUVA with systemic drugs.

Saltwater baths:
- Climatotherapy has also been used as a therapy for psoriasis, where, bathing in sea water is combined with sun exposure.
- Balneophototherapy involves use of salt water baths with artificial UV exposure.

Adverse effects associated with phototherapy include both acute adverse effects and cumulative, dose-related effects that occur with prolonged use. Early adverse effects associated with BB- and NB-UVB phototherapy are typically limited to erythema and drying of the skin, with maximal erythema occurring between 8 and 24 hours following exposure. Blistering is more common with BB-UVB phototherapy compared to NB-UVB due to the lower erythemogenicity of NB-UVB.

Late adverse effects due cumulative UVB dose include premature aging (photo aging), wrinkling, and leathery appearance, increased fragility of the skin, and increased risk of photo carcinogenesis.

Folate deficiency which is a theoretical possibility following UV exposure, more with UVA, than UVB has not been proved beyond doubt in psoriasis patients treated with phototherapy. In vitro study, exposure of plasma to UVA led to a 30–50% decrease in the serum folate level within 60 minutes. However, folate deficiency secondary to UVA exposure has not been proven to occur in vivo.

Units with a built-in controlled prescription timer (CPT) are advisable to reduce, unauthorized use or inappropriate use.

Warning About Phototherapy
- Patient should avoid exposure to risky levels of ultraviolet rays for fear of developing cancer.
- Proper protection should be given to the other parts of body that does not require radiation with sunscreen or clothing.
- All photosensitizing products including drugs and perfumes should be avoided during phototherapy.
- Periodic examination is mandatory to check for signs of skin cancer.

Due to ultraviolet radiation patients might have photodermatitis as it damages the ultraviolet-induced DNA damage that results in activated oncogenes or suppression of tumor suppression genes, which in turn associated with skin squamous cell carcinoma and melanoma. So, pros and cons of the phototherapy should be clearly explained by the consultant dermatologist.

LASER

Excimer laser is another development in ultraviolet therapy for psoriasis and involves use of a high energy 308 nm excimer laser. The laser allows treatment of only involved skin; thus, considerably higher doses of UVB can be administered to psoriatic plaques at a given treatment compared with traditional phototherapy. LASER therapy results in faster responses than conventional phototherapy. UV-induced hyperpigmentation is a common sequel of excimer laser therapy which resolves after the discontinuation of treatment. A pilot study has reported 308 nm excimer lasers to be a safe and effective treatment for localized psoriasis in children as in adults.[20]

Flash lamp pumped pulsed dye laser first used by Hacker and Rasmussen in 1992 with a 586–589 nm wavelength, that concentrates the chromophore HB and damage vessels, for congenital and vascular lesions this PDL is preferred one. PDL is indicated mainly in treating nail psoriasis and targeted for treating superficial cutaneous vascular lesions. In one study done in 2009, 62 nails were treated with PDL with 34% development after 18 weeks and 56% after 25 weeks based on NAPSI score.

Cold laser also known as low level light laser therapy has also been applied in treating psoriasis. A study suggests that near infrared that is with wavelength of 830 nm and visible red light of 630 nm emitted by LED is useful in treating recalcitrant psoriasis with wavelength ranging between 630 and 1,070 nm.

In conclusion, artificial light has the efficacy to provide greater dose regimen radiation to the selected areas of skin in minimal period can be a possible mechanism. So, combining different monochromatic lights acting on various targets could be an innovative approach in refining net result of phototherapy in near future.

SYSTEMIC THERAPIES

Specific systemic therapy is rarely used in childhood psoriasis. Systemic therapy including retinoids, methotrexate, and cyclosporine, biologic is only used in severe forms of the disease such as erythrodermic, pustular, and arthritic psoriasis. All these therapeutic options can be used as monotherapy or in various combinations.

The indication for systemic therapy is one or more of the following:
- Involvement of BSA > 20%
- Psoriasis area and severity index > 10
- Erythrodermic psoriasis, with or without metabolic complication
- Generalized pustular psoriasis
- Psoriatic arthropathy
- Localized disease not responding to topical therapy alone or with significant psychological morbidity

Specific systemic therapy is rarely used in childhood psoriasis. Systemic therapy including retinoids, methotrexate, and cyclosporine, biologic is only used in severe forms of the disease such as erythrodermic, pustular, and arthritic psoriasis. All these therapeutic options can be used as monotherapy or in various combinations.

The indication for systemic therapy is one or more of the following:
- Involvement of BSA > 20%
- Psoriasis area and severity index > 10
- Erythrodermic psoriasis, with or without metabolic complication
- Generalized pustular psoriasis
- Psoriatic arthropathy
- Localized disease not responding to topical therapy alone or with significant psychological morbidity

Retinoids[21]

- Family of common and artificial analogs of Vitamin A
- *Etretinate*: Etretinate is a drug that is particularly lipophilic therefore, accumulates in subcutis.
- *Half-life*: 80 days
- *Dosage*: 0.75 mg/kg/day, to begin with, maintenance dosage is 0.5-0.75 mg/kg/day
- It vanishes from plasma in 1 week, but stays in subcutis and is discernible in subcutis for months.[1]
- Because of the above mechanism this has been replaced by *acitretin*.
- Etretinate has been gauged in children with uncontrollable pustular psoriasis and for palmoplantar pustulosis even though there was a relapse seen after stopping the treatment.[2]

Acitretin

Acitretin: It is a nonselective retinoid with activity on three retinoic acid receptors. It is less lipophilic than etretinate.

Half-life of acitretin: It is 50-60 hours.

It is the safest systemic drug accessible and hence the number one choice unless there are any other reasons to prevent its usage.

Experimental data show esterification into *etretinate*—the reaction is seen to be increased and intensified with alcohol.

Dosage: 0.25-1 mg/kg/day

It is available as 10 mg and 25 mg capsule. Once daily consumption with meal increases the bioavailability of the drug.

Initially on starting acitretin, in some patients, the disease may get worse by increase in erythema and lesions thus to avoid this "dose escalation strategy" is advised—Initial dose is 25-30 mg/day and then increased up to 50 mg/day.

After the response to treatment is achieved, that is about 12-16 weeks of treatment, maintenance dose is again reduced to of 25-50 mg/day. Improvement is seen gradually after 3-6 months.

It is the drug of choice for palmoplantar pustulosis. Both skin and joint expressions of psoriasis with association of HIV infection have been reported to respond to acitretin.

Indications for retinoid therapy:
- Pustular psoriasis
- Erythrodermic psoriasis
- Generalized psoriasis
- *Psoriasis vulgaris*: It is best treated by retinoids in alloy with concomitant usage of other methods or modalities to reduce the required dosage of retinoid.

In children with generalized or psoriatic erythroderma, treatment of choice may be retinoids rather than steroids or methotrexate.

Even though acitretin is only abjectly effective as monotherapy, it is very effective for plaque psoriasis.

For pretreatment evaluation of patients to be started on acitretin, refer **Flowchart 1**.

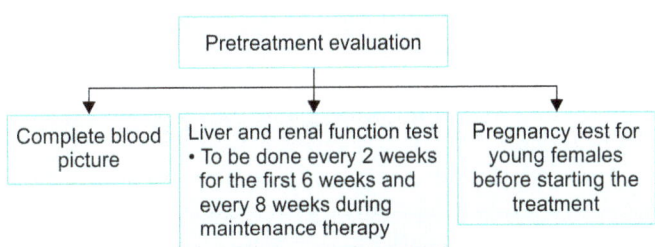

FLOWCHART 1: Pretreatment evaluation for acitretin.

Response to Therapy

Therapeutic benefits of oral retinoids in psoriasis are well documented; however, majority of patients relapse within 2 months of stopping the therapy.

Adverse Effects of Retinoids

Teratogenicity: These drugs are pregnancy category X drugs. Hence, they should not be given to young women in reproductive age group. They are also not recommended during pregnancy and in lactating mothers.

Contraindications and side effects of retinoids:
- Hyperlipidemia: Retinoids cause elevated serum lipid levels with derangement of liver enzymes.
- Active liver disease
- Special caution has to be taken in patients with diabetes, alcoholics, and obese patients.
- Renal impairment
- Dryness of mucosa with fissuring (most common cutaneous side effect) with staphylococcal infection
- Thinning of hair
- Burning sensation
- Skin atrophy
- Palmoplantar desquamation
- Increased bruising
- Widespread erythema
- Purulent paronychia
- Lethargy and headache
- Excessive granulation tissue formation
- Nodular prurigo-like lesions
- Conjunctivitis and ocular irritation
- Rarely intracranial hypertension and papilledema
- Gastrointestinal adverse effects include:
  - Nausea
  - Dysentery

Caution with Use of Retinoids

Retinoids are very effective hence sometimes the side effects are overlooked. Cheilitis can be seen in about 75% of patients; however, it can be treated with emollients and lip balms. Lipid abnormalities can be managed by reduction in the dosage of acitretin.

Mechanism of Action of Retinoids

The exact mode of action of retinoids is unknown, but it is believed to interact with retinoic acid nuclear receptors. They act by regulating the abnormal epidermal proliferation and differentiation. It stimulates the granular cell layer formation thus leading to a more orderly and uniform keratinocyte differentiation.

Retinoids also have anti-inflammatory action along with its effect on cell proliferation and differentiation. They interfere with cytokine synthesis and decrease inflammation in the epidermis and dermis. In <2 weeks of treatment polymorphonuclear leukocytes are reduced in number within the horny layer and the epidermis. The acanthotic component of the disease decreases by the third or fourth week.

Combination Therapy

Retinoids can be used along with vitamin D analogs and phototherapy as it prevents photocarcinogenesis. Initially, there may be a flare-up reaction on addition of retinoids in the form of increased surface area of skin lesions; however, this is followed by significant improvement. Combination therapy is most useful for the cases of pustular psoriasis and erythrodermic psoriasis. Acitretin can be used with the combination of UVB and PUVA especially in patients resistant to either treatment. Topical dithranol can be used with etretinate in patients with plaques previously resistant to dithranol.

Drug Interactions

Simultaneous use of:
- Tetracycline causes increase in photosensitivity.
- Minocycline causes pseudotumor cerebri.
- Alcohol causes hepatotoxicity.
- Vitamin A causes hypervitaminosis.
- Corticosteroids cause hyperlipidemia, pseudotumor cerebri.

Cyclosporine[22-24]

It is a cyclic undecapeptide, derived from a fungus called *Tolypocladium inflatum* Gams.

Mechanism of Action

Cyclosporin acts essentially by causing inhibition of T-cells. Mechanism of action is done by immunosuppression of the intraepidermal cytotoxic T-cell response by destroying the liberation of IL-1 and IL-2 which play a significant part in the proliferation and of the other T-lymphocytes. It is orally active and highly lipophilic and metabolized in liver by CYP450 enzyme. Cyclosporine can cause renal damage. The possible mechanisms are given in **Flowchart 2**. This drug

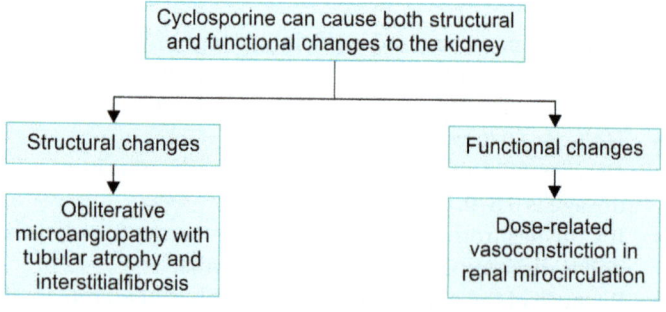

FLOWCHART 2: Cyclosporine structural and functional changes.

is majorly used in patients with severe form of disease that has not responded to other forms of treatment. Cyclosporine is an important component of many combination therapies but relapse is common on stopping the drug.

Indication to the cyclosporine treatment:
- Erythrodermic
- Generalized pustular psoriasis
- Localized forms of pustular psoriasis
- Psoriatic arthritis
- Nail dystrophy
- Scalp psoriasis
- Psoriatic arthropathy
- Patients who are in a need of sudden termination of another systemic medication

Pretreatment evaluation:
- Blood pressure determination
- Kidney function test—to check baseline serum creatinine levels
- Liver function tests
- Complete blood count
- Human immunodeficiency virus serology
- Chest radiology
- Electrolytes, blood urea nitrogen (BUN), and lipids
- Uric acid

Dosage of Cyclosporine

Initial administration: 2.5 mg/kg/day to maximum of 4 mg/kg/day

A dose of 3–5 mg/kg/day should preferably not be exceeded.

If the improvement is not seen even after 2 weeks of the therapy, dosage can be increased by 1 or 0.5 mg/kg/day at fortnightly gaps making sure that the maximum dose does not exceed 5 mg/kg/day.

Response to Therapy

Intermittent short course can be tolerated very well and it gives effective control of plaque psoriasis. The PISCES study shows that discontinuous short course treatment of cyclosporine controls moderate to severe psoriasis producing long term suspension of the disease and decreases the burden of side effects.

A higher starting dose produces more rapid response. Once the desired response is achieved drug can be either stopped or alternative therapies can be used with less severe cases or dose can be gradually tapered. Continuous treatment with cyclosporine for about 1 year or more is not recommended, relapse flares or re-emission is usual after stopping the treatment.

Contraindications:
- Renal disease
- Hypertension that is uncontrolled
- Previously diagnosed or presently diagnosed malignancy
- A known case of epilepsy
- Acute form of infections:
  - Relative contraindications:
    - Immunodeficiency
    - Noncompliant patient
    - Simultaneously using any nephrotoxic drugs
    - Liver functional diseases
    - Ladies that a pregnant or planning to conceive

Monitoring of therapy: According to the recommendations of consensus conference on cyclosporine microemulsion for psoriasis:
- Serum creatinine to be measured every 2 weeks for 6 weeks and then every month
- Diastolic blood pressure, if persistently >90 mm Hg requires a dose reduction if necessary, calcium-channel blockers need to be added.
- If malignancy occurs, cyclosporine should be withdrawn.

Side effects:
- Dose-related hypertension
- Nephrotoxicity
- Cutaneous melanoma skin cancers—squamous cell carcinoma
- Increased risk of lymphoproliferative disorders
- Altered LFTs
- Mild degree of normochromic and normocytic anemia
- Gum hyperplasia
- Tremors
- Hyperkalemia is a manifestation of renal impairment
- Increased blood pressure is seen even with short courses (for cyclosporine induced hypertension nifedipine is used)
- High lipids
- High potassium
- Lower levels of magnesium
- High levels of urea can occur but mild
- Increased serum cholesterol level
- Arthralgia
- GI disorders include:
  - Nausea
  - Abdominal pain
  - Diarrhea
  - Gingival hyperplasia
- Neurological side effects:
  - Headache
  - Paresthesia's
  - Tremors
- Gum hypertrophy
- Hypertrichosis

Drug interactions: Drug interactions with cyclosporin occur because they are related to induction and competitive inhibition of the microsomal p450 cytochrome 3A enzymes.

Drugs decreasing the cyclosporin levels:
- Anticonvulsants: Phenobarbital, phenytoin, carbamazepine
- Antibiotics: Rifampicin, trimethoprim-sulfamethoxazole
- Phenylbutazone[11]

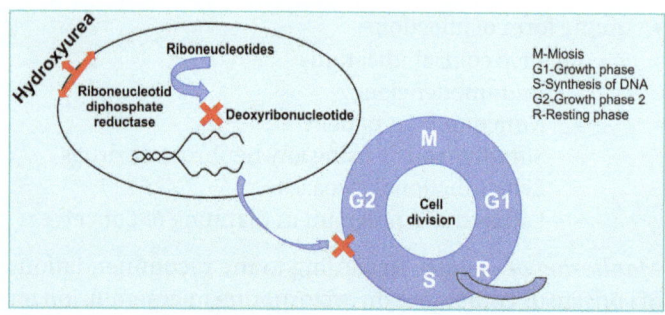

FIG. 1: Mechanism of action of hydroxyurea.

Drugs that increase the cyclosporin levels:
- Antibiotics: Doxycycline and erythromycin
- Antifungal drugs
- CCB: Verapamil and diltiazem
- Steroid hormones and diuretics: Frusemide and thiazides

Hydroxyurea

Hydroxyurea can be used in patients or can be reserved for patients who are resistant to methotrexate and require systemic treatment or develop adverse effects. Mechanism of action of hydroxyurea is depicted in **Figure 1**.

Dosage of Hydroxyurea

Usual dosage is 500 mg twice or thrice daily. Duration should be minimum for 2 months.

Side effects:
- Myelosuppression
- Anemia
- Pancytopenia
- Cutaneous vasculitis
- Diffuse hyperpigmentation
- Nail and skin hyperpigmentation

Razoxane

It is an antimitotic drug effective in treatment of psoriasis mostly in erythrodermic pustular psoriasis and psoriatic arthritis. Razoxane is not hepatotoxic, therefore, it can be given in patients with recalcitrant psoriasis and cirrhosis. Common complication seen with razoxane is neutropenia. Other adverse effects include acute myeloid leukemia and B-cell lymphoma.

Mycophenolate Mofetil

Mycophenolate mofetil acts by inhibiting the enzyme "inosine monophosphate" dehydrogenase that helps in transformation of xanthosine monophosphate from inosine monophosphate. Mycophenolic acid is a specific inhibitor or guanine synthesis and consumes nucleotides of guanine, which are used to block DNA that prime the RNA synthesis eventually blocking the proliferative response of T and B lymphocytes. In vitro, drug is a strong inhibitor of DNA synthesis and cell proliferation similar to methotrexate. Therapeutic response in patients may be because of inhibition of leukotatic factors, leukotriene B4 and 12-hydroxyeicosatetraenoic acid in psoriatic skin. Side effects may include vomiting, diarrhea, and UTI like urgency and frequency of micturition during therapy.

Methotrexate[25-27]

Methotrexate (MTX) is a folic acid antagonist. Low-dose MTX can be used successfully for treating rheumatoid arthritis (RA) and psoriasis. In the past 25 years, MTX has become the gold standard of care in treating the two diseases.

Mechanism of Action

The effects of MTX have been eventually detailed as antiproliferative, because of its inhibitory effects on methionine purine and thymidylate synthesis, and by doing so it inhibits DNA synthesis. MTX is transported through either by passive diffusion or with the help of a folate carrier and it is polyglutamated the time it enters into the cells. The half-life of MTX is 5–8 hours, MTX polyglutamates are retained in the cells and tissue for several weeks and months. Indications for use of MTX and dose are given in (**Flowchart 3 and Box 3**).

Pretreatment laboratory test while on therapy include:
- Complete blood picture
- Liver function tests
- Kidney evaluation

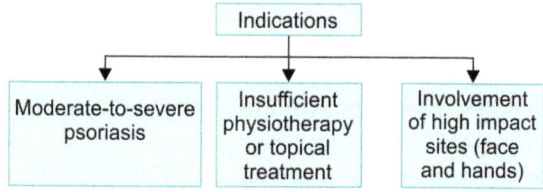

FLOWCHART 3: Indications of methotrexate (MTX).

> **BOX 3:** Dose (as per *Danish Expert Meeting*).
>
> - Initially 15 mg/week can be increased up to 25 mg/week
> - Reduced dose is recommended for elderly patients—10 mg/week
> - Patients with bone marrow dysfunction or renal impairment—2.5–5 mg/week

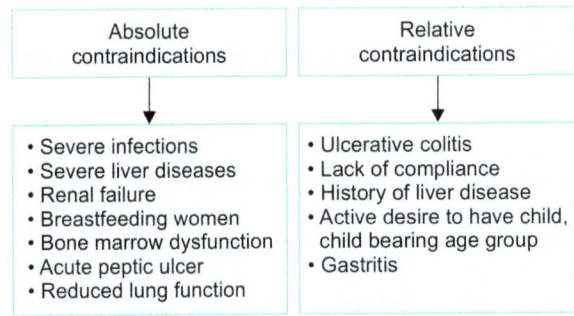

FIG. 2: Contraindications of methotrexate (MTX).

> **BOX 4: Methotrexate use in children with psoriasis.**
>
> - The MTX doses used in psoriasis are 0.2–0.4 mg/kg/week, even higher doses are to be used but up to a maximum dose of 20 mg/week
> - Methotrexate in children may be given orally or subcutaneously
> - Subcutaneous administration of MTX is preferred more in children because it has lesser side effects and gives the leverage to use higher doses. Also by doing so, the bioavailability is higher and more stable

Contraindications of methotrexate (MTX) and its use in children with psoriasis are given in **Figure 2** and **Box 4** respectively.

Drug interactions with MTX (**Box 4**):
- There is an increased liver dysfunction with—retinoids, ethanol.
- There is a decrease in elimination of MTX through kidneys when—NSAIDs, Colchicine, sulfonamides, and penicillin are used simultaneously.
- Increased risk of GI toxicity—ethanol, chloramphenicol
- Interactions with plasma protein bindings—NSAIDs, sulfonamides, barbiturates

Newer Small Molecular Therapy

Small molecules are a group of agents with a low molecular weight (<1 KD) that act by modulating the proinflammatory cytokines. Owing to their ease of administration either orally or through a topical route with an excellent safety profile they are emerging as therapeutic options for inflammatory dermatosis and other systemic conditions (**Fig. 3**).

Apremilast[28]

Apremilast is a phosphodiesterase-4 (PDE4) inhibitor that is administered orally. Apremilast was approved in 2017 by the FDA for managing psoriatic arthritis and certain type of plaque psoriasis. Apremilast can also be used for managing psoriasis at difficult sites such as scalp, nails, and palmoplantar pustular psoriasis (PPP).

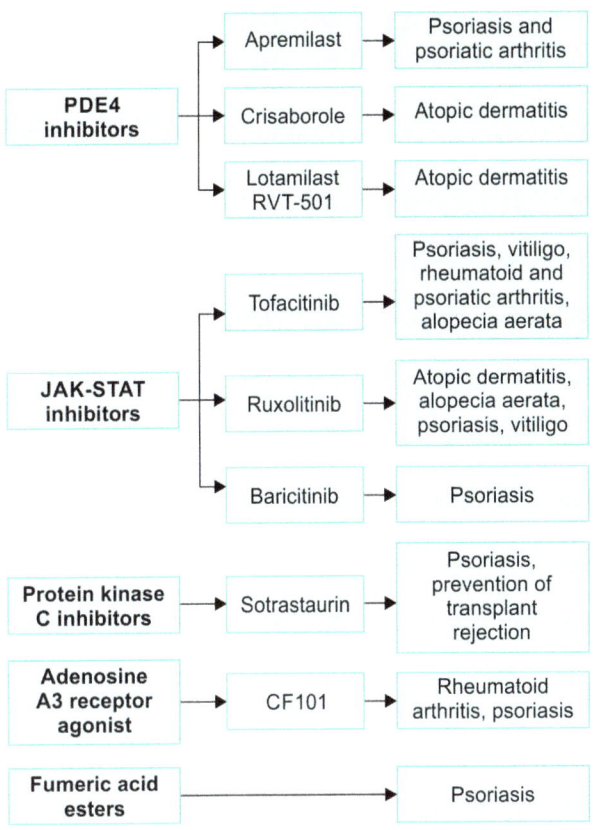

FIG. 3: Newer small molecules.

Mechanism of Action of Apremilast

Refer **Box 5**.

Dosage of Apremilast

In elderly psoriatic patients and patients with psoriatic arthritis recommended dosage—30 mg twice daily, orally. The regime usually starts with 10 mg in the morning on Day 1 with a daily addition of 10 mg till the 6th day.[19] This helps in minimizing the gastrointestinal side effects. For nail psoriasis, a new kind of nail lacquer is now available as well.

Adverse effects (**Figs. 4A and B**): A retrospective review of medical records was conducted of all patients across India who were prescribed apremilast for an entire 16 weeks. The primary endpoint was the percentage of patients achieving the PASI 75 at 16 weeks. The secondary endpoints were (i) change in mean PASI; (ii) change in mean BSA; (iii) percentage of patients who achieved PASI 50, 90, and 100; and (iv) adverse events (AEs) reported.

The records of 105 patients were analyzed. Mean age was 41 years and mean disease duration was 6.75 years. All the patients had previously received some forms of systemic treatment. Forty-three patients (41%) achieved ≥ PASI 75 of which four patients (3.8%) and five patients (4.76%) achieved

> **BOX 5: Mechanism of action of apremilast.**
>
> Apremilast represses the intracellular PDE4 leading to accumulation of cAMP within the cell that modifies the downstream signaling pathway in cells of the innate immune system such as monocytes and adaptive immune system, T cells and other non-immune cells, keratinocytes and synovial fibroblasts.
>
> As a results of PDE4 inhibition, the levels of tumor necrosis factor-alpha, IL-23 which are proinflammatory cytokines are decreased an IL-10 is increase.
>
> Apremilast is extensively metabolized by oxidative mechanism of CYP, mainly CYP3A4 and also by non-CYP mediated hydrolysis. The serum levels and its efficacy may be decreased by the coadministration of potent CYP enzyme activators such as:
> - Rifampicin
> - Carbamazepin
> - Phenytoin

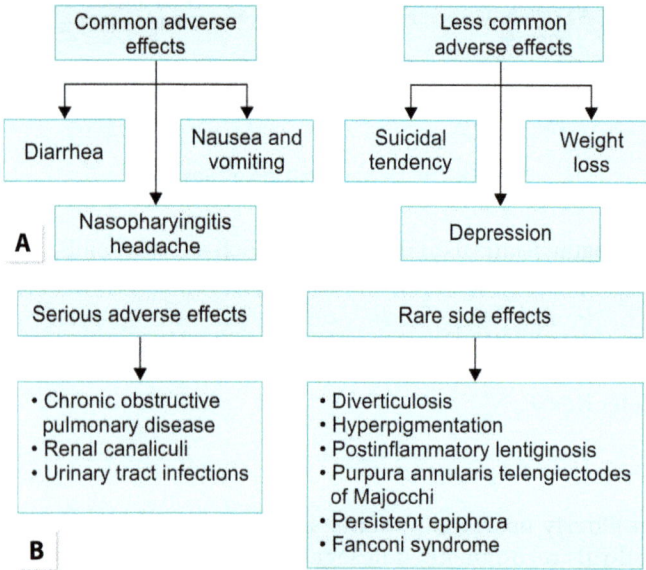

FIGS. 4A AND B: Adverse/Rare side effects of dosages of apremilast.

PASI 100 and PASI 90, respectively at week 16. Moreover, 28 patients (26.7%) demonstrated PASI 50 response. Baseline mean PASI score of 14.78 reduced to 4.5 (–69.55%), whereas mean BSA score of 24.4 reduced to 8.24 (–66.3%). Most AEs were mild to moderate in severity.

These results, from a real-world setting in India, confirmed the effectiveness and tolerability of apremilast as seen in clinical trials.

Tofacitinib[29]

The Janus kinase (JAK) intracellular signaling pathway is involved in the pathological process associated with inflammatory diseases and also some of the immune-mediated conditions. The same has also been in psoriasis.

Tofacitinib is an oral JAK inhibitor and interferes with JAK1 and JAK 3 mainly. The efficacy and safety of tofacitinib was investigated in placebo-controlled and head-to-head randomized clinical trials in patients with moderate-to-severe chronic plaque psoriasis. In two similarly designed Phase III placebo-controlled studies, higher response rates were seen with the 10 mg bid dosage regimen of tofacitinib. Decrease of hemoglobin, neutrophil, and lymphocyte counts, and increase from baseline in creatinine and alanine aminotransferase may occur, as well as dyslipidemia. Most of these abnormalities are transient and reversible either spontaneously or with discontinuation of the drug. On the whole, this drug has been found to be a useful systemic agent treating psoriasis.

BIOLOGICAL THERAPY OF PSORIASIS[30-33]

Biological agents offer a crucial therapeutic opportunity for patients suffering from severe to moderate psoriasis, especially if their comorbidities contraindicate the regular systemic therapies. To this date, the US-FDA has approved 12 different drugs for the treatment of psoriasis and psoriatic arthritis which are divided into different classes depending on their target molecule **(Flowchart 4)**. The four anticytokine agents include, etanercept, infliximab, adalimumab and ustekinumab.

Some of the available biological agents for use in psoriasis, their mechanism of action and route of administration are described below. The eligibility criteria are given in **(Fig. 5)**.

IL-23 inhibitors are used for both plaque psoriasis and psoriatic arthritis **(Flowchart 5)**.

Guselkumab

Guselkumab is a complete human immunoglobulin G1 lambda (IGIλ) monoclonal antibody that targets the p19 subunit of IL-23 **(Flowchart 6)**. Dosage of guselkumab: 100 mg of guselkumab is given subcutaneously at 0 weeks and 4 weeks, followed by every 8 weekly. It is indicated in moderate to extensive plaque psoriasis.

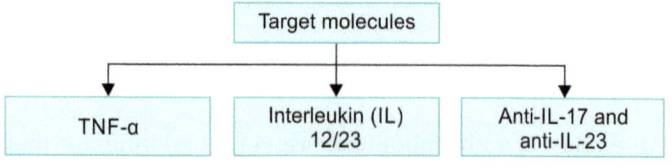

FLOWCHART 4: Target molecules.

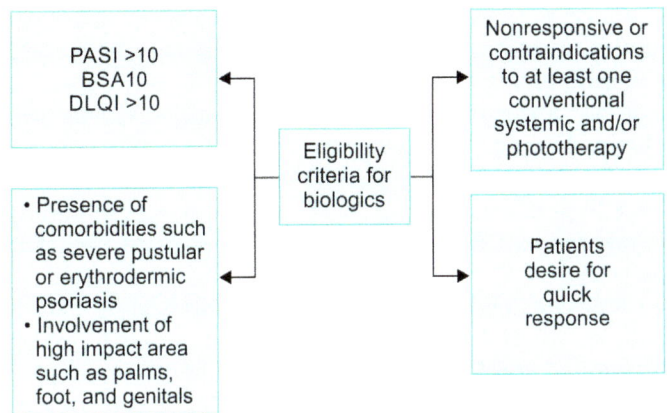

FIG. 5: Eligibility criteria for biological agents.
(BSA: body surface area; DLQI: dermatology life quality index; PASI: psoriasis area and severity index)

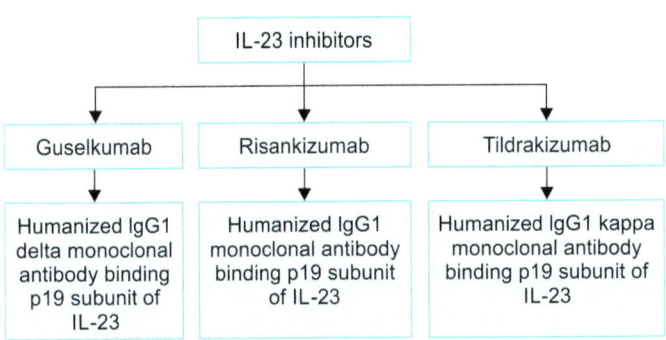

FLOWCHART 5: Interleukin-23 (IL-23) inhibitors.

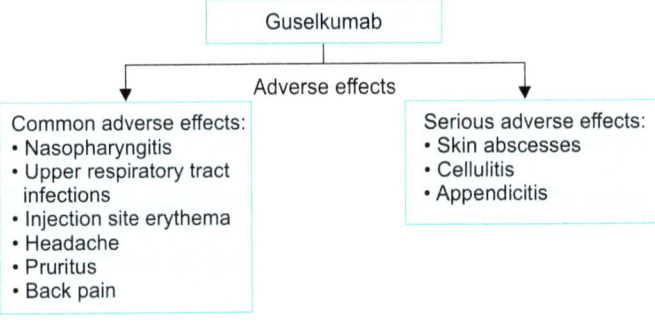

FLOWCHART 6: Adverse effects of guselkumab.

Tildrakizumab

Tildrakizumab is a humanized form of IgG1k monoclonal antibody that binds to the p19 subunit of IL-23 and inhibits it.

Dosage of tildrakizumab: 100 mg of tildrakizumab is given subcutaneously at 0 weeks and 4 weeks later, followed by every 12 weeks. It is used for treating moderate to extensive plaque psoriasis.

Adverse Effects

- Common side effects include catarrh, migraine, and reaction where the injection is given.
- Serious adverse effects are rarely seen even with 3 years of continuous treatment.

Risankizumab

Risankizumab is monoclonal antibody that is humanized IgG-1 directed against the p19 subunit of IL-23.

Dosage of risankizumab: 150 mg is given subcutaneously at 0 and 4 weeks and every 12 weeks thereafter to treat moderate-to-severe plaque psoriasis.

Adverse Effects

The common adverse effects include:
- Upper respiratory (UTI) infections
- Diarrhea, and
- Joint pains

Interleukin-17 Inhibitor Agents (Flowchart 7)

Multiple clinical trials have shown the importance of anti-IL-17 agents in psoriasis. It has been seen that the IL-17 micro-RNA expression is a little more in the skin lesions when compared to the nonlesional skin in psoriasis. The IL-17 levels also correspond to the severity of the disease. Blocking of IL-17 is associated with reduction of the T-cell infiltration into the dermis and keratinocyte hyperproliferation.

Secukinumab

Secukinumab approved in 2015 for treating moderate-severe plaque psoriasis. It is a human recombinant monoclonal immunoglobulin G1 (IgG1)/κ antibody that specifically targets IL-17α and blocks the interaction with IL-17 receptors.

Thus, by inhibiting the proinflammatory cytokine pathway and downstreaming its effects, it interferes with the pathological pathway of psoriasis thereby encourages normalizing of the immune functions and its skin cytology. When used at the therapeutic doses for the treatment, this

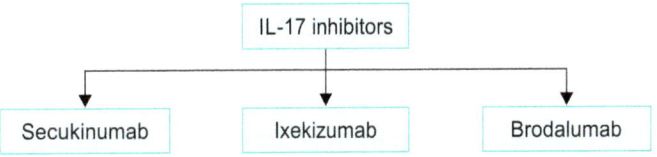

FLOWCHART 7: Interleukin-17 (IL-17) inhibitor agents.

drug fully counteracts IL-17α and does not interfere with the functions of IL-17F. This is associated with much less side effects. The data collected from the phase III randomized trials shows that this drug at doses of 150–300 mg is very safe and successful in treating moderate-to-severe psoriasis up to 52 weeks. It also has a dynamic and long-lasting effect in patients who receive the optimal dosage of treatment every 4 weeks.

Dosage of Secukinumab

It is given subcutaneously at a dosage of two 150–300 mg injections at 0, 1, 2, 3, and 4 weeks followed by 300 mg every 4 weeks.[32,33]

Ixekizumab

Ixekizumab is a monoclonal antibody that is humanized immunoglobulin G4 that selectively blocks IL-17A. A multicenter study stated that this drug shows considerable efficiency in treating moderate-to-severe plaque psoriasis and has sustained results for up to 156 weeks.

It also shows considerable improvement in case of nail psoriasis, scalp psoriasis, and palm psoriasis.

Dosage of Ixekizumab (Flowchart 8)

Two 80 mg (160) injections given subcutaneously on week 0. Then, in the weeks 2, 4, 6, 8, 10, and 12—80 mg once 2 weeks. Then, from week 16–80 mg once every 4 weeks.

Brodalumab

Brodalumab is an IgG2k human monoclonal antibody that is directed against human IL-17 RA (receptor A) that targets IL-17AA, IL-17AF, IL-17FF, IL-17C, and IL-17E. It is expressed in a Chinese Hamster ovary (CHO) and is made up of 1,312 amino acids. Brodalumab brings a quick improvement in histological, and clinical hallmarks of the disease by the 12th week.

A real-life retrospective observational study on the treatment of moderate to severe psoriasis conducted on pediatric (<18 years) and geriatric (≥65 years) psoriasis patients treated with anti-TNF biosimilar agents. Two young patients (19%) and 7 old patients (31%) had accompanying psoriatic arthritis. Concerning comorbidities, elderly was obviously more affected than young [21/23 (91.3%) vs. 1/11 (9.1%), $p < 0.001$], and the most commonly reported were hypertension, dyslipidemia, and diabetes in elderly compared to inflammatory bowel diseases in pediatric patients.

Study included total number of 11 children and 23 elderly patients where 6 children (55%) were under adalimumab biosimilar and 5 children (45%) were under etanercept biosimilar. In geriatric age group, 15 (65%) were treated with adalimumab and 8 (35%) were treated with etanercept biosimilar. All the patients were monitored by regular follow-ups on week 12, 24, 48, and 72 thorough hematological and clinical assessments and side effects were noted down.

Previous treatments included topical therapies in all participants (100%); NB-UVB phototherapy was the most utilized treatment for children while methotrexate for the elderly. Previous biologic failure was more common in elderly compared to pediatric group though not significantly.

For the first group, mean PASI reduced from 16.1 ± 4.7 to 2.1 ± 2.7 by week 72. Similarly, BSA reduced from 26.4 ± 12.1 to 2.9 ± 2.7. For the second group, mean PASI was 15.7 ± 5.4 at baseline and reached 1.9 ± 1.4 by the end of the study, while mean BSA improved by around 90%. No significant adverse effects were reported and none of the study groups discontinued the treatment. Adalimumab and etanercept were found to be equally effective and safe for up to 72 weeks.

AGENTS TARGETTING THE T-CELL

Alefacept[34]

Alefacept is a fusion protein which is full dimeric in nature that consists of an extracellular portion of LFA-3 human leukocyte function antigen-3 fused to the Fc portion of the immunoglobulin G1 **(Fig. 6)**.

Alefacept attaches competitively to the T-cells CD2 locus with the LFA-3 protein part of its molecule and interferes

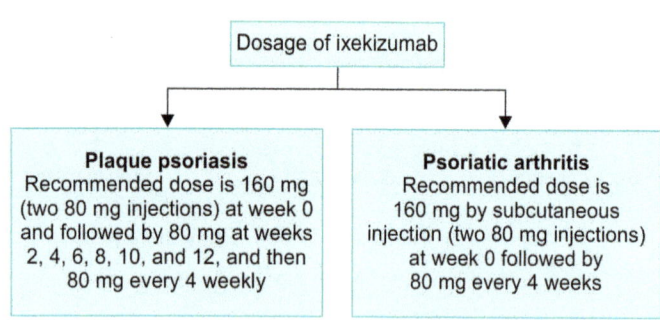

FLOWCHART 8: Dosage of ixekizumab.

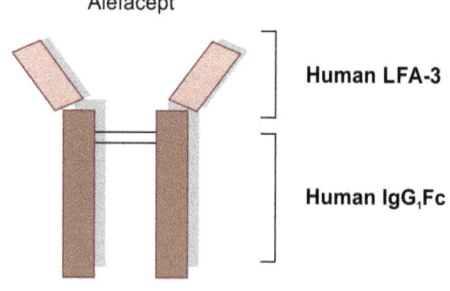

FIG. 6: Structure of alefacept.

with the T cell activation. The Fc portion of the molecule interacts with the IgG receptor on the surface of NK cells and results in programmed cell death of certain memory T cells.

Alefacept binds mainly to memory T-cells because CD2 expresses more on memory T-cells than that of naïve T-cells and then induces apoptosis by selective reduction of specific T-cells. Therefore, by the above mechanism alefacept can selectively deplete memory T-cells and also inhibit T cell activation.

Dosage of Alefacept

- 7.5 mg once weekly (IV) given as a bolus (or)
- 15 mg once a week (IM) for 12 weeks followed by an intermission of 12 weeks void of any treatment in between the doses.

IM administration is easier to administer, however, the site needs to be regularly examined due to higher chance of local reaction as compared to IV administration.

The injections are given by the managing physician and thus ensures regular compliance, clinical response assessment.

Side Effects and Contraindications

T cell plays a very important role as a defender cell of the immune system. Alefacept selectively reduces a specific T cell subset therefore, this might predispose the patients to a variety of reactions and septicemia. There is also a risk of developing malignancies, therefore, CD4+ T-cell count needs to be checked every 2 weeks throughout this 12-week regimen.

CD4+ lymphocyte count must be >400 cells/μL before initiating the treatment. If the counts are <250 cells/μL, alefacept dose must be lowered and monitored weekly, if low counts are recorded persistently for a month the treatment regimen has to be discontinued.

If a patient on alefacept treatment develops any malignancies the treatment has to be withheld. This drug is contraindicated in all patients with any past history of systemic malignancies such as leukemia.

Alefacept in Psoriatic Arthritis

Alefacept given in patients with psoriatic arthritis showed an improvement in clinical picture as well as a change of inflammation in synovial tissue after treatment. About 7.5 mg (IV) of alefacept was administered at weekly intervals for 12 weeks. Clinical evaluations were done at 4 and 12 weeks which included an examination of joints for swelling and tenderness, morning stiffness and pain. Arthroscopic synovial biopsies were also taken.

Alefacept in Palmoplantar Pustular Psoriasis

Palmoplantar pustular psoriasis is characterized by recurrent crops of sterile pustules on the palms and soles over months or years. Many different treatments have been used but none has been particularly effective. After treatment with a total of 17 doses of alefacept, the lesions on palms and soles showed much improvement. Erythema was well as the number of pustules were clearly regressive. Nearly all the lesions were cleared after 12 weeks of treatment.

Alefacept in Nail Psoriasis

Psoriatic nail disease can be refractory to treatment because therapeutic options are limited. Up to 15 patients with moderate-to-severe disease treated with alefacept showed a median decrease of severity by 38%.

Efalizumab[33]

Lymphocyte activation and trafficking to skin plays an important in the pathophysiology of chronic plaque psoriasis. In psoriatic skin, ICAM-1 cell surface expression is upregulated on endothelium and keratinocytes. Efalizumab binds to CD11a, the α subunit of leukocyte function antigen-1 (LFA-1) on all leukocytes, and thus decreases the cell surface expression of CD11a. It also inhibits the binding of LFA-1 to ICAM-1, thereby inhibiting the adhesion of leukocytes to other cell types. Interaction between LFA-1 and ICAM-1 contributes to activation of T lymphocytes, adhesion of T lymphocytes to endothelial cells, and migration of T lymphocytes to sites of inflammation including psoriatic skin. Thus, efalizumab acts by obstructing the action of LFA1 dependent activation of T cells and also migration of these into the inflamed skin.

Pharmacodynamics of efalizumab: Efalizumab pharmacodynamic properties were investigated in several phases both following IV and SC routes either administered as weekly or as a single-dose therapy. Efalizumab-bound cells are demarginated and blocked from entry into the tissues, therefore, decreasing the lymphocyte count. The full pharmacodynamic effect is achieved with an intravenous dose of 0.3 mg/kg used.

At a plasma concentration of 5 μg/mL of efalizumab, there is complete maintenance of CD11a and complete saturation of CD11a was achieved. This requires a weekly dosage of 0.6 mg/kg intravenously. The effect of efalizumab given as 1 mg/kg/week subcutaneously observed on lymphocytes were compared to the effects after intravenous dosing.

Several histological changes are seen in patients of plaque psoriasis with efalizumab (**Flowchart 9**).

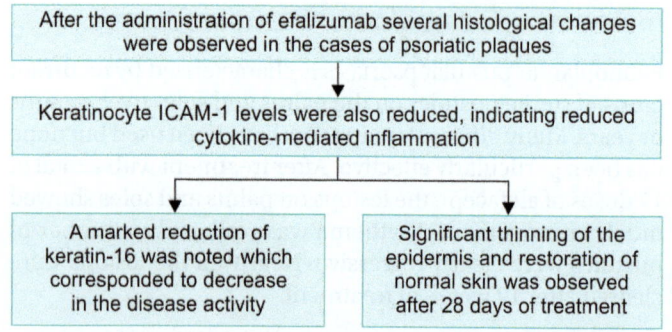

FLOWCHART 9: Histological changes observed after efalizumab.

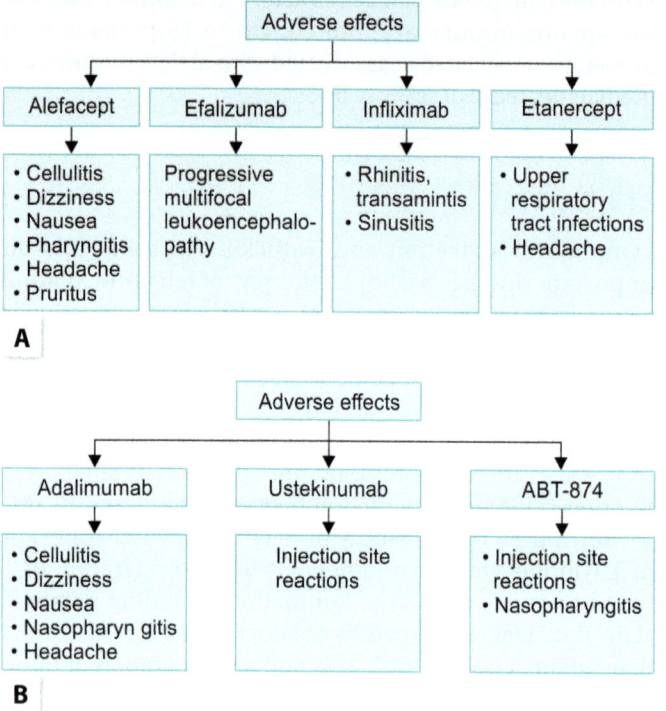

FLOWCHARTS 10A AND B: Adverse effects of biologics.

ADVERSE EFFECTS OF BIOLOGICAL THERAPIES

Refer **Flowchart 10A and B**.

CORTICOSTEROIDS (FLOWCHART 11)

Systemic corticosteroids are very helpful and can sometimes even be lifesaving, having said that they can also carry a high risk of several side effects. Side effects could include the development of rebound flare, tachyphylaxis, and precipitation of generalized pustular psoriasis.

Psoriasis may remain unstable, resistant, and persistent for several days even after withdrawing corticosteroids. The mitotic index is decreased in psoriatic epidermis by systemic corticosteroids.

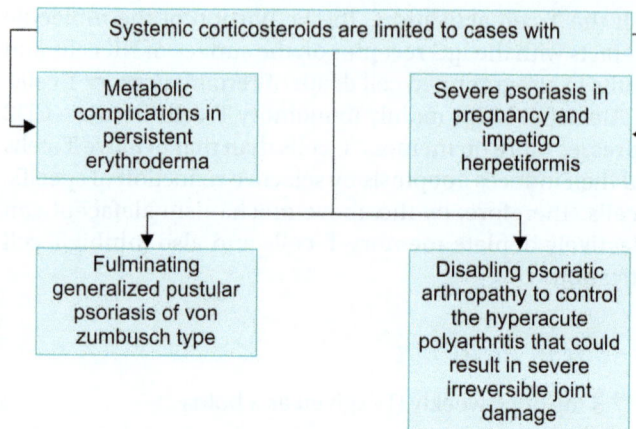

FLOWCHART 11: Systemic corticosteroid limitations.

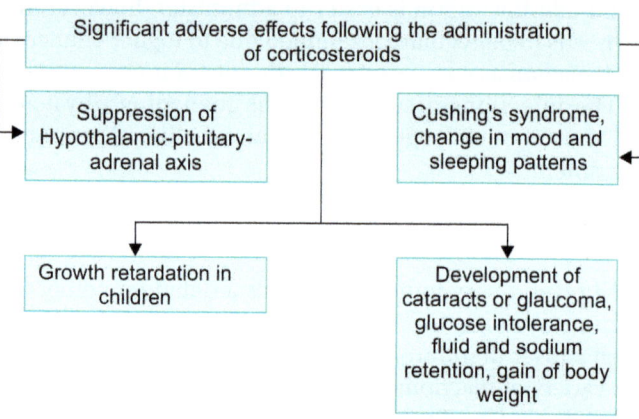

FLOWCHART 12: Significant adverse effects following corticosteroids administration.

The effectiveness is significant but the potential for toxicity and chances of recurrence after cessation of the therapy is a drawback (**Flowchart 12**). In conditions where there is an acute exacerbation or when there is a need to change to other drugs or even waiting for those to start taking any effect, systemic corticosteroids can be used. Adverse effects increase with the prolonged administration therefore, corticosteroids must not be used for a longer period of time.

OTHER SYSTEMIC DRUGS

The following are the other systemic drugs used in the treatment of psoriasis:
- Auranofin oral
- Colchicine
- Zidovudine
- The antithyroid drugs: Methimazole
- Oral tacrolimus
- Oral 2-chloro-deoxyadenosine
- Fumaric acid esters
- 6-mercaptopurine

- Sulfasalazine
- Fish oil (omega-3 fatty acids)
- Antiestrogen therapy
- Antimicrobial therapy of psoriasis
- Liarozole is an imidazole compound.
- Thalidomide
- Rifampicin

Auranofin

Auranofin, lipophilic, organogold compound has a dose-dependent inhibitory effect on RNA, DNA, and protein synthesis in vitro. It is available as tablet and ointment forms.

Oral Colchicine

Colchicine oral dose is 0.5–1 mg twice daily for about 1–6 weeks.

It is effective in treating pustulosis palmaris et plantaris. Colchicine is an anti-inflammatory agent and its effect disrupts the polymorphonuclear leukocyte function.

Zidovudine

Zidovudine was reported to clear psoriasis in HIV-patients.

Dosage of zidovudine: 1,200 mg/day.

Zidovudine may be less effective in HIV-negative patients. It is believed to decrease the proliferative rates of an epidermal cell in vitro as a result may at first hand effect the generation. All though the drawback for the treatment with zidovudine is that there are high chances of relapse and associated arthritis does not improve.

Antithyroid Drugs

Methimazole and Propylthiouracil

The exact mechanism of action of oral thyroid drugs for the treatment of psoriasis is not known, postulated mechanisms include:
- Direct inhibition of epidermal growth
- Alterations in immunology
- Reduced T-cell activation by scavenging of free radicals

Recently topical propylthiouracil (5% lotion) also has been found to be effective in psoriasis.

The dosage of methimazole and propylthiouracil is given in **Figure 7**.

Oral Tacrolimus

Tacrolimus is a macrolide antibiotic used in patients who have undergone a liver transplant for prophylaxis of allograft rejection. There are isolated studies of its effectiveness for treating extensive psoriasis. Tacrolimus has antilymphocytic activity henceforth making is structurally different from cyclosporine.

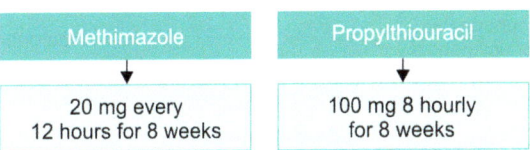

FIG. 7: Dosage of methimazole and propylthiouracil.

Azathioprine

It has been tried with success in some cases of psoriatic arthritis and psoriasis.

Dosage of azathioprine: 50–300 mg daily.

Fumaric Acid Esters[35]

Even though fumaric acid esters have poor absorption they have been shown to be effective in psoriasis. Fumaric acid esters used are a mixture of dimethyl fumarate and hydrogen fumarate.

Mechanism of Action

The Th1-type response in psoriasis is shifted to a Th2 type pattern, IL-10 inhibits Th1 cytokine IL-2, IL-12, and IFN-γ. Lab tests required during therapy with fumaric acid include leukocyte count, liver enzymes, renal function tests including urine sediment. Treatment should be discontinued when leukocyte count falls below 3,000/μL or lymphocyte count below 500/μL **(Fig. 8)**.

Contraindications:
- Pregnancy
- Lactation
- Malignant diseases
- GI diseases
- Bone marrow disease

Side effects:
- Flushing
- GI complications, resulting in dropouts

6-thioguanine

6-thioguanine is a close analog of 6-mercaptopurine which is used as an anticancer drug. It is a useful alternative drug for recalcitrant generalized psoriasis because of its activity against T-cells.

Dosage of 6-thioguanine: Drugs have to be started at a low dose of 20 mg to be given twice a week. It may cause sudden and severe bone marrow toxicity, hepatic, and GI dysfunction, therefore should always be started at a very low dose.

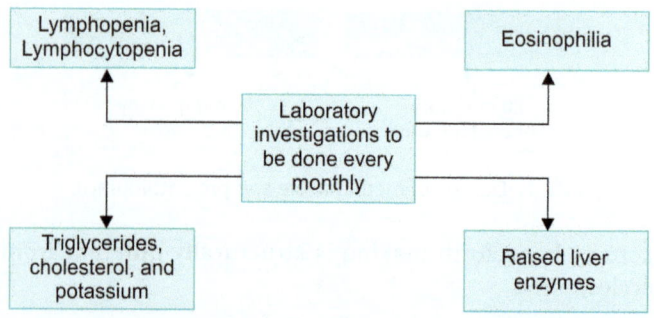

FIG. 8: Laboratory investigations recommended to be done every month in patients treated with fumaric acid ester.

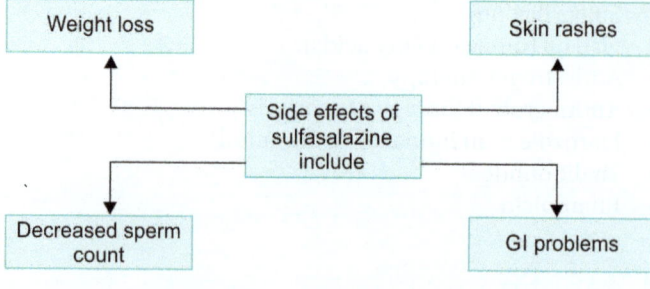

FIG. 9: Side effects of sulfasalazine.

Sulfasalazine

Sulfasalazine was initially used for the treatment of rheumatoid arthritis. It acts by inhibiting arachidonate-5-lipoxygenase pathway. The side effects are given in **(Fig. 9)**.

Dosage of sulfasalazine: 1 g four times a day was found to produce a marked improvement in about 87.5% cases.

Fish Oil

Fish oil, i.e., the omega-3 fatty acids, consists of eicosatetraenoic acid and docosahexaenoic acid. It acts by inhibiting arachidonic acid metabolism.

Antiestrogen Therapy

Antiestrogen therapy is useful in some cases of psoriatic arthritis. In patients who are unresponsive to the treatment with MTX, responded with the use of tamoxifen.

Antimicrobial Therapy

Antimicrobial therapy is useful as several microbial agents are incriminated in the pathogenesis of psoriasis. These organisms include *Malassezia, Candida, Streptococci, Helicobacter*, and gram-negative rods. Therefore, drugs directed against these organisms can be used for the treatment of psoriasis and they have been found helpful. These drugs include:
- Ketoconazole
- Penicillin
- Amoxicillin
- Omeprazole

Liarozole

Liarozole acts by inhibiting CV P450-mediated metabolism of all the trans-retinoic acid. It is an imidazole compound.

Antihistamines

Antihistamines are mainly used as an adjuvant. They help in reducing itching and also help in decreasing ICAM-1 expression in keratinocytes. Most commonly used antihistamines are:
- Cetirizine
- Ranitidine
- Cimetidine

Rifampicin

Rifampicin may be used in psoriasis, especially in its eruptive form. Its therapeutic effect is most probably because of its immunosuppressive property.

MULTIMODALITY THERAPEUTIC STRATEGIES

Refer **Flowchart 13**.

COMBINATION THERAPY[36]

Combination therapy includes two therapeutic agents being used simultaneously in smaller doses in order to attain better results with reduced toxicities **(Tables 1 and 2)**. One of them being or acting as an accelerator, e.g.,
- Cyclosporine
- Ultraviolet B
- MTX

And the other agent being the maintainer, e.g.,
- Psoralen with ultraviolet A
- Acitretin

In this combination therapy, the accelerator is tapered after reaching the maximal therapeutic response but the maintainer is continued. After the clearance of psoriasis, the agent with the maximum safer index is continued as the

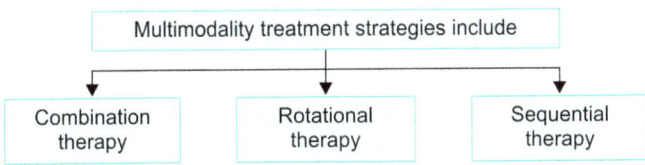

FLOWCHART 13: Multimodality treatment strategies.

TABLE 1: Systemic and topical agents.	
PUVA + Topical steroids	This requires smaller total UVA dose but higher relapse rate. It provides rapid clearing
Methotrexate + Topical steroids	Very beneficial during maintenance therapy
Retinoids + Topical steroids	This will let us use smaller doses of retinoids
UVB + Topical steroids	No added efficacy
Cyclosporine + Topical steroids	Allows the usage of low dosage of cyclosporine and irritate topical agents because the inflammation is suppressed by cyclosporine
PUVA + Topical calcipotriol	Reduces the total UVA dosage and shows rapid clearance
UVB + Tazarotene	Faster clearance than UVB alone
PUVA + Retinoid	• Retinoid to be started 1–2 weeks prior to PUVA • This reduces the number of PUVA treatment by almost 50%
UVB + Retinoids	This helps in achieving clearance by lower dose of UVB
PUVA + UVB	Number of PUVA treatment reduced by 30%
PUVA + Cyclosporine	This combination is as effective as RE-PUVA but overall exposure to UVA is considerably higher
UVB + Methotrexate	This is effective in clearing psoriasis but ineffective in maintaining the clearance
PUVA + Methotrexate	Even though it reduces the total UVA exposure by half, the combination increases the risk of skin cancer and phototoxicity induced by methotrexate
Methotrexate + Cyclosporine	This combination is generally not recommended as they cancel each other's actions. But, it can be used with precautions in patients with psoriatic arthritis
Methotrexate + Retinoids	This may cause hepatotoxicity but can be used with precaution
Methotrexate + Sulfasalazine	This also causes hepatotoxicity but can be used with precaution
Sulfasalazine + PUVA	This is generally not recommended because it causes sulfasalazine-induced phototoxicity

TABLE 2: Combination therapy with biologics.	
Etanercept + Methotrexate	It is used and has been effective in treatment of recalcitrant psoriasis with no additional side effects. It has also been effective in arthritis
Etanercept + Acitretin	Effective in recalcitrant psoriasis with no additional side effects
Etanercept + Cyclosporine	It is used and has been effective in treatment of recalcitrant psoriasis with no additional side effects. It has also been effective in arthritis
Alefacept + UVB	This helps in rapid onset of action with no additional toxicity than compared to alefacept monotherapy
Alefacept + Immunosuppressants	This combination therapy shows no altered frequency or spectrum of adverse events or any serious infections in terms of usage of concomitant methotrexate, cyclosporine, etanercept, or prior use of immunosuppressants such as leflunomide, mycophenolate mofetil, and infliximab

maintenance therapy and the other agent is discontinued. The indication of combination therapy includes:
- Failure of monotherapy
- Emergency of toxicity to single agent
- And to taper a patient from an individual drug

One must carefully select the combinations to avoid adverse effects. Before choosing the combination therapy one must always look into the severity of the disease, patients' expectations, compliance to the therapy and previous experience of the patient with the drugs regarding the side effects all of these need to be considered.

ROTATIONAL THERAPY (TABLE 3)

In order to prevent the cumulative toxicity of an individual drug, the therapeutic agents are rotated at regular interval (2 years) from one agent to another. In rotational therapy, different regimens are rotated before significant toxicity to individual drug is developed. There may be a brief period of overlap during the transition between medications.

Rotation with hydroxyurea is beneficial when patient with psoriasis develops severe toxicity with other drugs, when the hydroxyurea is started as the primary drug, it can be stopped abruptly without the risk of rebound. There is an increased risk of bone marrow if hydroxyurea is used just before or after MTX.

SEQUENTIAL THERAPY (FLOWCHART 14)

The fact that some therapeutic agents produce fast results, even though others are suited for maintaining remission,

TABLE 3: Rotational therapy.	
Methotrexate to PUVA	• PUVA is a better alternative, but it should not be given on the days. Methotrexate is given • Methotrexate can be withdrawn when the effect of PUVA becomes evident
Methotrexate to cyclosporine	Liver dysfunction induced by methotrexate will not be affected by cyclosporine. However, the rotation should be done carefully
Methotrexate to retinoid	Retinoids should be started 2–3 months before the primary drug is stopped. Retinoids have a less toxic effect on the liver
Retinoids to other agents	Retinoids can be stopped abruptly without producing a rebound
Cyclosporine to methotrexate	• Renal function has to be carefully monitored during rotation • If the renal function does not return to normal stop methotrexate
Cyclosporine to phototherapy	During this rotation, there is a slight concern for increased risk of skin cancer as immunosuppression is induced by prior cyclosporine

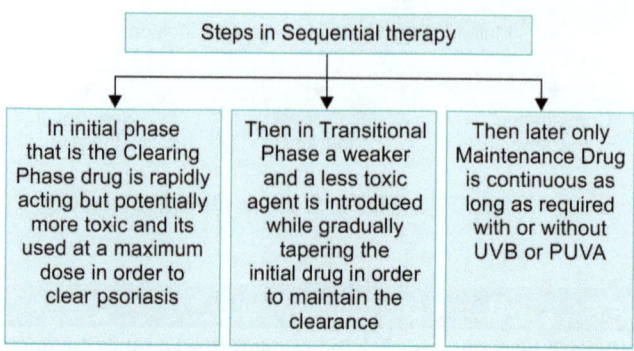

FLOWCHART 15: Steps involved in sequential therapies.

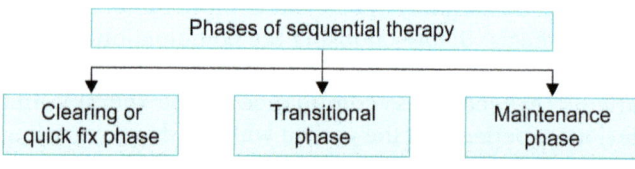

FLOWCHART 14: Three steps of sequential therapy.

the drugs are used in a very deliberate sequence, moving gradually from one therapy to another with a brief period of overlap.

Sequential therapy can be applicable for both topical and systemic therapies. The aim is to produce a fast remission along with minimizing long-term toxicity and maintaining a prolonged disease-free state. For example, use of topical clobetasol propionate and calcipotriol twice a day in phase one, followed by steroid in transitional phase is used on weekends and calcipotriene on weekdays, and then in a maintenance phase, calcipotriene is continued as long as required with gradually tapering off **(Flowchart 15)**.

Dietary Supplement

Fish oil, rich in omega-3 fatty acids, is the best-known dietary supplement. Oral and intravenous supplementation of omega-3 and, less effectively, omega-6 fatty acids have been found effective in psoriatic adults, possibly through alterations in production and alterations in arachidonic acid (20:4 omega 6) and docosapentaenoic acid.

Indigo naturalis, a traditional Chinese medicine, can be formulated into topical ointment with anecdotal reports of good results in childhood psoriasis when used for 8 weeks.[37]

TREATMENT ACCORDING TO TYPE AND SITE OF PSORIASIS

Treatments must be tailored to the age of the patient, quality of life issues, type of psoriasis, and surface area affected. Patients may be grouped into mild, moderate, and severe disease categories. Limited, or mild-to-moderate, skin disease can often be managed with topical agents, while patients with moderate-to-severe disease may need systemic therapy. The location of the disease and the presence of psoriatic arthritis and other comorbidities will also affect the choice of therapy. Psoriasis of the hand, foot, or face can be debilitating functionally or socially and may deserve a more aggressive treatment approach. Moderate-to-severe psoriasis is typically defined as involvement of >5–10% of the BSA (the entire palmar surface, including fingers, of one hand is ~1% of the BSA or involvement of the face, palm or sole, or disease that is otherwise disabling). Patients with >5–10% BSA affected are generally candidates for systemic therapy.

Application of topical agents other than emollients, to a large area is not usually practical or acceptable for most patients. The chances of treatment failure are high due to added cost, and inadequate clinical response which can lead to frustration in the patient-clinician relationship. The management of patients with extensive or recalcitrant disease is a challenge even for experienced dermatologists.

This portion will discuss the treatment of following types:
- Plaque type psoriasis
- Guttate psoriasis
- Pustular psoriasis
- Scalp psoriasis
- Inverse psoriasis

- Palmoplantar psoriasis
- Nail psoriasis
- Mucosal psoriasis

Plaque Type Psoriasis

Anthralin is an effective treatment of plaque psoriasis either with or without topical steroids. With the advent of newer drugs, the frequency of its use has come down. Topical steroids, calcipotriol, and tazarotene are useful and safe if used properly. Salicylic acid can be used along with steroids in thick plaques. Systemic agents like methotrexate and phototherapy may be needed in moderate to severe recalcitrant disease.

Guttate Psoriasis

Oral antibiotics are found to be useful in the treatment of guttate psoriasis. Systemic agents and phototherapy may be needed in moderate to severe disease. It should be remembered that guttate psoriasis can evolve into psoriasis vulgaris and hence the child should be followed up regularly.

Short-term antibiotic treatment is not effective in cases of acute guttate psoriasis. However, long-term antibiotic treatment seems to be more effective in controlling psoriatic relapse. This might be due to the elimination of antigenic stimulation caused by carried micro-organisms.

In patients with acute guttate psoriasis, antibiotics can be added to conventional psoriasis treatment only if the presence of a streptococcal infection or a carrier state has been identified based on laboratory results. If there is no clinical or bacteriological evidence of an infectious episode precipitating the episode antibiotic treatment is unnecessary due to the lack of evidence supporting its benefits. Tonsillectomy can be advised if there is definite evidence of tonsillitis which correlates with exacerbation of the disease, as tonsillectomy was shown to be effective only in uncontrolled studies.

Although both antibiotics and tonsillectomy have frequently been advocated both for patients with guttate psoriasis and for selected patients with chronic plaque psoriasis, there is to date no good evidence that either intervention is beneficial.

Topical emollients, drugs like coal tars, steroids, or vitamin D creams are useful. Regular moisturizing should be encouraged. UVB therapy is to be considered if the conventional treatment fail. Counseling is very important as most of the guttate psoriasis evolve into psoriasis vulgaris in future.

Pustular Psoriasis

If the disease is localized, topical agents like steroids will suffice. Treatment of palmoplantar pustulosis is dealt with under palmoplantar psoriasis.

All patients with generalized pustular psoriasis should be treated as inpatients. Maintenance of nutrition, fluid electrolyte balance prevention of organ failure should be stressed. Multidisciplinary approach is mandatory depending on the extent of systemic involvement. Acitretin/isotretinoin (better avoided in adolescent girls), and Dapsone can be tried depending on the biochemical parameters. Oral steroids are used only to tide over the acute crisis or in pregnant woman with impetigo herpetiformis. Generalized pustular psoriasis responds well to methotrexate in children.[38]

Scalp Psoriasis

Topical steroid with or without salicylic acid as lotion applied at night followed by steroid/ketoconazole-based shampooing in the morning is helpful. For resistant plaques, tar-based shampoos will help. A combination with narrow-band UVB/targeted phototherapy will give better results.

Inverse Psoriasis

Scientific evidence shows that involvement of the genital skin occurs in 29–40% of patients with psoriasis.

Short-term intermittent application of low-to-medium potent topical corticoids is useful as a first-line treatment option, which can be combined with vitamin D analogs or mild tar preparations. Mild topical coal-tar preparations are the second most advised topical therapy in adults and the first choice for children with napkin plaque psoriasis with or without topical steroids. Skin atrophy due to steroid and irritation or folliculitis due to tar preparation should be looked for and avoided. Zinc oxide and tacrolimus or 1% pimecrolimus cream are regarded as third-line treatment options which can be used with safety in children. If used for a longer period, complications, such as local irritation, stinging, irritant or allergic contact dermatitis, candidiasis, and viral infections are the potential side effects. Topical cyclosporine is beneficial in genital psoriasis of the glans, penis, and prepuce. If concurrent bacterial or fungal infections are present, they should be treated with topical antibiotics or antifungal drugs. Emollients should be advised to prevent friction and possible Koebner effect. Local treatment with topical dithranol and tazarotene should be avoided in the genital area. Systemic therapies are not used for isolated genital psoriasis. Dapsone has been shown to be an effective and convenient alternative for the treatment of inverse psoriasis in genital skin folds, which can provide effective control of the disease.

Palmoplantar Psoriasis

Patients with palmoplantar psoriasis should be encouraged to wear good footwear made from natural fibers should avoid minor trauma, resting the affected area where possible. Mild psoriasis of the palms and soles may be treated with topical treatments such as emollients, keratolytic agents, steroids, dithranol, and vitamin D analog.

Emollients frequent application of thick, greasy barrier creams or ointments will moisturize the dry, scaly skin, and help to prevent painful cracking.

Keratolytic agents such as urea or salicylic acid and tar will help to remove thick scaling skin.

Topical steroids ultrapotent ointment applied initially daily for 2–4 weeks, if necessary under occlusion, to reduce inflammation, itch, and scaling. Maintenance use should be confined to 2 days each week (weekend pulses) to avoid thinning the skin and causing the psoriasis to become more extensive.

Calcipotriol ointment is not very successful for palmoplantar psoriasis and may cause an irritant dermatitis on the face if a treated area inadvertently touches it. Dithranol is too messy for routine use on hands and feet.

Note: UVB and 308-nm excimer laser are found very useful in the treatment of palmoplantar psoriasis.

More severe palmoplantar psoriasis usually requires phototherapy or systemic agents.

PUVA, acitretin, methotrexate, and cyclosporine are useful for severe palmoplantar psoriasis. A variety of other medications that can help some subjects include colchicine, dapsone, and tetracycline antibiotics.

Biologics are occasionally effective when used for severe palmoplantar psoriasis. However, TNF-α inhibitors such as infliximab, etanercept, and adalimumab may sometimes induce palmoplantar pustulosis as a side effect of treatment.

Acupuncture is found useful in the management of palmoplantar psoriasis. Refined form of trauma, induced by needle piercing at certain points in acupuncture therapy, may possibly be working through reverse Koebner's phenomenon.[39]

Nail Psoriasis

Psoriasis nail will frequently have super-added fungal infection after treatment of which, topical corticosteroids, tazarotene, or calcipotriene can be applied to the paronychial skin. Intralesional triamcinolone can also be used in the same region to reduce the subungual inflammation. Calcipotriol or tazarotene under occlusion covering the nail folds, plate, and under the nail plate are useful.

Mucosal Psoriasis

No therapy is usually needed; however, topical steroids in an oral base can be used when needed. Candidal overgrowth is a common side effect which should be kept in mind while prescribing steroids topically.

ERYTHRODERMIC PSORIASIS

Patients with erythrodermic psoriasis require hospitalization. Some of these patients may have unstable psoriasis and require close monitoring before deciding on the specific therapy. All such patients are preferably managed in the intensive care unit to take care of the fluid electrolyte balance and nutrition. A multi-disciplinary approach is essential depending on the extent of system involvement. Emollients, wet dressings, and oatmeal baths can be used in concordance with systemic treatment to manage symptoms Long-term maintenance therapy for psoriasis is required.

There is no high-quality evidence to support specific recommendations for the management of erythrodermic psoriasis. Patients with severe and unstable disease should be treated with cyclosporine or infliximab due to the rapid onset and high efficacy of these agents. Patients with less acute disease can be treated with acitretin or methotrexate as first-line agents. Systemic glucocorticoids should be avoided except in cases of erythroderma due to impetigo herpetiformis where other drugs are contraindicated due to the potential for these drugs to induce a flare of psoriasis upon withdrawal of therapy. Infliximab is reported to be effective in erythrodermic psoriasis. Etanercept, adalimumab, and ustekinumab are other biologic agents found useful in erythrodermic psoriasis.

ARTHROPATHIC PSORIASIS

Early diagnosis and treatment can help to slow the disease and preserve joint function and range of motion. The following are early indicators of severe disease:
- Onset at a young age
- Having many joints involved
- Spinal involvement

Good control of the skin disease is an important factor in the management of psoriatic arthritis. Exercise and physical therapy are useful in better control of disease and may reduce requirement of drug intake. Treatments such as heat, exercise, and physical therapy may also help to relieve the pain and stiffness associated with psoriatic arthritis.

Drugs for the treatment of psoriatic arthritis are divided into three main categories:
1. Nonsteroidal anti-inflammatory drugs (NSAIDs)
2. Disease-modifying antirheumatic drugs (DMARDs)
3. Biologics

Treatment varies depending on the level of pain. Those with very mild arthritis may require treatment only when their joints are painful and may stop therapy when they feel better.

Nonsteroidal anti-inflammatory drugs such as ibuprofen or naproxen are used as initial treatment. It is also worth remembering that NSAIDs such as brufen and indomethacin themselves can worsen skin lesions of psoriasis.

If the arthritis does not respond, disease modifying anti-rheumatic drugs are to be prescribed. These include sulfasalazine, methotrexate, cyclosporine, and leflunomide. Sometimes combinations of these drugs may be used together. The anti-malarial drug hydroxychloroquine is better avoided as it can cause a flare of psoriatic skin lesions. Azathioprine may help those with severe forms of psoriatic arthritis.

Like methotrexate, the antitumor necrosis factor agents such as adalimumab, etanercept, golimumab and infliximab have the advantage of reducing both the skin lesion and joint involvement. Ustekinumab has been recently approved by the FDA to be used alone or in combination with methotrexate for the treatment of adult patients (18 years or older) with active psoriatic arthritis. The approval was supported by findings from two pivotal Phase III trials.

Certolizumab pegol has also been approved recently for the treatment of patients with active and progressive adult onset of psoriatic arthritis. Patients treated with certolizumab pegol 200 mg every other week demonstrated greater reduction in radiographic progression compared with placebo-treated patients at week 24. It also resulted in improvement in skin manifestations in patients with PsA.

For swollen joints, corticosteroid injections can be useful. Surgery can be resorted to repair or replace badly damaged joints

In children with psoriatic arthropathy methotrexate is the drug of choice.

TREATMENT OF PSORIASIS IN SPECIAL POPULATIONS

The treatment of psoriasis in pregnant women and patients with hepatitis B, hepatitis C, human immunodeficiency virus infection, latent tuberculosis, and malignancy can be challenging.

Treatment of Psoriasis in Pregnancy and Lactation

Psoriasis is known to be associated with metabolic syndrome. Comorbidities such as diabetes, obesity or hypertension in pregnancy may worsen psoriasis and vice versa. Therefore, the management of psoriasis in such patients means medical, dermatological, and obstetric challenge which has to be borne in mind while treating a pregnant woman with psoriasis. It is also possible that some women experience spontaneous improvement of psoriasis during pregnancy.

Topical Therapies for Psoriasis in Pregnancy and Lactation

- Simple emollients appear safe to use in pregnancy.
- Salicylic acid is absorbed through the skin (10–25%). It is proved that oral salicylates are associated with bleeding and are harmful to the baby it is better to avoid topical salicylic acid over large areas of the body for prolonged periods.
- Coal-tar products are considered safe if used for short periods or on localized areas such as the scalp. Though the risk of coal tar and injury to the baby is unknown, it is better to avoid their use over large areas of the body for prolonged periods as they contain potentially hazardous polycyclic aromatic hydrocarbons.

Since dithranol/anthralin is not absorbed through skin, the risk in pregnancy is unknown but the drug is not frequently advised due to its irritant nature.

- Topical corticosteroids appear to be safe during pregnancy if used judiciously. Mild- to moderate-potency topical corticosteroids should be preferred to more potent corticosteroids during pregnancy. Potent to very potent topical corticosteroids should be used only as second-line therapy for as short a time as possible. They are better avoided over high-absorption areas like the eyelids, genitals, and flexures. Whether the newer potent lipophilic topical corticosteroids (e.g., mometasone, fluticasone, and methylprednisolone) are associated with less risk to fetus is not fully determined.
- Mild, moderate, and potent topical corticosteroids are also considered safe to use when breastfeeding. Patient should be instructed to wash off any steroid cream applied breasts before feeding. It is advisable that very potent topical corticosteroids are not recommended to use over the chest while breastfeeding.
- Calcipotriol, a Category B drug, with 6% systemic absorption should be used with caution though the risk in pregnancy is unknown. Dose should not exceed 100 g/week, and should not be applied over the chest area, if the mother is breastfeeding.
- Calcineurin inhibitors such as tacrolimus and pimecrolimus belong to Category C and their risk in pregnancy is unknown
- Tazarotene, although topical, is a category X medication therefore, is to be strictly avoided in pregnancy

Phototherapy for Psoriasis in Pregnancy and Lactation

Phototherapy with broadband UVB and narrowband UVB appears as safe in pregnancy as at other times. The risk of topical PUVA in pregnancy is considered very low, but oral PUVA should be avoided during pregnancy.

Systemic Therapies for Psoriasis in Pregnancy and Lactation

Systemic therapies for psoriasis in pregnancy: It is always better to avoid systemic therapy in pregnancy. Most of the systemic drugs used in the treatment of psoriasis are unsafe in pregnancy and lactation. Cyclosporin and biologics are the only drugs relatively safe in pregnancy coming under category C **(Box 6)**.

Though cyclosporine belongs to category C drug, it may cause high blood pressure and kidney damage, which might harm the baby. If treatment is essential, it must be monitored carefully. It is best not to breastfeed during treatment as cyclosporin passes into the milk.

Biologics, the category C drugs are better avoided during pregnancy and breastfeeding as little information is available about their safety in pregnancy and lactation.

The appropriate treatment for psoriasis in a woman who is pregnant, or who plans pregnancy, will depend on the extent and severity of the skin condition.

Topical therapy can be used with confidence, but large quantities of salicylic acid, calcipotriol, topical steroids, and calcineurin inhibitors should be avoided for long periods of time.

UVB phototherapy is safe for pregnant women with more severe psoriasis. If there is a need to prescribe cyclosporine, blood pressure and kidney function should be monitored very prudently.

Impetigo Herpetiformis

Impetigo herpetiformis can be successfully treated with topical and systemic corticosteroids. Antibiotics may be indicated for secondary bacterial infection. Fluid and electrolytes especially calcium should be monitored and normalized. Unresponsive cases can be given cyclosporine, narrowband ultraviolet B (NBUVB), psoralen ultraviolet A (PUVA), clofazimine or induction of early delivery]. During the postpartum period, oral retinoid can be given. Treatment is imperative due to the life-threatening nature of the disease. The treatment of choice in pregnancy is prednisone 15–30 mg/day. Cyclosporine is used only if the potential benefits justify the potential risk to the fetus. As the fetal mortality is high, even when the disease appears well controlled with corticosteroids, fetal well-being should be monitored using biophysical profile and umbilical artery Doppler studies. If fetal or maternal conditions deteriorate, pregnancy should be terminated by induction of labor or cesarean section, as indicated. Though maternal mortality is less with the advent of treatment options available, stillbirth and intrauterine growth retardation may occur even when the disease appears to be controlled with corticosteroids. Low-dose methotrexate can be substituted in the postpartum period to prevent rebound of rashes, but is contraindicated in pregnancy and lactation. The disease remits after delivery but may recur in successive pregnancies.

Psoriasis and Hepatitis

There are enough studies to show that psoriasis is associated with hepatitis C virus infection and not hepatitis B virus infection. Treating psoriasis in patients with concomitant hepatitis C virus (HCV) infection presents a special challenge. Not only is psoriasis exacerbated by interferon therapy, the standard of care for HCV, but many psoriasis therapies are potentially hepatotoxic, immunosuppressive, or both, which has been generally thought to be a contraindication in chronic infections such as HCV.

In limited psoriasis with HCV infection, topical therapies are first-line therapy and UVB phototherapy will be the second-line treatment. In moderate-to-severe disease, UVB phototherapies in combination with topical therapies are first line and systemic therapies, such as acitretin and etanercept, are considered second line. Apart from screening for liver enzymes screening for hepatocellular carcinoma must be performed in all patients with hepatitis C infection being treated with biologic therapies. Oral PUVA can be considered provided the liver functions can be maintained.

Patients with hepatitis B virus infection should not be given methotrexate. As there are reports showing viral reactivation, in patients treated with tumor necrosis factor (TNF) inhibitors; it is advisable to screen all patients for HBV before initiating treatment with these biologics. For patients found to be seropositive, antiviral treatment is recommended with close follow-up.

HIV-positive patients who have psoriasis typically have severe symptoms, and particular care must be taken with any immunosuppressive therapy in this group. Studies thus far have not found serious adverse events in HIV-positive patients given TNF inhibitors, but the suitability of this treatment remains a matter of dispute.

Psoriasis in TB Patient

All the TNF-α inhibitors are associated with an increased risk of developing active disease in patients with latent tuberculosis infection, because of TNF-α playing a key role against *Mycobacterium tuberculosis*. Hence, exclusion of active tuberculosis and treatment of latent tuberculosis infection are clinical imperatives prior to starting this therapy. Apart from topical therapy, UVB and acitretin seem

---

BOX 6: Systemic drugs in pregnancy.

- Methotrexate: Category D
- Acitretin: Category X
- Cyclosporin: Category C
- Hydroxyurea: Category D
- Mycophenolate mofetil: Category D
- Biologics: Category C

to be safer drugs in the treatment of psoriasis in a patient with tuberculous infection.

Psoriasis and Human Immunodeficiency Virus

Psoriasis occurs with at least undiminished frequency in HIV-infected individuals. The behavior of psoriasis in HIV disease is of interest, in terms of pathogenesis and therapy because of the background of profound immunodysregulation. It is paradoxical that, while drugs that target T lymphocytes are effective in psoriasis, the condition should be exacerbated by HIV infection.

Psoriasis in the setting of HIV disease may be mild, moderate, or severe. Standard therapies and zidovudine are effective in management. Survival does not seem to be adversely affected by the presence of psoriasis or its therapy.

Mild-to-moderate disease: Topical therapy is the first-line recommended treatment.

UVB can be considered as a second-line therapy.

Moderate-to-severe disease: Phototherapy is the recommended first-line therapeutic agent.

Oral retinoids may be used as a second-line treatment.

Refractory, severe disease: Cyclosporine, methotrexate, hydroxyurea, and TNF-α inhibitors may be considered and used with extreme caution. Since skin lesions of patients with therapy-resistant AIDS associated psoriasis have been reported to clear with oral zidovudine, and this drug may be considered as retinoid-resistant AIDS-associated psoriasis, where, methotrexate, cyclosporin and PUVA may be contraindicated.

Oral gold was found to be safe and useful in a woman in the treatment of disabling psoriatic arthritis with human immunodeficiency virus (HIV) infection, in whom CD4 count during oral gold therapy showed a significant, sustained increase in CD4 cells.

Psoriasis and Malignancy

PUVA, when given long term, is associated with increased risks of cutaneous squamous cell carcinoma and malignant melanoma. MTX, CsA, and MMF—are associated with an increased risk of lymphoproliferative disorders. TNF-α inhibitors may cause a slightly increased risk of cancer, including nonmelanoma skin cancer and hematologic malignancies. The increased risk of malignancy associated with psoriasis itself is a confounding factor. Topical therapy and UVB remain safe options for the treatment of psoriasis in patients with malignancy.

TREATMENT OF CHILDHOOD PSORIASIS

Psoriasis in children is more or less similar to that in adults. However, there are some real differences between treating a child and an adult. Many of the systemic drugs used for adults may not be appropriate for children due to long term or delayed side effects. Treatment should be carefully tailored according to the type and severity of the psoriasis, the areas of the skin affected and the patient's age and past medical history giving due importance to the family history as well.

Infants: Treatment should be very conservative. Moisturizers can be a good first step. Oatmeal baths and anti-itch creams can help to relieve the itching. The disease must be allowed to evolve before embarking on any specific therapy.

Children: For mild psoriasis, in addition to emollients, topical agents like steroids of appropriate strength, formula, and dose should be the ideal choice. Other drugs such as vitamin D analog, calcineurin inhibitors are used where steroids are contraindicated. For moderate cases, regular broad-band or narrow-band UVB therapy can help to clear the lesions. Antibiotics may help to clear the bacteria that could have triggered the psoriasis only if there is clinical or laboratory evidence. Undue usage of antibiotics in children should be avoided. Severe psoriasis can be treated with systemic drugs under careful monitoring.

Adolescent: Can be treated as above. One should always bear in mind that antimitotics like methotrexate should not be used as a routine in this age group. Being an emotionally turbulent stage of life, a lot of time should be spent counseling these patients as well as their parents and caregivers.

REFERENCES

1. van de Kerkhof PC, Barker J, Griffiths CE, Kragballe K, Mason J, Mentor A, et al. Psoriasis: Consensus on topical therapies. J Euro Acad Dermatol Venereol. 2008;22:859-70.
2. Del Rosso J. Pharmacotherapy updates: Current therapies and research for common dermatologic conditions. The many roles of salicylic acid. Skin Aging. 2005;13:38-42.
3. Volden G, Kragballe K, van de Kerkhoffe PC, A berg K, White RJ. Remission and relapse of chronic plaque psoriasis treated once a week with clobetasol propionate occluded with a hydrocolloid dressing v/s twice daily treatment with clobetasol propionate occluded with a hydrocolloid dressing v/s twice daily treatment with clobetasol propionate alone. J Dermatol Treat. 2001;12:141-4.

4. Patel T, Bhutani T, Busse KL, Koo J. Evaluating the efficacy and safety of calcipotriene/betamethasone ointment occluded with a hydrogel patch: A 6-week bilaterally controlled, investigator-blinded trial. Cutis. 2011;88:149-54.
5. Bourke JF, Berth-Jones J, Hutchinson PE. Occlusion enhances the efficacy of topical calcipotriol in the treatment of psoriasis vulgaris. Clin Exp Dermatol. 1993;18:504-6.
6. Vakirlis E, Kastanis A, Ioannides D. Calcipotriol/betamethasone dipropionate in the treatment of psoriasis vulgaris. Their clin risk Manag. 2008;4:141-8.
7. Berth-Jones J, Chu AC, Dodd WA, Ganpule M, Griffiths WA, Haydey RP, et al. A multi centre, parallel-group comparison of calcipotriol ointment and short-contact dithranol therapy in chronic plaque psoriasis. Br J Dermatol. 1992;127:266-71.
8. de Korte J, van der Valk PG, Sprangers MA, Damstra RJ, Kunkeler AC, Lijnen RL, et al. A comparison of twice-daily calcipotriol ointment with once-daily short-contact dithranol cream therapy: Quality-of-life outcomes of a randomised controlled trial of supervised treatment of psoriasis in a day-care setting. Br J Dermatol. 2008;158:375-81.
9. Tzaneva S, Honigsmann H, Tanew A. Observer blind, randomised, intrapatient comparison of a novel 1% coal tar preparation (Exorex) and calcipotriol cream in the treatment of plaque psoriasis Br J Dermatol. 2003;149:350-3.
10. Smith CH, Jackson K, Chinn S, Angus K, Barker JN. A double blind, randomised, controlled clinical trial to assess the efficacy of a new coal tar preparation (Exorex) in the treatment of chronic, plaque type psoriasis. Clin Exp Dermatol. 2000;25:580-3.
11. Mahrle G. Dithranol. Clin Dermatol. 1997;15:723-37.
12. Ramsay B, Lawrence CM, Bruce JM, Shuster S. The effect of triethanolamine application on anthralin-induced inflammation and therapeutic effect in psoriasis. J Am Acad Dermatol. 1990;23:73-6.
13. Loffler H, Effendy I, Happle R. Skin susceptibility to dithranol: Contact allergy or irritation? Eur J Dermatol. 1999;9:32-4.
14. Runne U, Kunze J. Short duration ('minutes') therapy with dithranol for psoriasis: a new out-patient regimen. Br J Dermatol. 1982;106:135-9.
15. Witman PM. Topical therapies for localised psoriasis. Mayo Clin proc. 2001;76:943-9.
16. Kaidbey K, Kopper SC, Sefton J, Gibson JR. A pilot study to determine the effect of tazarotene gel 0.1% on steroid-induced epidermal atrophy. Int J Dermatol. 2001;40:468-71.
17. Napolitano M, Patruno C. Aryl hydrocarbon receptor (AhR) a possible target for the treatment of skin disease. Med Hypotheses. 2018;116:96-100.
18. Lebwohl M, Stein Gold L, Strober B, Armstrong A, Chih-Ho Hong H, Kircik L, et al. Tapinarof cream 1% QD for the treatment of plaque psoriasis: Efficacy and safety in two pivotal phase 3 trials. Skin J Cutan Med. 2020;4(6):s75.
19. Nolan BV, Yentzer BA, Steven R, Feldman SR. A review of home phototherapy for psoriasis. Dermatol Online J. 2010;16(2):1.
20. Pahlajani N, Katz BJ, Lozano AM, Murphy F, Gottlieb A. Comparison of the efficacy and safety of the 308 nm excimer laser for the treatment of localized psoriasis in adults and in children: A pilot study. Pediatr Dermatol. 2005;22:161-5.
21. Pang ML, Murase JE, Koo J. An updated review of acitretina systemic retinoid for the treatment of psoriasis. Expert Opin Drug Metab Toxicol. 2008;4:953-64.
22. Perrett CM, Ilchyshyn A, Berth-Jones J. Cyclosporin in childhood psoriasis. J Dermatolog Treat. 2003;14(2):113-8.
23. Alli N, Góngφr E, Karakayali G, Lenk N, Artóz F. The use of cyclosporin in a child with generalized pustular psoriasis. Br J Dermatol. 1998;139:7545.
24. Pereira TM, Vieira AP, Fernandes JC, Sousa-Basto AJ. Cyclosporin A treatment in severe childhood psoriasis. Eur Acad Dermatol Venereol. 2006;20:651-6.
25. Kumar B, Dhar S, Handa S, Kaur I. Methotrexate in childhood psoriasis. Pediatr Dermatol. 1994;11(3):271-3.
26. Collin B, Vani A, Ogboli M, Moss C. Methotrexate treatment in 13 children with severe plaque psoriasis. Clin Exp Dermatol. 2009;34(3):295-8.
27. Kalb RE, Strober B, Weinstein G, Lebwohl M. Methotrexate and psoriasis: 2009 National Psoriasis Foundation Consensus Conference. J Am Acad Dermatol. 2009;60:824-37.
28. Reich K, Gooderham M, Bewley A, Green L, Soung J, Petric R, et al. Safety and efficacy of apremilast through 104 weeks in patients with moderate to severe psoriasis who continued on apremilast or switched from etanercept treatment: Findings from the LIBERATE study. J Eur Acad Dermatol Venereol. 2018;32:397-402.
29. Tian F, Chen Z, Xu T. Efficacy and safety of tofacitinib for the treatment of chronic plaque psoriasis: a systematic review and meta-analysis. J int med res. 2019;47(6):2342-50.
30. Boehncke WH, Prinz J, Gottlieb AB. Biologic therapies for psoriasis. A systematic review. J rheumatol. 2006;33(7):1447-51.
31. Yang K, Oak ASW, Elewski BE. Use of IL-23 Inhibitors for the Treatment of Plaque Psoriasis and Psoriatic Arthritis: A Comprehensive Review. Am J Clin Dermatol. 2021;22(2):173-92.
32. Boehncke WH. Efalizumab in the treatment of psoriasis. Biol: targets ther. 2007;1(3):301-9.
33. Castelo-Soccio L, Van Voorhees AS. Long-term efficacy of biologics in dermatology. Dermatol ther. 2009;22(1):22-33.
34. Jenneck C, Novak N. The safety and efficacy of alefacept in the treatment of chronic plaque psoriasis. Therap clin risk manage. 2007;3(3):411-20.
35. Harries MJ, Chalmers RJ, Griffiths CE. Fumaric acid esters for severe psoriasis: a retrospective review of 58 cases. Br J Dermatol. 2005;153:549.
36. Kirby B, Marsland AM, Carmichael AJ, Griffiths CE. Successful treatment of severe recalcitrant psoriasis with combination infliximab and methotrexate. Clin experiment dermatol. 2001;26(1):27-9.
37. Lin YK, Yen HR, Wong WR, Yang SH, Pang JH. Successful treatment of pediatric psoriasis with Indigo naturalis composite ointment. Pediatr Dermatol. 2006;23:507-10.
38. Parimalam K, Nithya P, Saratha KP, Mythili PC, Manoharan K. Effect of methotrexate in juvenile generalised pustular psoriasis. J Applied Med Surg. 2012;1(3):28-31.
39. D'Souza PV. Beating palmoplantar psoriasis away. Indian J Dermatol. 2012;57(3):241-2.

Complications and "The Psoriatic March"

INTRODUCTION

Complications in psoriasis by themselves are though rare, they may result from the persistence of inflammation. Association of certain diseases themselves can be considered as complication, as they at times worsen, as psoriasis worsens. Complications in psoriasis can be viewed as:
- Cutaneous complications
- Metabolic and systemic complications
- Arthropathic complications
- Ocular complications
- Psychosocial complications
- Complications due to treatment.

CUTANEOUS COMPLICATIONS

Secondary infection of psoriatic lesions is rarely a problem except during. However, staphylococci are carried by 50% of psoriatics, especially on the lesions. Carriage of staphylococci may prove to be a problem, if a surgical procedure is to be carried out through a psoriatic plaque. Because of exfoliation, these patients may disseminate infections in hospital wards. Fissuring in flexural psoriasis may get secondarily infected. Itching can be considered as a symptom, which by itself in some individuals can be very severe, especially in unstable forms. Whereas pustular and erythrodermic patterns are accompanied by sensations of burning or tightness. One must also remember that itching may reflect the emotional state of the patient and, if severe, may be a symptom of anxiety or depression.

METABOLIC AND SYSTEMIC COMPLICATIONS (BOX 1)

- Obesity, diabetes, hypertension, dyslipidemia are common comorbidities resulting from psoriasis.
- A significant incidence of hyper- and hypothyroidism and the presence of thyroid antibodies have been found in association with palmoplantar pustulosis (PPP).

> **BOX 1: Metabolic and systemic.**
> - Obesity
> - Diabetes
> - Hypertension
> - Dyslipidemia
> - Liver disease
> - Hyper- and hypothyroidism
> - Folate deficiency
> - Arthropathies
> - Chronic recurrent multifocal osteomyelitis
> - Antigliadin antibodies
> - Nephritis and renal failure
> - Organ failure in erythroderma
> - Apical pulmonary fibrosis
> - Secondary amyloidosis
> - Subfertility

- A greater tendency to develop diabetes has also been documented.
- Various arthropathy are also associated, including chronic recurrent multifocal osteomyelitis, sternoclavicular involvement, pustular arthro-osteitis, axial and peripheral arthritis.
- Some patients have antigliadin antibodies.
- Patients with severe psoriasis can develop folate deficiency.
- *Nephritis and renal failure*: The role of streptococcal infection, especially in the throat, in provoking acute guttate psoriasis is well known, a case of concomitant onset of diffuse psoriasis and mesangiocapillary glomerulonephritis has been reported. Renal failure due to acute tubular necrosis may rarely result from the oligemia after loss of albumin into and from the skin in acute pustular psoriasis.
- *Hepatic failure*: Severe abnormalities of liver function may occur in erythrodermic or pustular psoriasis, and are likely to be related to drugs, alcohol intake and oligemia.
- Apical pulmonary fibrosis has been established as a nonarticular complication of psoriatic spondylitis as well

as chronic plaque psoriasis. Secondary amyloidosis is a rare sequel of arthropathic, generalized pustular and severe nonpustular forms which may be an additional cause of renal failure in association with psoriasis.

- The prevalence of polycystic ovary syndrome (PCOS) in women with psoriasis is remarkably greater than in age- and body mass index (BMI)-matched control women. Psoriasis is linked with metabolic syndrome (MS), insulin resistance (IR) and nonalcoholic fatty liver diseases (NAFLD), which are also common features found to be associated with PCOS.

Whether, there is a missing link between psoriasis and subfertility is to be probed and explored.

Generalized pustular psoriasis is known to develop complications and morbidity more frequently than other forms of psoriasis. Occasionally, acute respiratory distress syndrome may complicate generalized pustular psoriasis.

Other complications in pustular psoriasis may include the following:
- Secondary bacterial skin infections, hair loss (telogen effluvium) and nail loss
- Malabsorption and malnutrition
- Hypoalbuminemia secondary to loss of plasma protein into tissues
- Hypocalcemia
- Renal tubular necrosis as a result of oligemia
- Liver damage as a result of oligemia and general toxicity
- Telogen effluvium
- Amyloidosis
- Inflammatory polyarthritis

Death in untreated pustular psoriasis may occur as a result of cardiorespiratory failure.

ARTHROPATHIC COMPLICATIONS

Approximately, one-half of patients with early onset psoriatic arthritis develop erosive joint damage within 2 years of onset. In addition, psoriatic arthritic patients have an increased mortality rate, with cardiovascular (CV) complications reported to be the most common cause of death. Psoriatic arthritis patients can experience sleep apnea and a reduced quality of life and increased functional disabilities compared with the general population, and the reduction in quality of life is greater in those with higher scores of psoriasis area and severity index (PASI).

OCULAR COMPLICATIONS

Ophthalmic complications of psoriasis affect almost any part of the eye. Psoriatic eye findings may include conjunctivitis, dry eye, episcleritis and uveitis, all of which may precede articular changes. Uveitis, seen in up to 25% of psoriatic arthritis patients, may be recognized by the presence of conjunctival injection, photophobia, pain, lid swelling, or otherwise unexplained visual changes.

A clinically distinct form of bilateral uveitis, that is prolonged, can develop in patients with psoriatic arthritis and in patients with psoriasis.

Ocular involvement of psoriasis may be easily missed. Early recognition is of paramount importance as the natural course may lead to loss of vision. Physicians should maintain a high index of suspicion that ophthalmic symptoms in patients with psoriasis may be related to their underlying disease, even though signs and symptoms are often vague.

PSYCHOSOCIAL COMPLICATIONS

Alcoholism is known to exacerbate psoriasis, however, heavy drinking was found significantly more commonly in male patients with severe psoriasis than in other groups with the disease and could be a symptom of stress caused by severe skin disease.

COMPLICATIONS DUE TO TREATMENT

- Topical therapy is considered relatively safe. However, they are not without causing side effect, if not properly used. Topical steroid therapy, under occlusive dressings, can lead to cutaneous atrophy and secondary infection with bacteria, fungi and virus.
- *Salicylic acid*: Percutaneous salicylate absorption leading to salicylism.
- *Tar*: Irritation, when combined with ultraviolet light in the Goeckermann regimen
- *Anthralin*: Irritation problems of normal skin surrounding lesions and staining of the skin
- *Vitamin D analog*: Burning and stinging sensation; hypercalcemia
- Tazarotene, although topical, is a category X medication. Side effects include desquamation, erythema, burning/stinging, dry skin, skin irritation, skin pain, irritant or contact dermatitis, photosensitivity.
- Systemic agents used in psoriasis are known for their adverse effects requiring judicious follow-up. Common side-effects of retinoid include xerosis, cheilitis, epistaxis and reversible alteration in liver enzymes and serum lipids. Premature closure of epiphysis limits its use in children.

The following drugs cause immunosuppression and hence lead to increased proneness for infection:
- Methotrexate can cause myelotoxicity, hepatotoxicity and pulmonary fibrosis
- Cyclosporine is known for its nephrotoxicity. It can also induce systemic hypertension.
- Biologics are found to be associated with increased risk of malignancies, including lymphoma, leukemia and development of new onset psoriasis. Reversible posterior

leukoencephalopathy syndrome and a lymphomatoid drug eruption and CV complications were reported with the use of ustekinumab.

THE PSORIATIC MARCH[1] (FIG. 1)

The "march of psoriasis" has been used to describe the process in a stepwise manner, beginning with genetic, and possibly, environmental factors that initiate disease-specific pathways involving the immune system. This leads to expression of psoriasis and subsequent comorbidities as a consequence of chronic inflammation. CV risk being the one most elaborately studied in this aspect. The common factor, the vasculature and the IR lead to a cascade of events marching to affect the corresponding effector organ, depending on the degree of resultant impairment.

The systemic inflammation associated with psoriasis enhances IR, causing endothelial dysfunction, atherosclerosis and eventual coronary events. The innate and adaptive immune responses are both responsible for disease pathology, resulting in changes to the epidermis and vasculature. Although the "march of psoriasis" is described in a stepwise manner, the inflammatory processes involved may drive the development of CV risk factors concomitantly with the presentation of psoriasis.

Biomarkers indicating a state of systemic inflammation have been observed to be elevated in the blood of psoriasis patients, including C-reactive protein (CRP), vascular endothelial growth factor (VEGF) and indicators of platelet activation, such as P-selectin. Of these, it was noted that VEGF never drops to levels as low as in nonpsoriatic controls, but remains somewhat elevated even in the absence of clinical signs of psoriasis. This persistently elevated levels of VEGF support the concept of psoriatic march even in the absence of clinical activity of the disease indicating that all psoriasis need to be treated vigorously in order to prevent organ damage. The elevated levels of resistin and leptin functioning as insulin antagonists lead to IR.

The resulting insult is simplified for better and easy understanding:

- Insulin resistance leads to hyperglycemia. With the beta-cells in the pancreas producing more of insulin, further contributes to hyperinsulinemia. This often remains undetected and can contribute to development of type 2 diabetes mellitus.

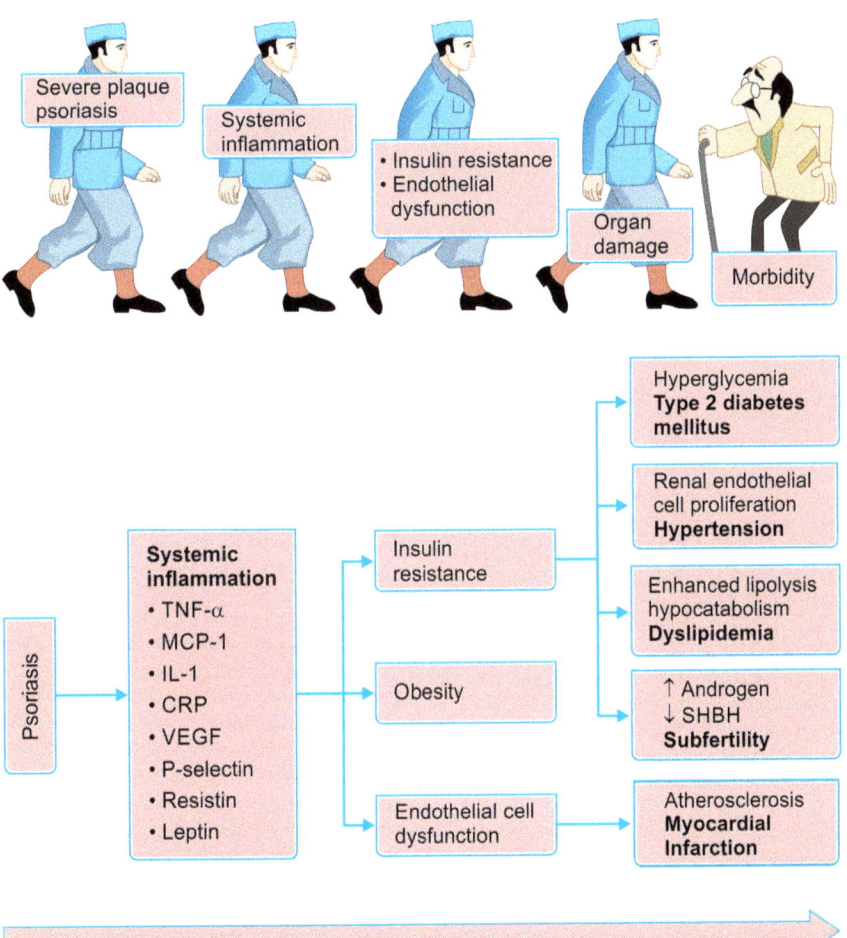

Fig. 1: The psoriatic march.
(CRP: C-reactive protein; IL-1: interleukin-1; MCP-1: monocyte chemoattractant protein-1; TNF-α: tumor necrosis factor-alpha: SHBG: sex hormone binding globulin; VEGF: vascular endothelial growth factor)

- Renal endothelial cell proliferation with extramedullary matrix deposit, induced by IR through a cascade of events, results in glomerular sclerosis and hypertension. Hypertension by itself can have its effect on all organs including the central nervous system leading to stroke.
- In insulin-resistance states, enhanced lipolysis and increased fatty acid flux from adipose tissue, hypersecretion and hypocatabolism of chylomicron (CM) and very low density lipoprotein (VLDL) remnants and *de novo* lipogenesis (DNL) are three major sources of triglyceride (TG), the main substrate regulating ApoB secretion as VLDL. Altered metabolism of TG-rich lipoproteins is crucial in the pathophysiology leading to dyslipidemia associated with IR.
- Insulin resistance and the resultant hyperinsulinemia via increased levels of androgenic enzymes and reduced sex hormone binding globulin (SHBG) leads to androgen excess. Anovulation and polycystic ovary caused by androgen excess may lead to subfertility.
- Endothelin are identified to be produced by keratinocytes. The levels of endothelin 1 are significantly elevated in psoriasis. This, along with the reduced production of nitric oxide creates an imbalance, predisposing the endothelium towards an atherogenic milieu.

Timely and appropriate systemic therapy will certainly reduce the pace of March, though cannot fully stop the progress and organ damage.

REFERENCE

1. Boehncke WH, Boehncke S, Anne-Marie Tobin, et al. The psoriatic march: a concept of how severe psoriasis may drive cardiovascular comorbidity. Exp Dermatol. 2011;20:303-7.

Psychological Aspects, Course and Prognosis, Follow-up, and Rehabilitation

PSYCHOLOGICAL ASPECTS

Living with psoriasis often has emotional and social consequences:
- Patients may feel embarrassed by having visible plaques and that can lead to depression to such an extent as to stay withdrawn from society **(Figs. 1 and 2)**.
- Symptoms may become so severe that patients have to leave their jobs, further increasing the risk of psychological and emotional problems, in addition to the economical strain.
- Several surveys have shown that a significant number of patients with psoriasis report a negative mental and physical impact that is similar to several chronic conditions including cancer, hypertension, heart disease, depression and diabetes.

QUALITY OF LIFE AND PSYCHOLOGICAL ASPECTS OF PSORIASIS

Although psoriasis generally does not affect survival, it certainly has a number of major negative effects on

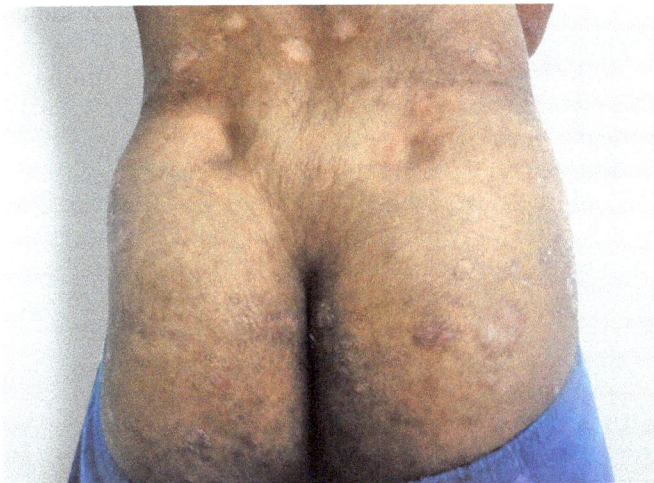

Fig. 2: Note the psoriatic plaques in the same patient as seen in **Figure 1**.

patients, demonstrable by a significant detriment to quality of life (QoL). Stress in the form of pathological worry has a deleterious effect in response to therapy. The exact mechanism by which psychological distress exacerbates or triggers psoriasis is poorly understood. May be that psychological stress has the potential to regulate the immune response and there is emerging evidence that abnormal neuroendocrine responses to stress may contribute to the pathogenesis of chronic autoimmune diseases, as has been described for rheumatoid arthritis. It is likely, that in some patients with psoriasis, there is an abnormal hypothalamic adrenal axis response to acute stress.

The "QoL" measures take into account the effect of the treatment on the patient. QoL data fulfils the role of measuring the intangible changes in a patient's life that determines "treatment success".

The Salford psoriasis index (SPI) provide an holistic assessment of overall disease severity:
- *S—Signs*: A 0-10 measure of physical severity derived from the psoriasis area and severity index (PASI)
- *P—Psychosocial disability*: Measured as 0-10 on a visual analog scale
- *I—Interventions*: A cumulative historical record of systemic therapies, episodes of erythroderma, etc.

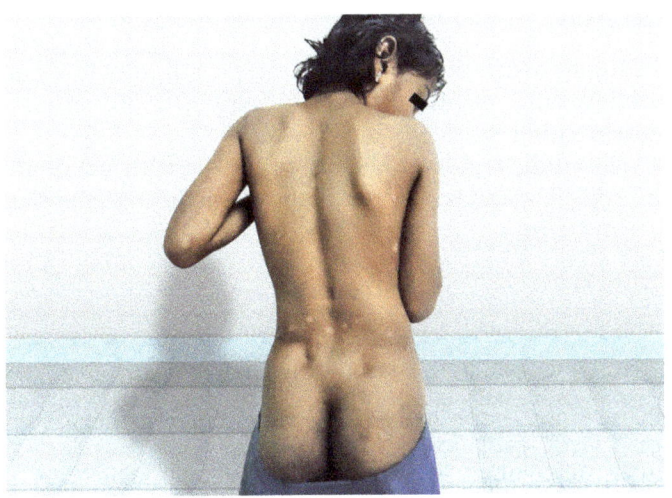

Fig. 1: Depression leading to social isolation in an adolescent with psoriasis.

The SPI is represented as three figures such as 9, 7, 6 and is a guide to the difficulty of treating any one patient at a certain time. There are many instruments to measure QoL for psoriasis and psoriatic arthritis. It does not appear that one will cover all the issues that QoL encompasses. Human leukocyte antigen (HLA)-Cw6 is found to be linked to depression in psoriatic patients.[1]

Not only dermatologists, but also general practitioners and other healthcare providers should assess the severity and impact the condition has on a person at first presentation, and before referral for specialist's advice.

This assessment should cover the impact the disease has on the physical, psychological and social well-being of those with the condition.

The severity of disease should also be assessed, as should the presence of comorbid conditions.

Risk factors for cardiovascular comorbidities should be discussed with people who have any type of psoriasis. The patient's caretaker or the parent, as the case may be, should be adequately informed about the consequences.

Tailored advice and healthy lifestyle information, and support for behavioral change should be provided. All possible measures must be taken to advice on lifestyle modification and to prevent comorbidity, especially obesity and type 2 diabetes mellitus.

COURSE AND PROGNOSIS

Course and prognosis of psoriasis still remains unpredictable despite the enormous development that has taken place in the understanding of the disease and its consequences. It is not possible to predict neither the duration of the disease nor the period of remission. Though guttate psoriasis tends to carry a better prognosis, most of them eventually end up in psoriasis vulgaris sooner or later.

At the other extreme, erythrodermic and pustular forms carry an appreciable mortality and arthropathic forms a considerable morbidity. Early onset and a family history of the disease appear to worsen the prognosis. Stress in any form seems to precipitate, exacerbate or worsen psoriasis.

Relapse is the rule, however completely the lesions are treated and by whatever method. Despite the advent of new biological agents, it has not been possible to assure any patient a complete cure. If only the clinician is able to prevent the march of psoriasis and reduce the incidence of resultant comorbidity, will there be justification in treating any given patient, be it an infant, child, adolescent or an adult young or old.

FOLLOW-UP AND REHABILITATION

Psoriasis by itself is a disease that causes a lot of psychological stress and vice versa.

Psoriasis was recently shown to have a great impact on QoL, even in affected children. Like atopic dermatitis, urticaria and acne, psoriasis in the pediatric age group can lead to a severe emotional burden to the extent of impairing the health-related QoL. A study on children and adolescents aged between 5 years and 16 years found that in children with psoriasis the values were as high as in children with atopic dermatitis, and higher than in children with urticaria or acne.[2]

The afflicted children must learn to cope with life and to adapt to their individual health situation. They must be counseled to choose a profession suitable for them in future. Rehabilitation of psoriatic children and adolescents can also supplement therapy and prevent the disease.[3]

Therapy goals of rehabilitation will include:
- Regular treatment of the skin under proper supervision clubbed with climate therapy, nutritional therapy and psychological interventions.
- Help in coping with the disease with respect to the psychosocial consequences of psoriasis.
- Help in finding an occupation.

Accurate assessment of people with psoriasis will ensure they can access the right treatment, as early as possible, whether in primary or specialist care.

Psoriasis patients must be given enough time in the consultation chamber, either by the physician or a counselor, who takes time to explain the patients to cope with the disease with ease and learn to live with the disease at the same time try to control it. This will not only improve the QoL of the patient but also reduce the financial burden in the form of treatment.

Following are some of the aspects that can be given importance:

Good Nourishment

A balanced protein rich diet and complete abstinence from alcohol will go a long way in maintaining the remission.

Effective Management of Day-to-day Stress

Regular meditation and or exercise will alleviate the anxiety and reduce stress thereby will prevent an exacerbation.
- Planning regular holidays to places with adequate sunshine and ample relaxation will help calm the skin and mind.

Wearing Ideal Clothing and to be Cautious during Winter

Loose fitting cotton cloth will be comfortable and help avoid friction due to tight fitting garments.
- To get exposed to sunlight as much as possible and using moisturizers liberally will help prevent an exacerbation.

To Build Self-esteem

Patients must be made to believe that they are not their disease. They should be helped to find a support group of people (locally or online) who are coping positively with their condition. Periodic meeting in person with such group will be beneficial to all in a positive manner.

We, the healthcare providers have the duty to see that every patient with psoriasis is helped to live his/her normal span of life in perfect health.

REFERENCES

1. Gudjónsson JE, Kárason A, Antonsdóttir AA, et al. HLA-Cw6-positive and HLA-Cw6-negative patients with Psoriasis vulgaris have distinct clinical features. J Invest Dermatol. 2002;118(2):362-5.
2. Beattie PE, Lewis-Jones MS. A comparative study of impairment of quality of life in children with skin disease and children with other chronic diseases. Br J Dermatol. 2006;155:145-51.
3. Sticherling M, Augustin M, Boehncke WH, et al. Therapy of psoriasis in childhood and adolescence: a German expert consensus. JDDG. 2011;9:815-23.

Dermoscopy in Psoriasis

INTRODUCTION[1,2]

Dermoscopy, a noninvasive diagnostic tool facilitates the diagnosis of "Psoriasis". It not only helps in the early detection of the disease but also in differentiating psoriasis from close mimickers. The use of "Dermoscopy" can be extended in assessing the response of the psoriatic plaques to topical and systemic drugs. By using dermoscopic findings one can detect subclinical side effects of topical steroids. Although diagnosis of psoriasis is clinical and does not require biopsy, atypical presentations, modified conditions like eczematized lesions pose diagnostic difficulty. Under such challenging situations, the diagnosis of psoriasis can be easily confirmed with the help of dermoscopy.[1] In this chapter, common dermoscopic findings of different types of psoriasis will be described. Trichoscopy and onychoscopy help in differentiating scalp and nail psoriasis from other common similar disorders of scalp and nail. Pink background, scales, and uniform red dots are the most common dermoscopic features of psoriasis as shown in **Figure 1**.[2]

FEATURES OF PSORIASIS OF SKIN[3-8] (FIGS. 2 TO 80)

Background

The background of psoriatic plaque is usually a pink homogenous background. However, it can be of different shades of pink or red. However, not demonstrable in all cases of palmoplantar psoriasis. Yellowish or gray-blue background can be observed when there is overlap or coexistence of eczema or lichen planus with psoriasis. Chronic plaque treated psoriasis can have a background of brown, black, or brownish black.

Different background colors observed in psoriasis are:
- Light pink
- Dull pink
- Dark pink
- Light red
- Dark red
- Yellowish
- Gray-blue

However, background color assessment is subjective and highly variable. The pressure of the instrument may to a great extent devascularize the plaque and modify the background color. This can be overcome by using computational methods which is in use for pigmented lesions.

Vascular Findings

The most frequent vascular findings of psoriasis involving skin include red dots and globules. Red dots and globules were demonstrated by both handheld dermoscope and video-dermoscope in nearly 97–100% of cases.

The distribution of these vascular structures varies from case-to-case and from plaque-to-plaque in the same patient. Following are some of the patterns of distribution of vascular dots:

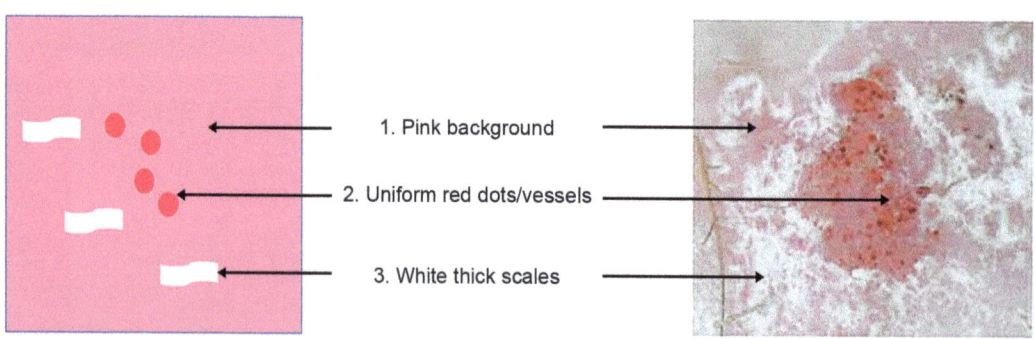

Fig. 1: Important dermoscopic findings of psoriasis.

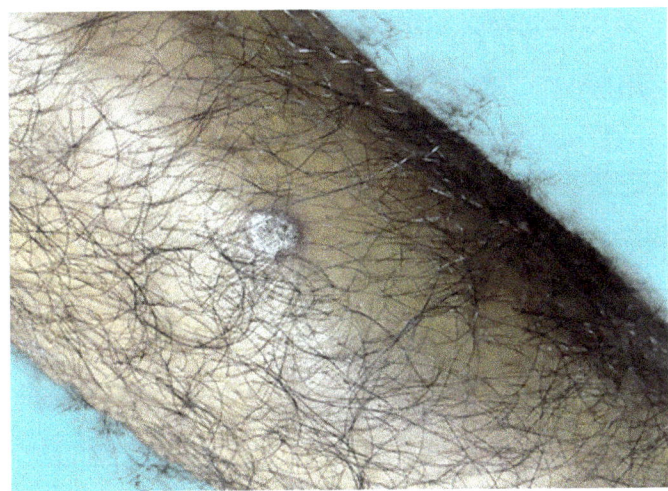

Fig. 2: Scaly plaque of psoriasis on hairy skin.

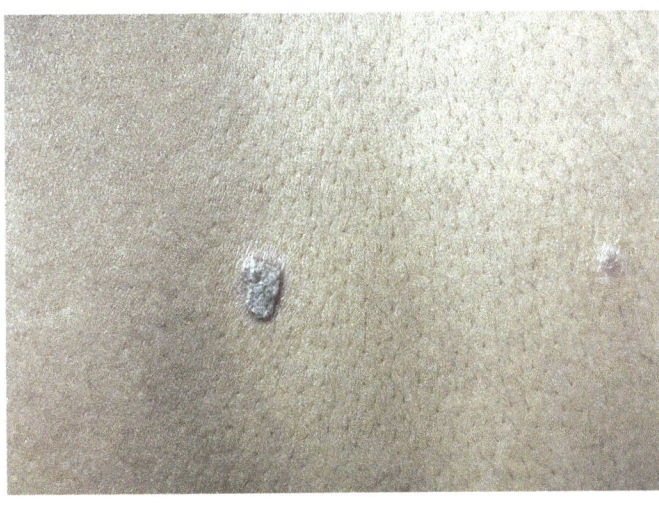

Fig. 5: Guttate psoriasis over back.

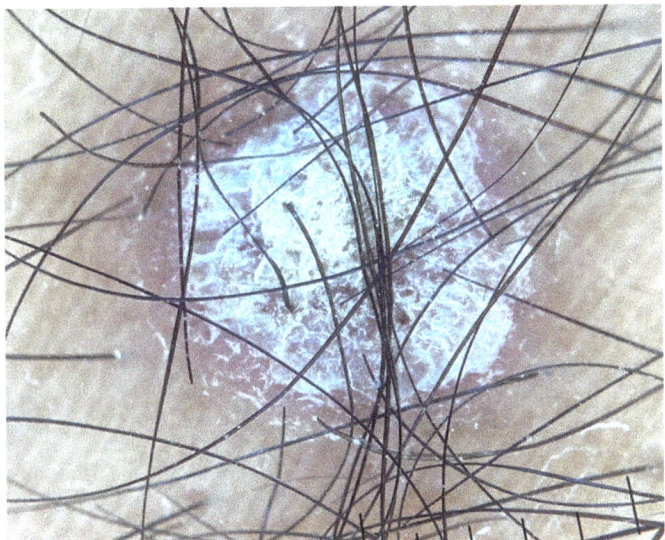

Fig. 3: Dermoscopy before removal of scale.

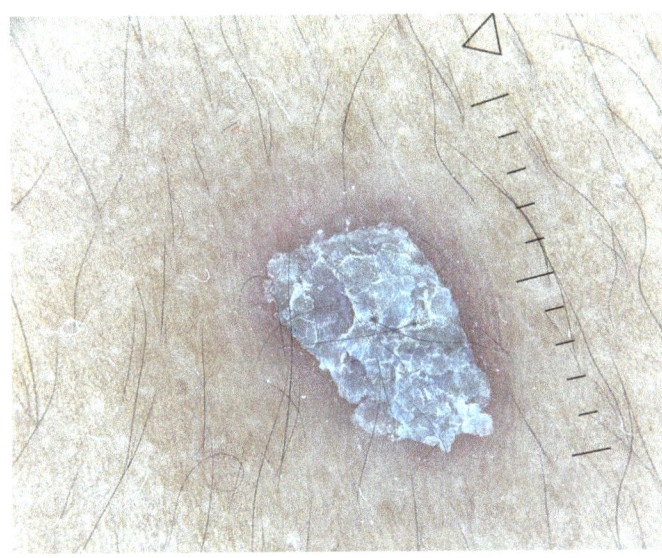

Fig. 6: Dermoscopy before removal of scales.

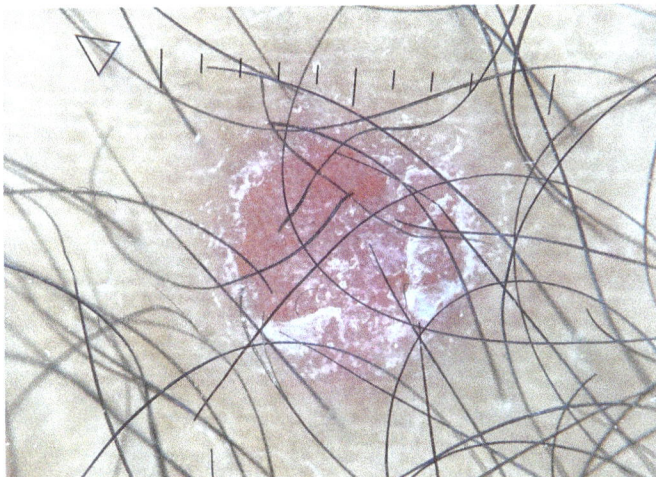

Fig. 4: Dermoscopy of plaque over hairy skin after removal of scale showing uniform pink.

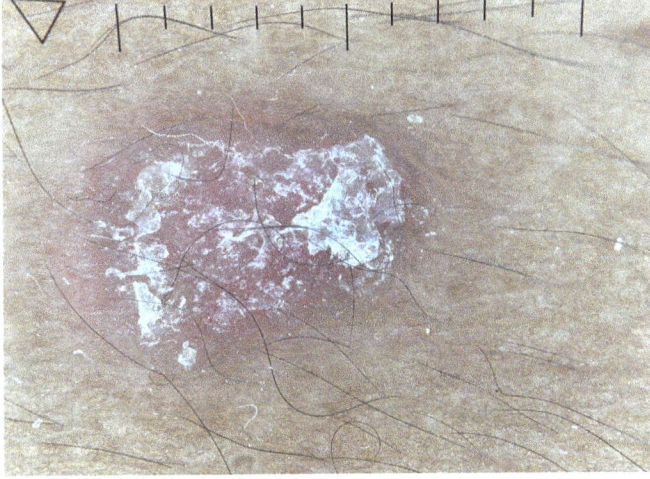

Fig. 7: Dermoscopy of plaque over nonhairy skin after removal of scale showing uniform pink.

CHAPTER 13 Dermoscopy in Psoriasis

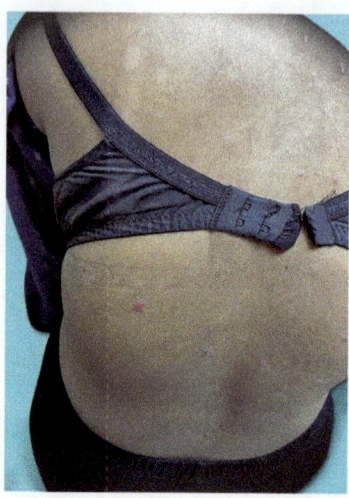

Fig. 8: Patient with early, evolved, and resolved psoriatic papule.

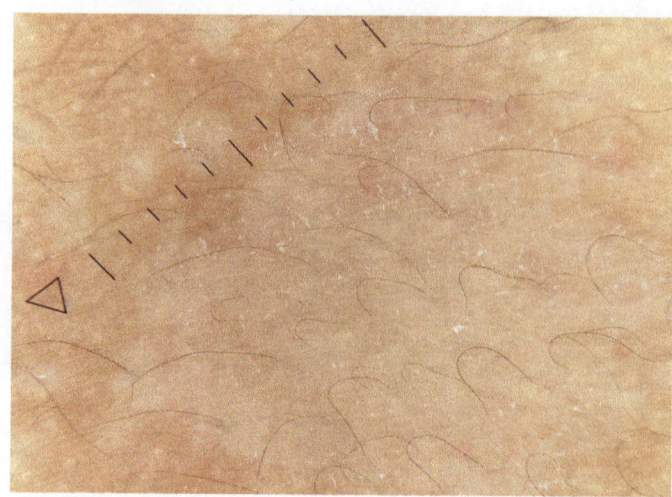

Fig. 11: Dermoscopy of resolved papule showing reduced pigment network.

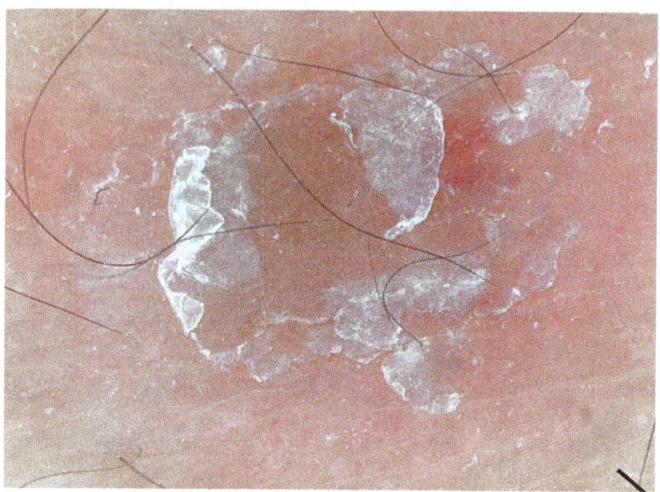

Fig. 9: Psoriasis early papule with pink background and scaling.

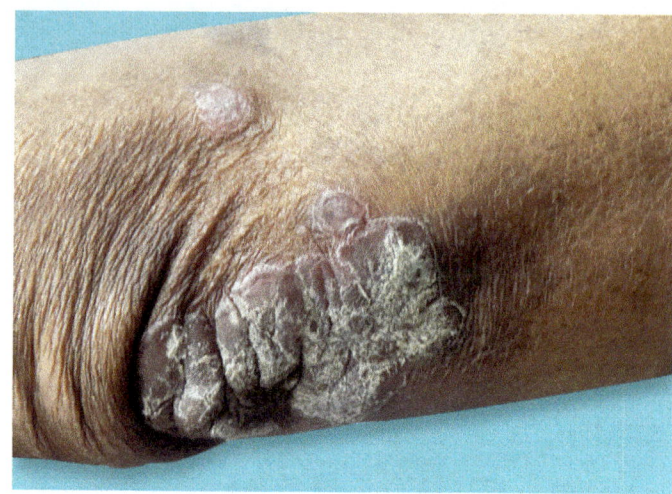

Fig. 12: Psoriasis elbow.

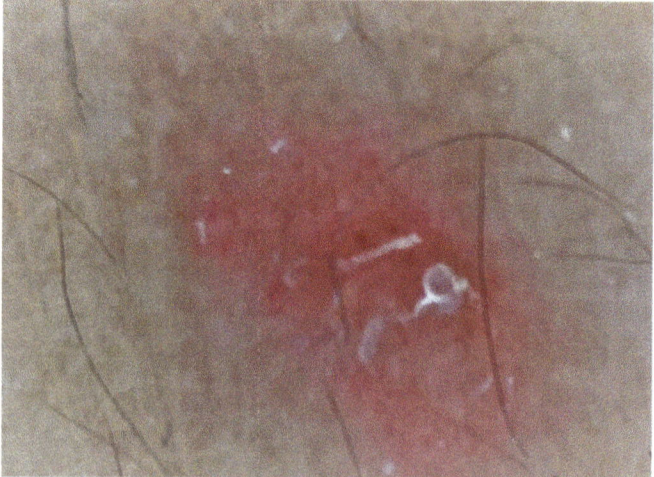

Fig. 10: Psoriasis evolved papule showing pink background scales and dotted vessels.

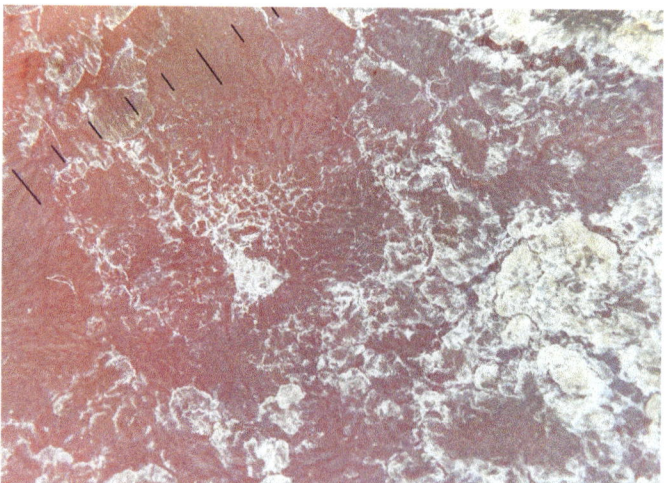

Fig. 13: Image showing pink background and diffuse scales with honeycomb pattern in some areas.

CHAPTER 13 Dermoscopy in Psoriasis **123**

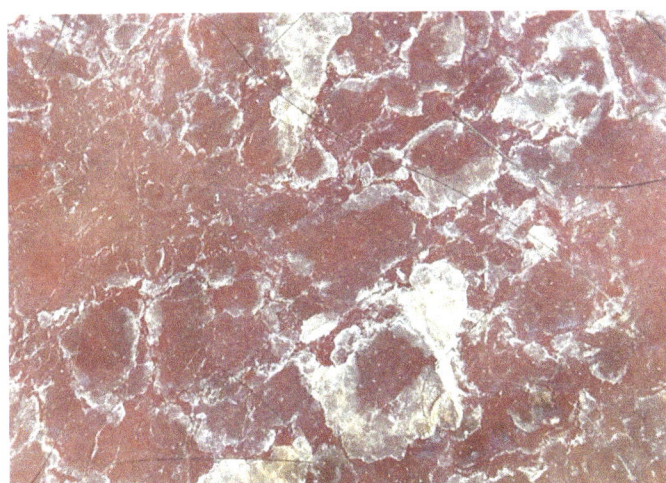

Fig. 14: Whitish patchy scales.

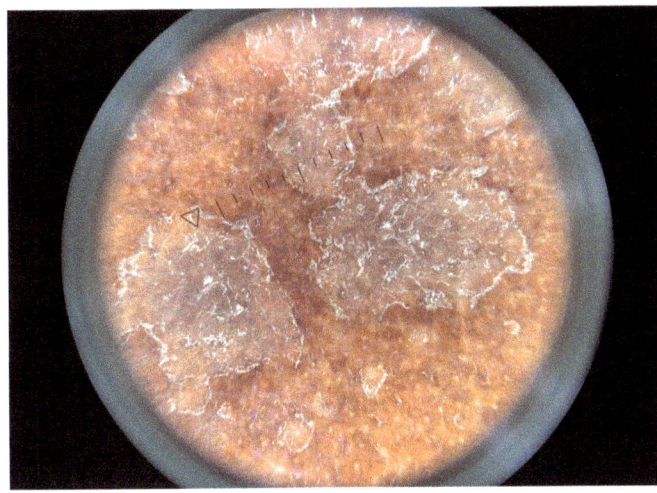

Fig. 17: Varying background and patchy scaling: Note white globules.

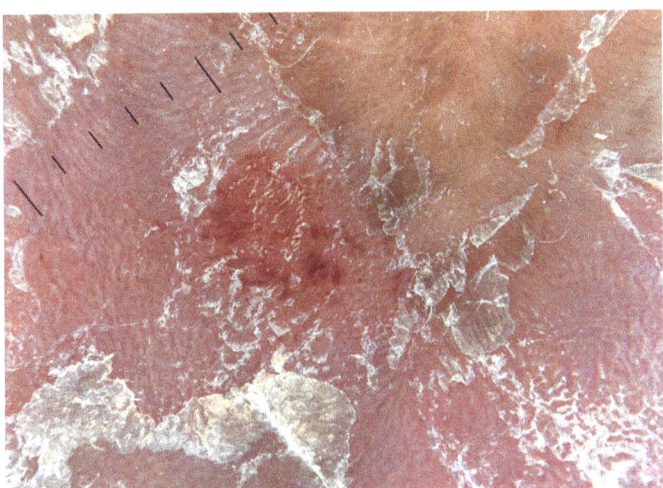

Fig. 15: Linear and dotted vessels.

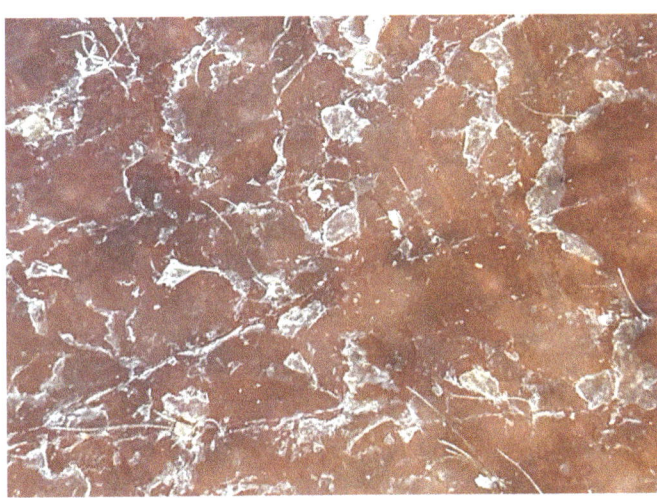

Fig. 18: White streak and diffuse scales.

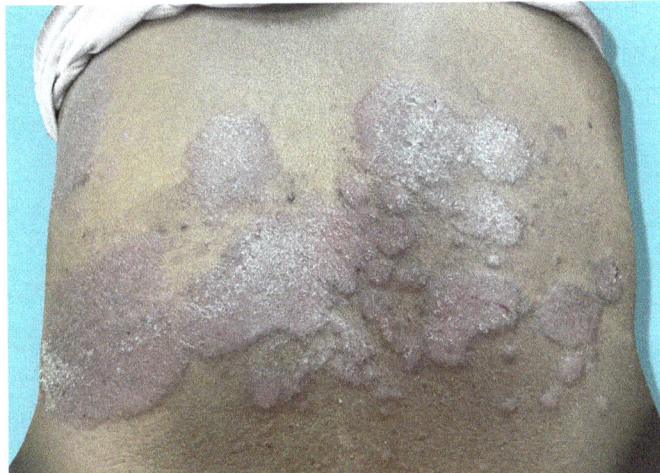

Fig. 16: Chronic plaque psoriasis.

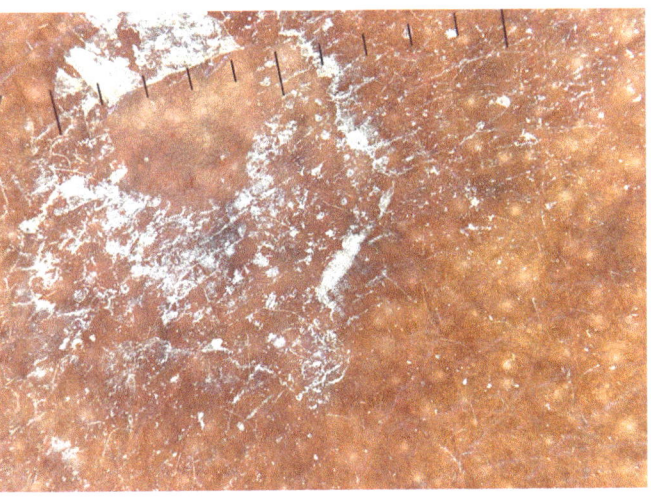

Fig. 19: Prominent eccrine opening white structureless areas.

CHAPTER 13 Dermoscopy in Psoriasis

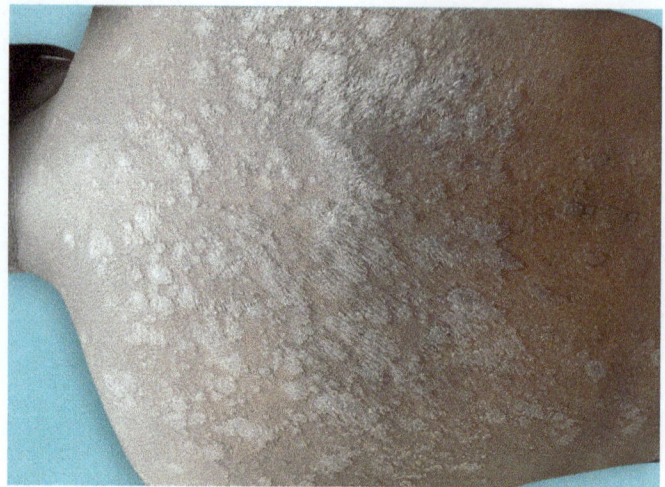

Fig. 20: Exacerbation of plaques over back.

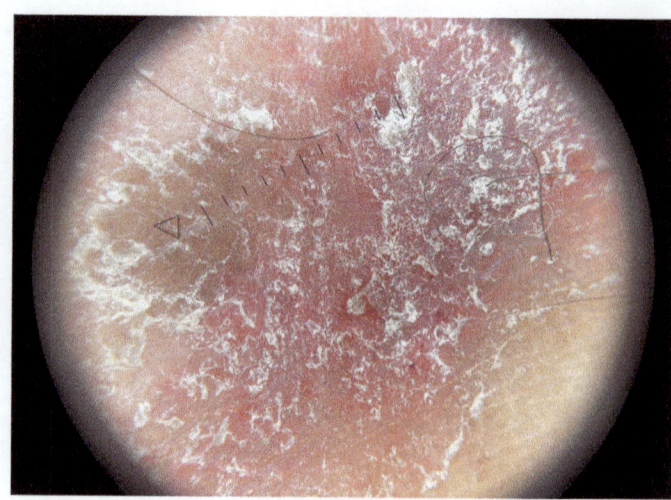

Fig. 23: Pink background with uniform white dotted vessels and scaling.

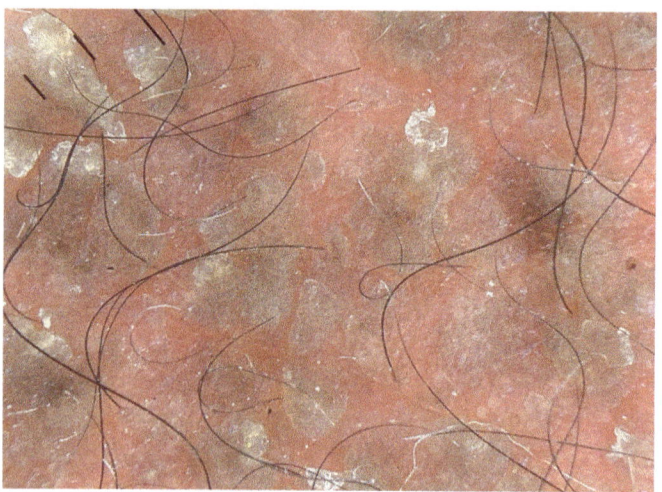

Fig. 21: Different types of scale in same site on pink background.

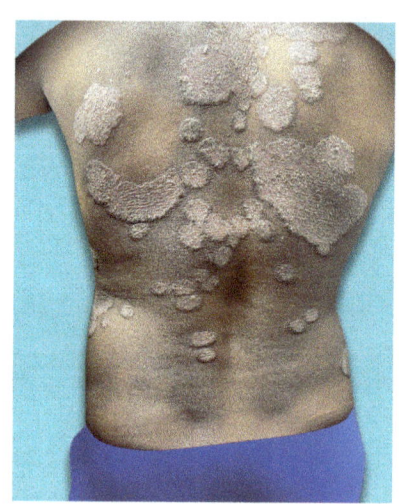

Fig. 24: Resistant plaque psoriasis.

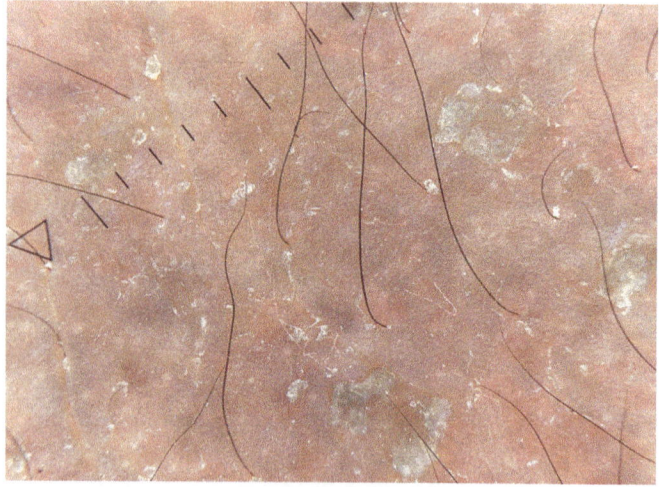

Fig. 22: Pink background dernd minimal scales.

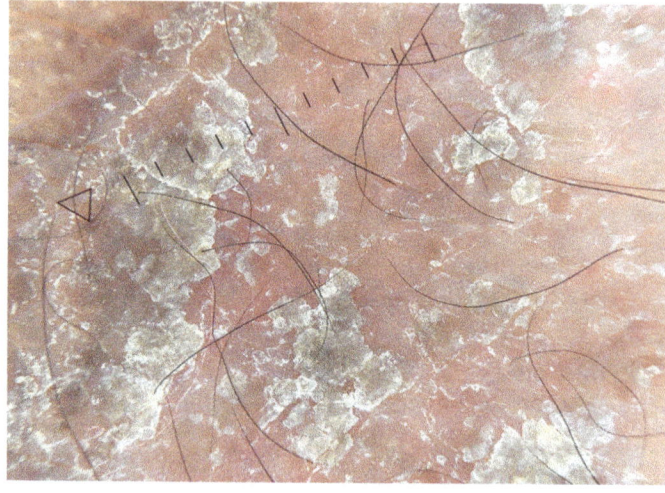

Fig. 25: Thick yellowish white scale masking other findings.

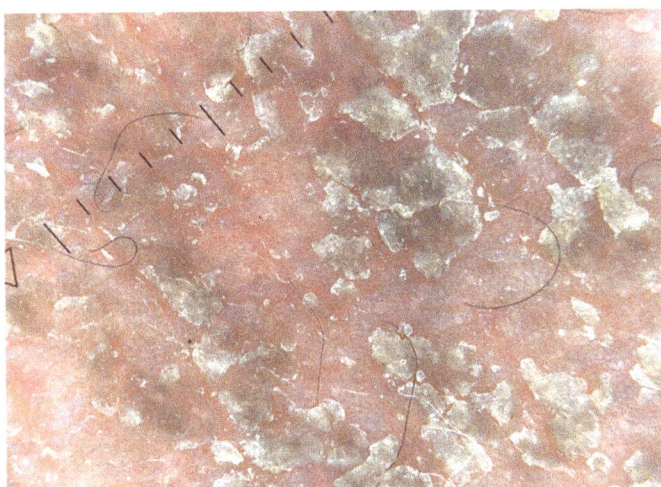

Fig. 26: Grayish and pink background with yellowish diffuse scaling.

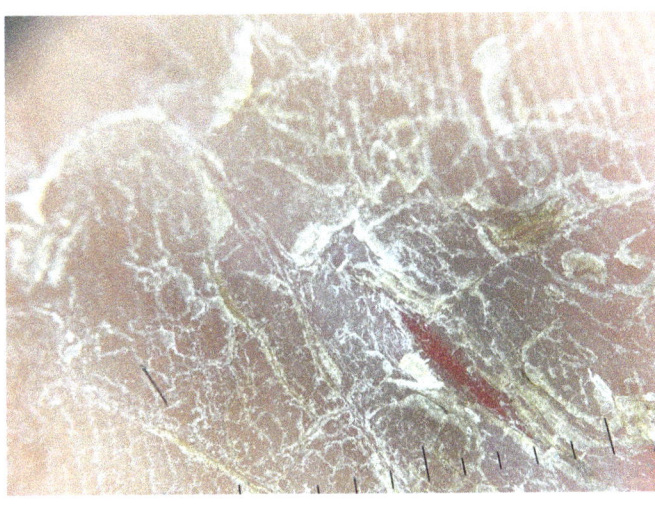

Fig. 29: Scaling and pink fissure. Note: Absent dotted vessels.

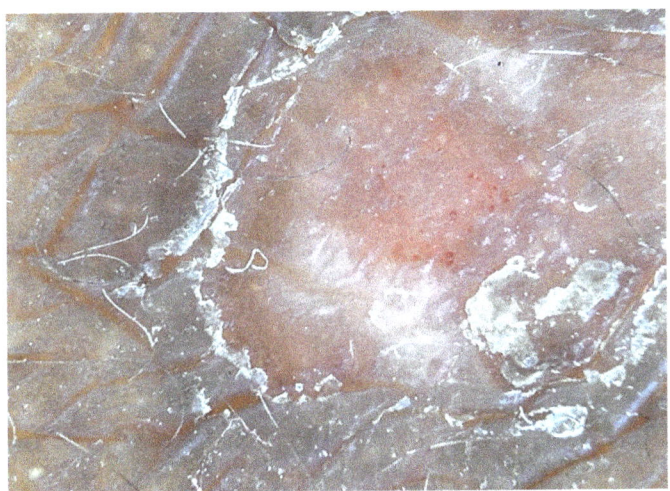

Fig. 27: Multiple dotted vessels and white structureless areas.

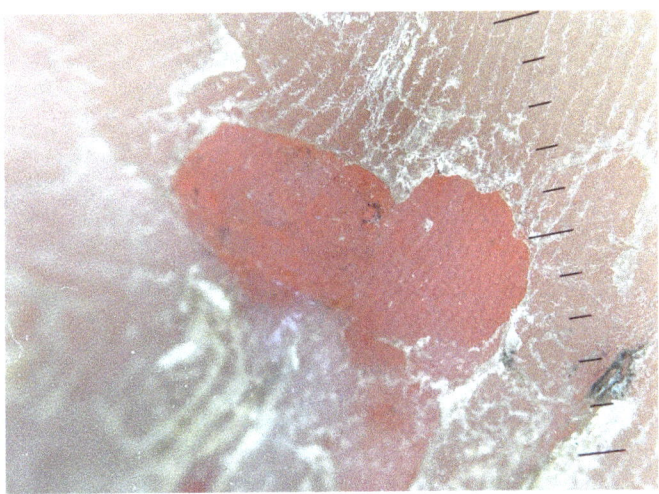

Fig. 30: Pink irregular erosion with few dotted vessels surrounding white scales.

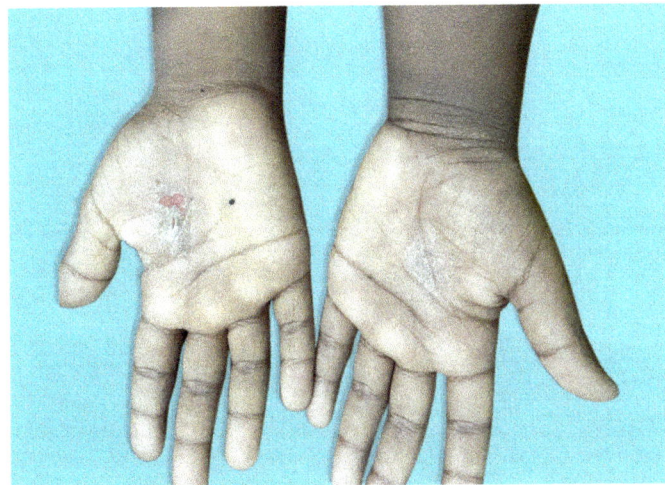

Fig. 28: Psoriasis of palm in a boy.

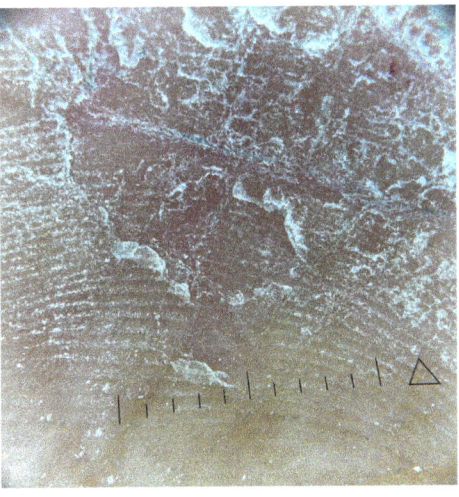

Fig. 31: Diffuse scaling on erythematous background; note the dotted vessel.

CHAPTER 13 Dermoscopy in Psoriasis

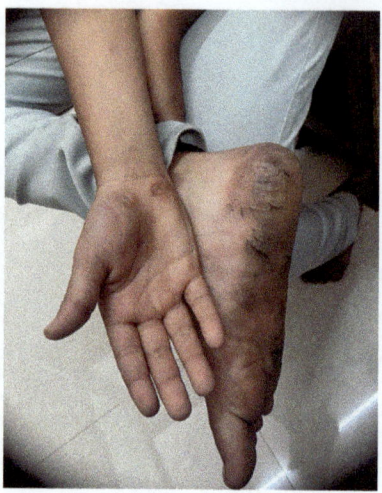

Fig. 32: Palmoplantar psoriasis adult.

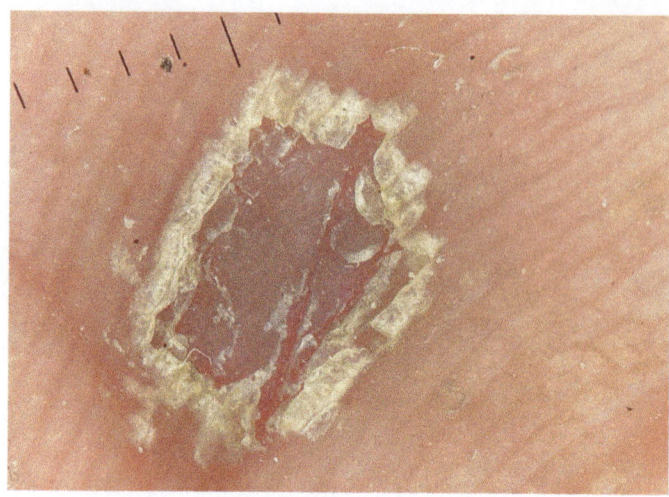

Fig. 35: Silvery white peripheral scales with linear fissure.

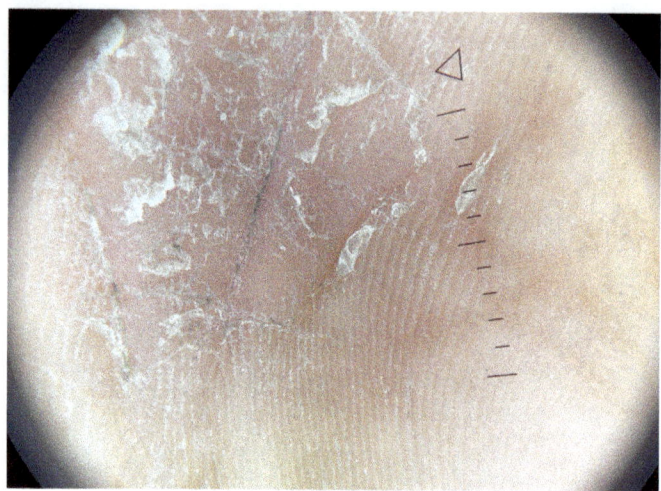

Fig. 33: Diffuse scaling surrounding normal skin lacks scaling.

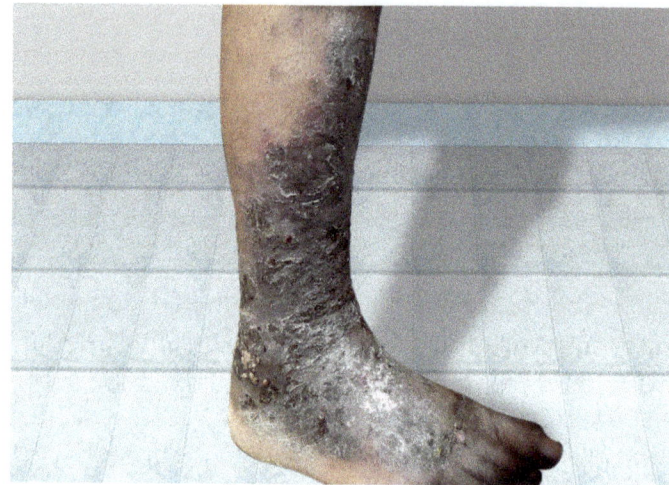

Fig. 36: Psoriasis: eczema overlap.

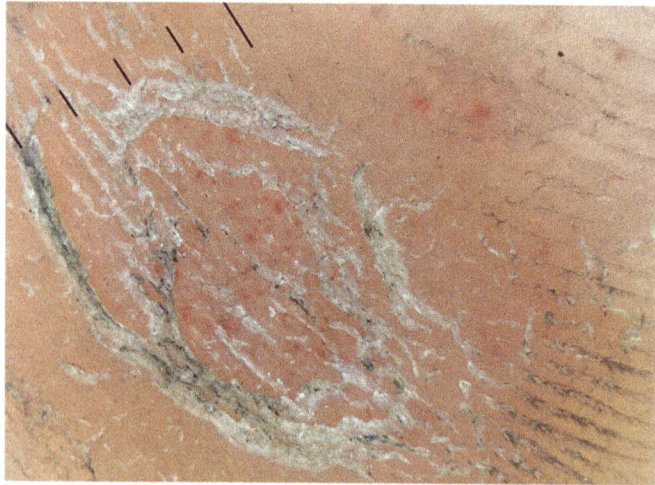

Fig. 34: Focal peripheral scaling.

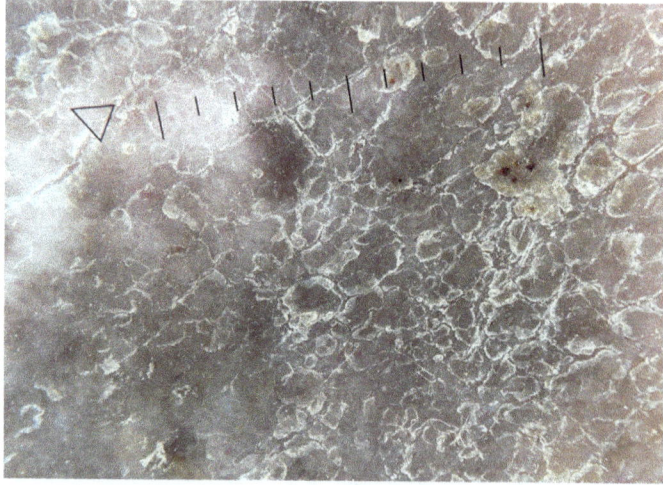

Fig. 37: Yellowish and grayish scales.

CHAPTER 13 Dermoscopy in Psoriasis 127

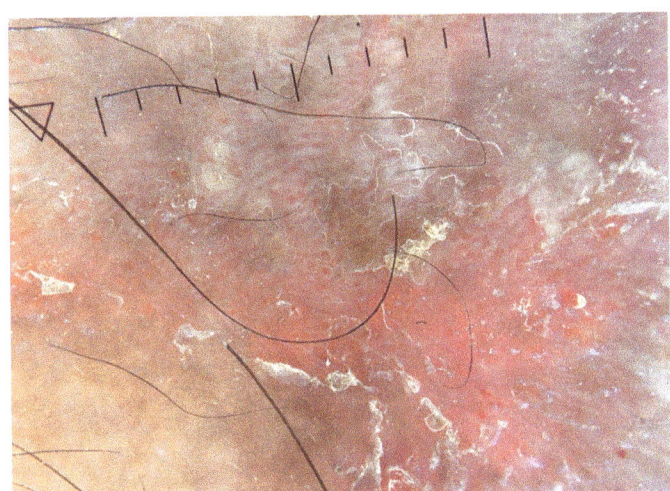

Fig. 38: Pink background white scales and dotted vessels.

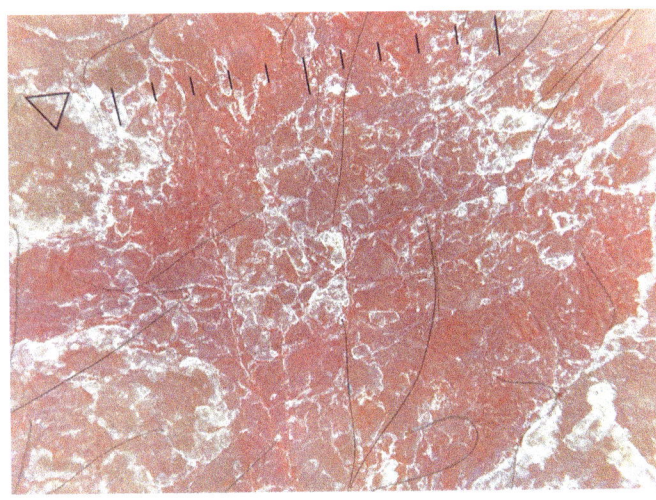

Fig. 41: Central erythema with regular dotted vessels and white scales.

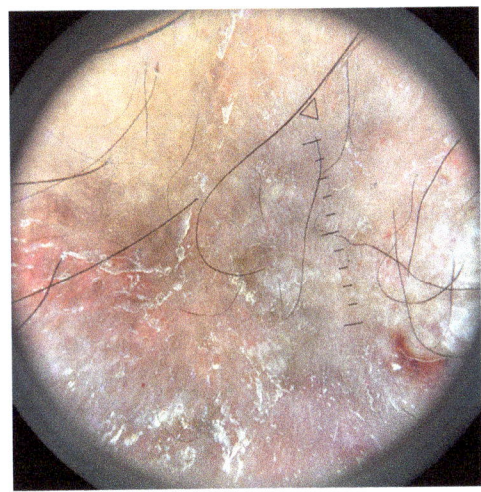

Fig. 39: Pink, yellow, and grayish background scattered dotted vessels.

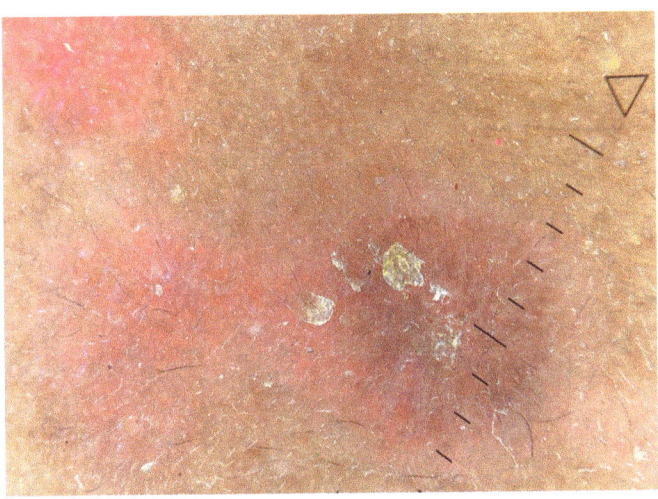

Fig. 42: Scattered dotted vessels and blotchy pink background.

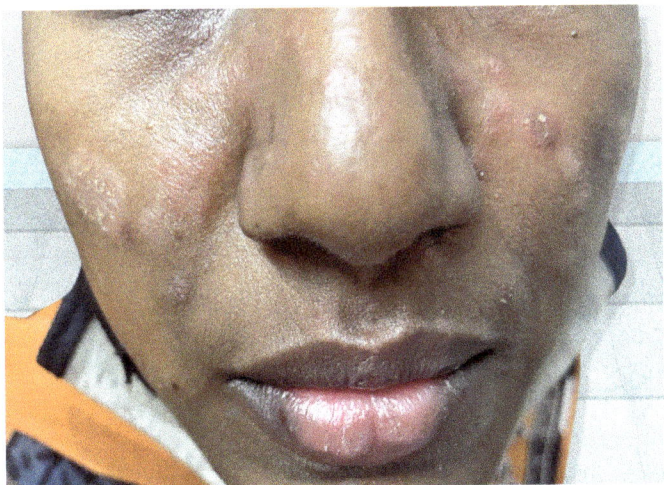

Fig. 40: Psoriasis: Over butterfly area.

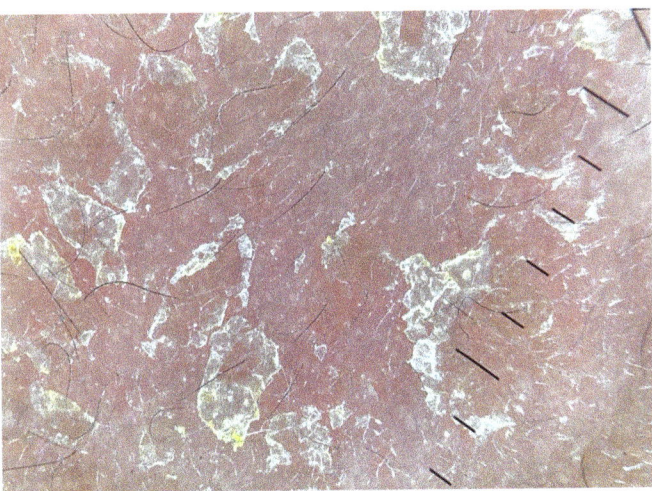

Fig. 43: Clustered scales and dotted vessels.

CHAPTER 13 Dermoscopy in Psoriasis

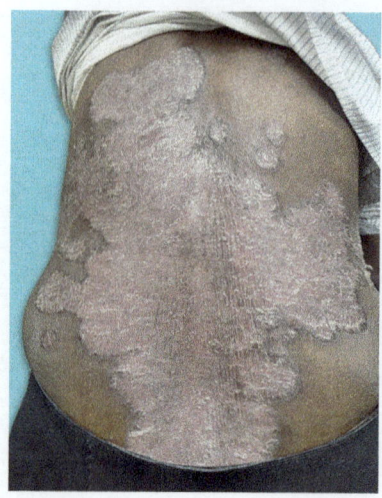

Fig. 44: Psoriatic plaque over back impending erythroderma.

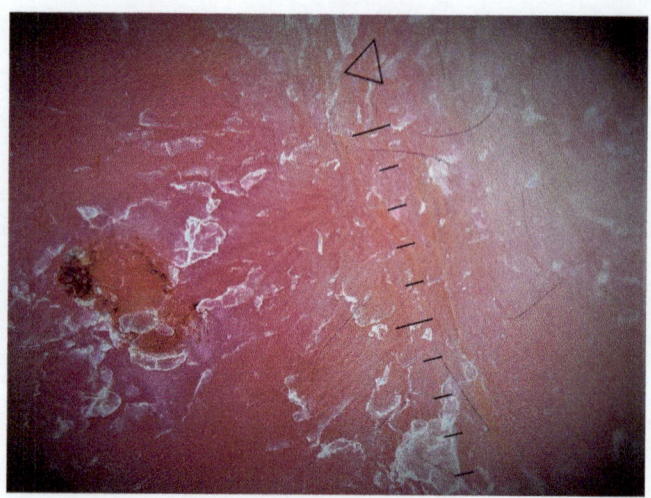

Fig. 47: Pinkish background hemorrhagic spots.

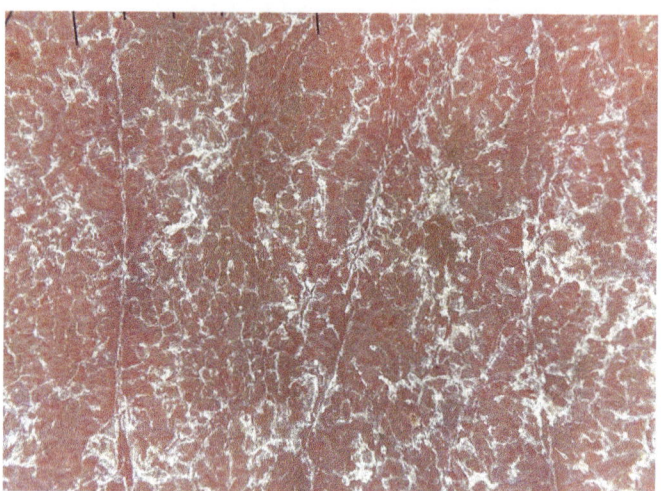

Fig. 45: Pink background diffuse scales white streaky lines.

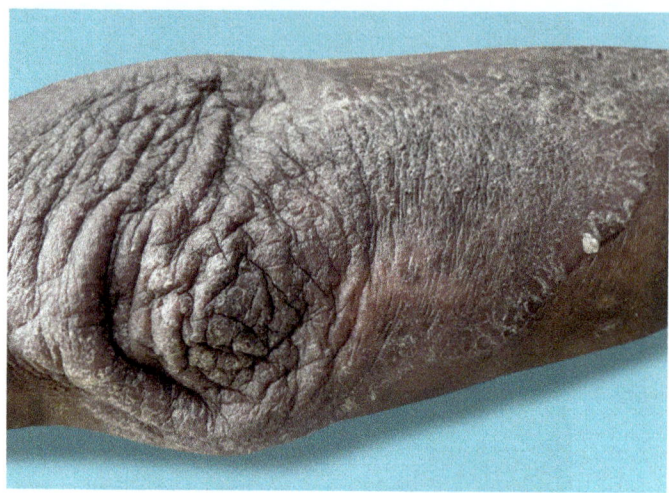

Fig. 48: Psoriatic plaque over elbow impending erythroderma.

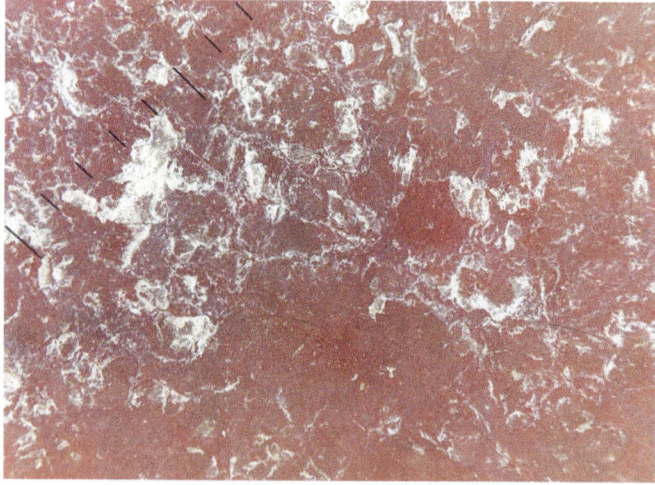

Fig. 46: Uniform pinkish red background dotted vessels in clusters.

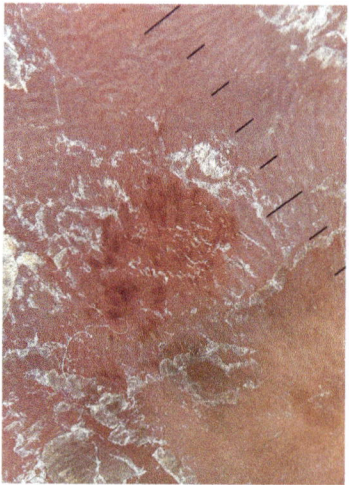

Fig. 49: Pink background ripple-like pattern linear hemorrhagic spots white scales.

CHAPTER 13 Dermoscopy in Psoriasis

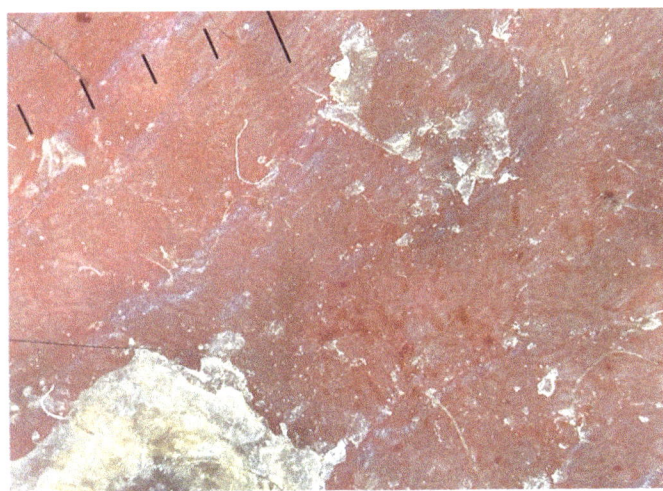

Fig. 50: Pink background thick and thin scales scattered dotted vessels.

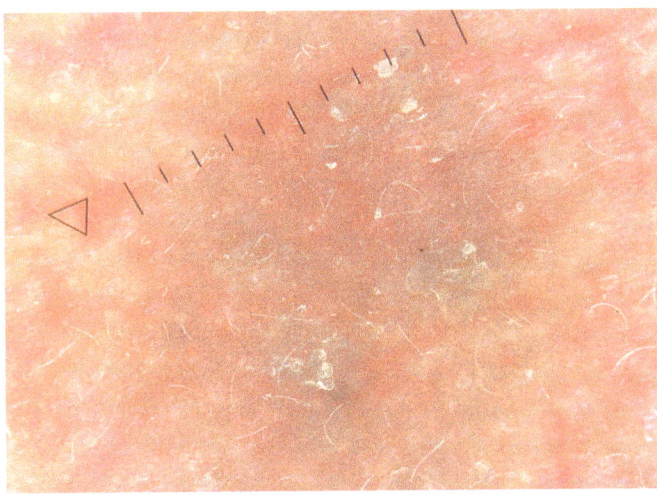

Fig. 53: Pink background scales, note there are no dotted vessels.

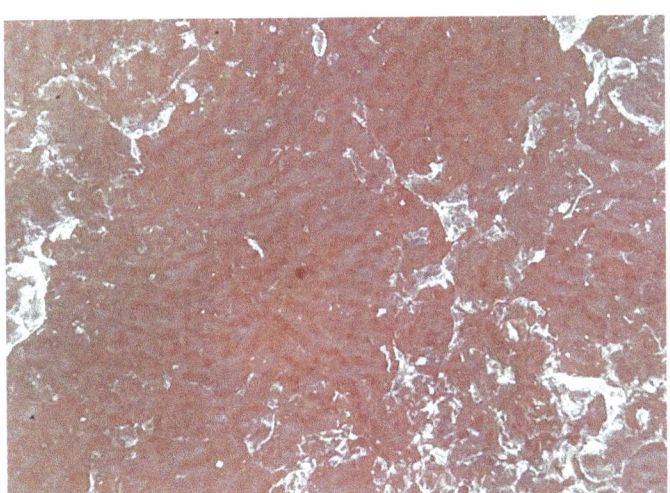

Fig. 51: Pink background ripple-like pattern dotted vessel.

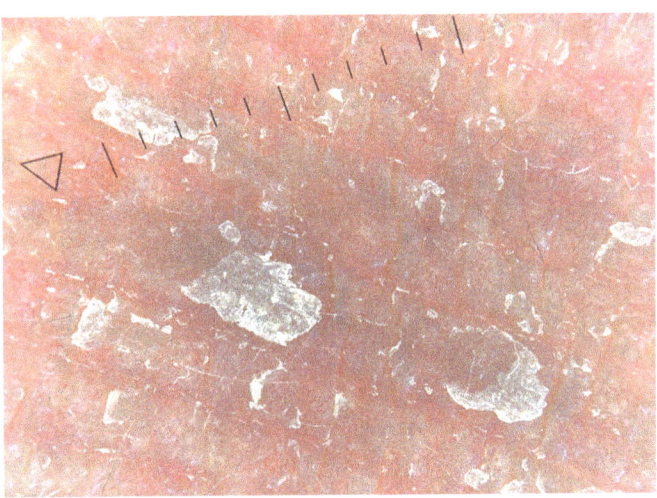

Fig. 54: Grayish background whitish scale.

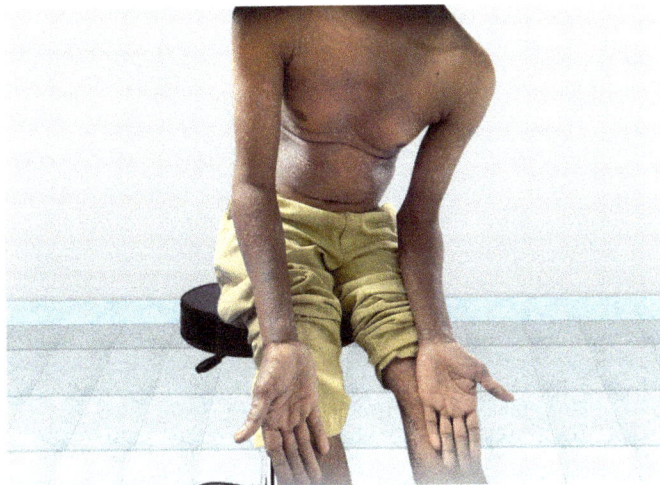

Fig. 52: Psoriatic erythroderma.

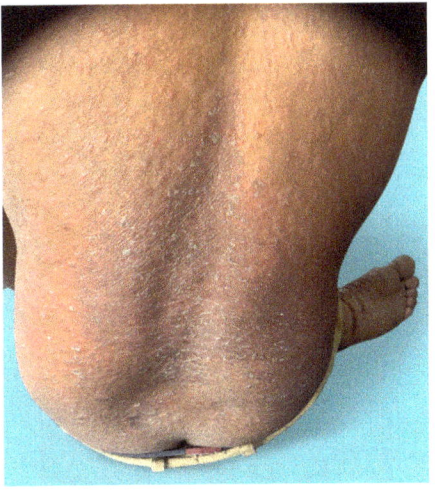

Fig. 55: Psoriatic erythroderma back.

CHAPTER 13 Dermoscopy in Psoriasis

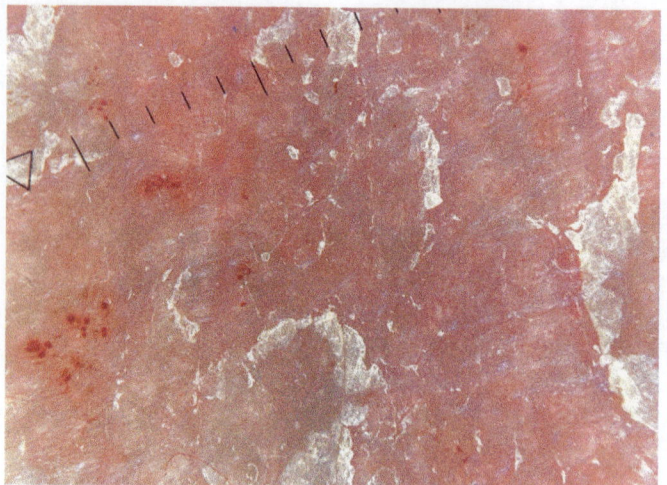

Fig. 56: Pink background dotted vessels hemorrhagic spots.

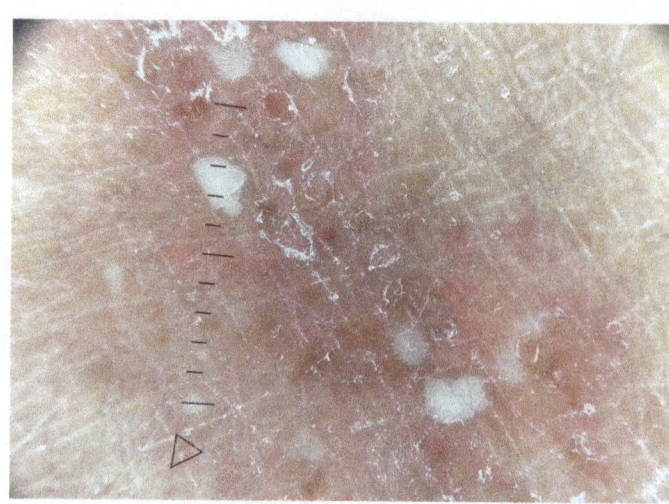

Fig. 59: Scattered pustule on pink background.

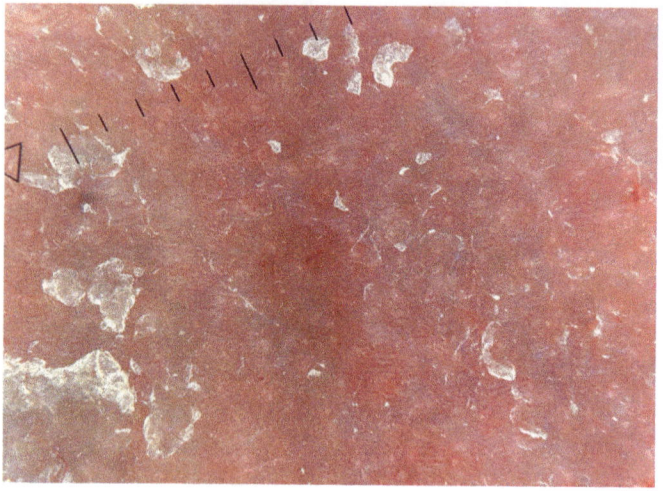

Fig. 57: Reddish background ripple-like pattern dotted vessels white scales.

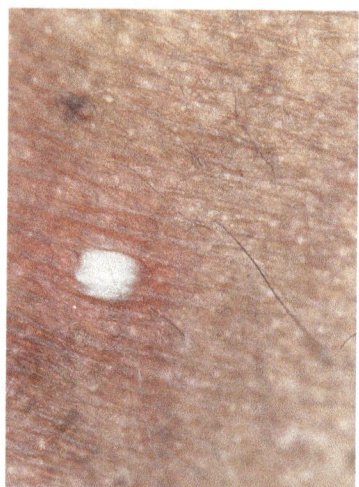

Fig. 60: Pustule with surrounding erythema.

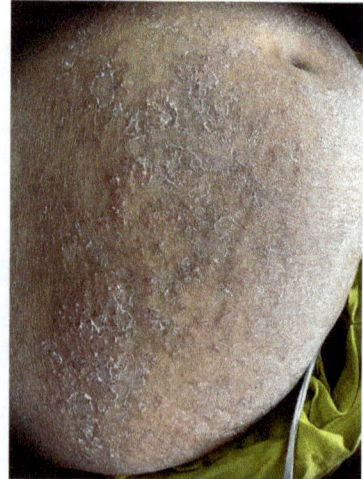

Fig. 58: Pustular psoriasis.

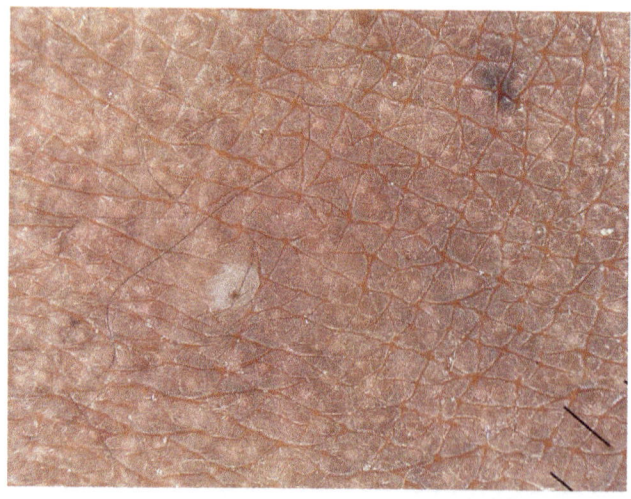

Fig. 61: Pustule with follicular localization indicating folliculitis.

CHAPTER 13 Dermoscopy in Psoriasis

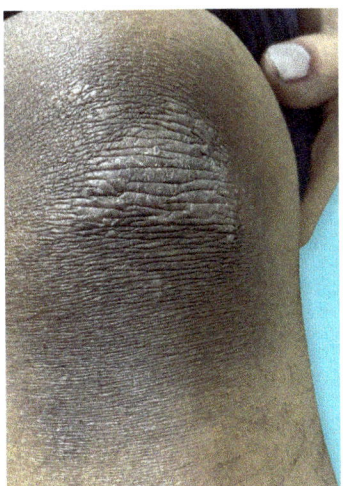

Fig. 62: Psoriasis before treatment.

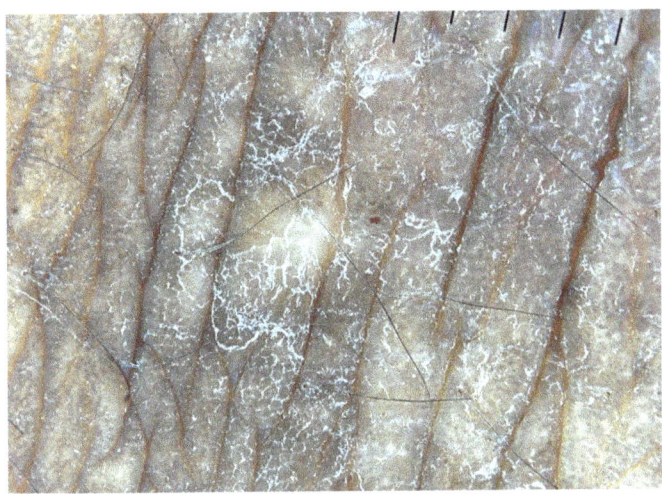

Fig. 65: 6 days after topical cortico steroid much reduction in scales single-dotted vessels.

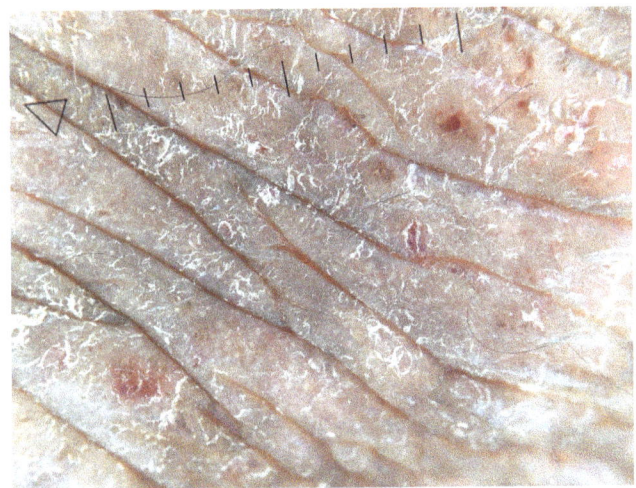

Fig. 63: Psoriasis before treatment greyish background dotted vessel hemorrhagic dot white structureless areas.

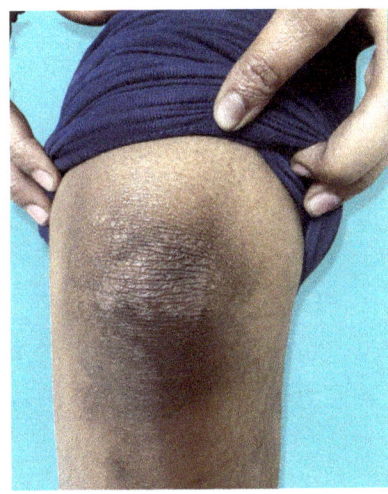

Fig. 66: 10 days after topical cortico steroid almost cleared.

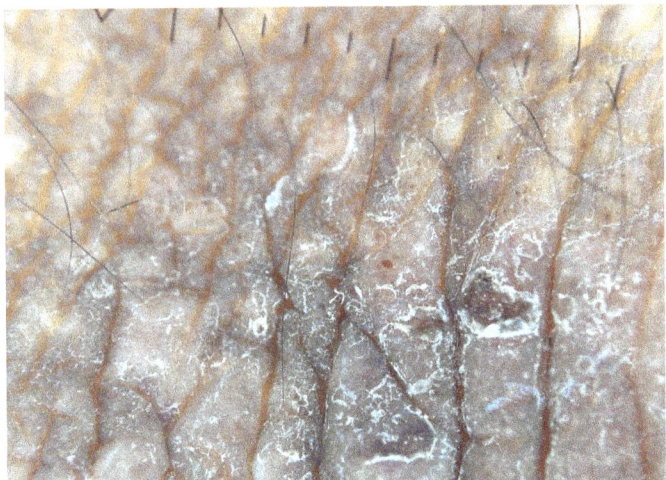

Fig. 64: 3 days after topical cortico steroid reduction in scaling and hemorrhagic vessels.

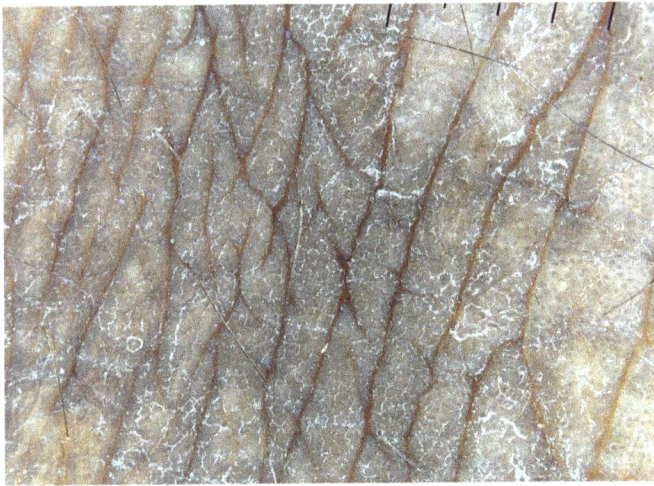

Fig. 67: 10 days after judicious use of topical cortico steroid no side effect.

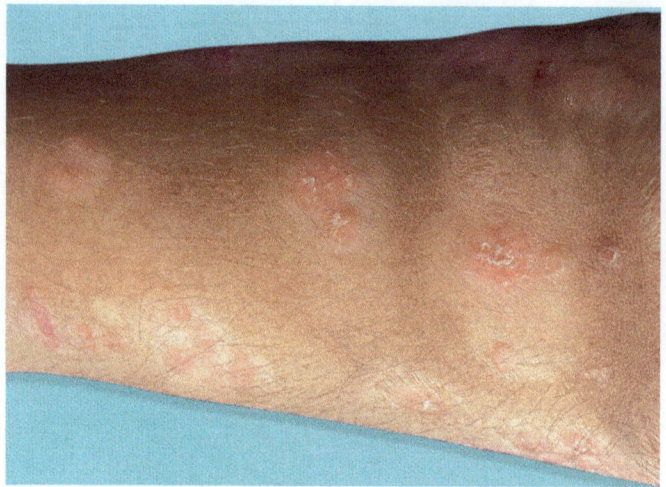

Fig. 68: Hypopigmentation and atrophy following topical corticosteroid.

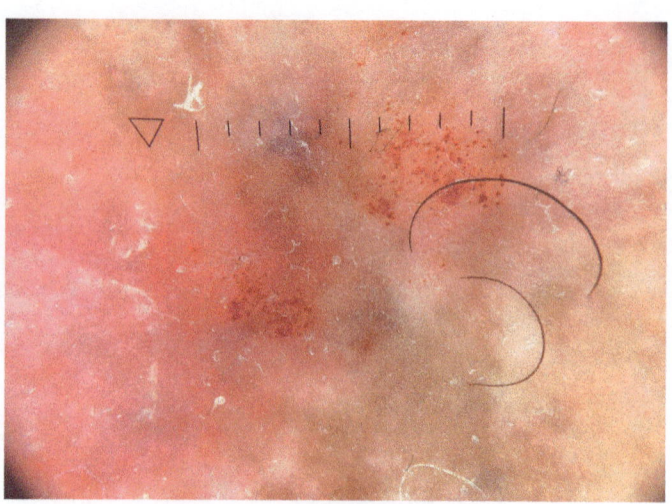

Fig. 71: Image showing multiple hemorrhagic vessels, an indicator of response to therapy (same patient as **Fig. 70**).

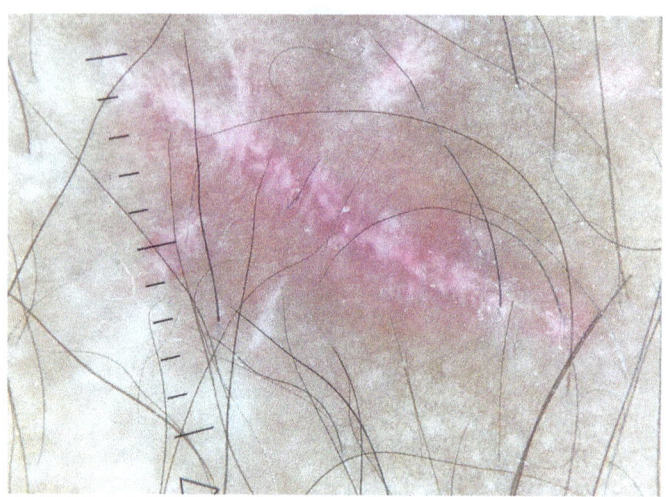

Fig. 69: Pink linear shiny structure indicating stria.

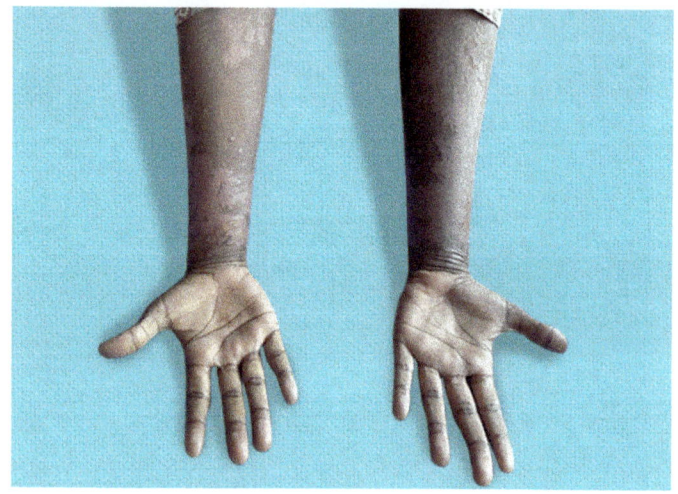

Fig. 72: Psoriasis on etanercept.

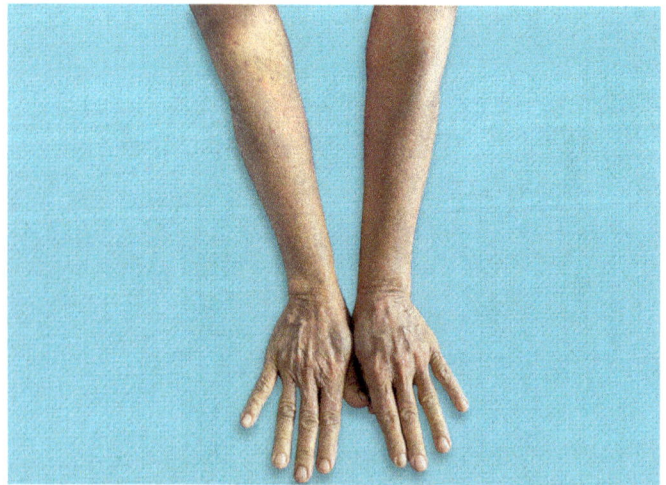

Fig. 70: Psoriasis on etanercept.

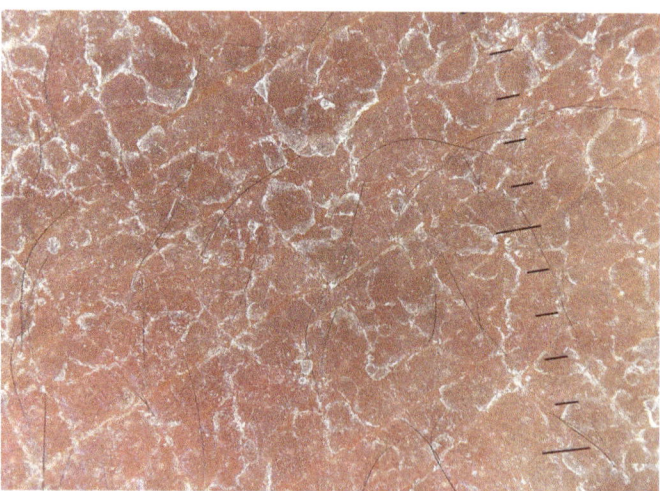

Fig. 73: Disappearance of pink background and dotted vessels (same patient as **Fig. 72**).

CHAPTER 13 Dermoscopy in Psoriasis **133**

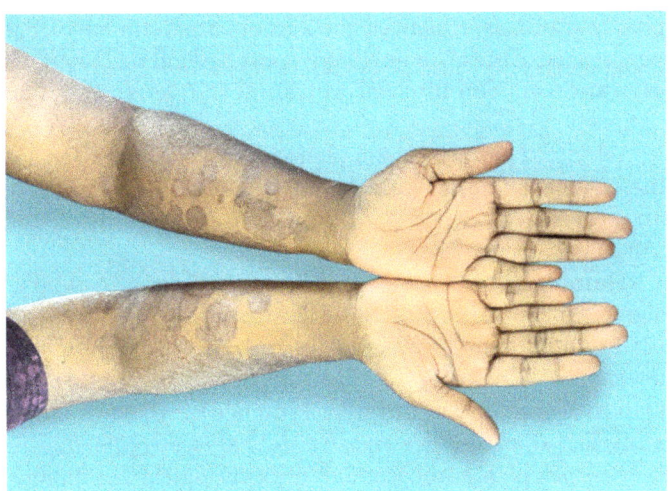

Fig. 74: Psoriasis etanercept.

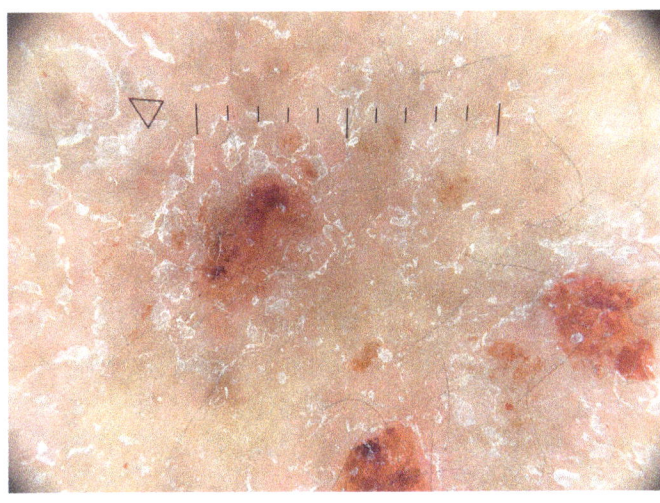

Fig. 77: Multiple hemorrhagic dots (same patient as **Fig. 76**).

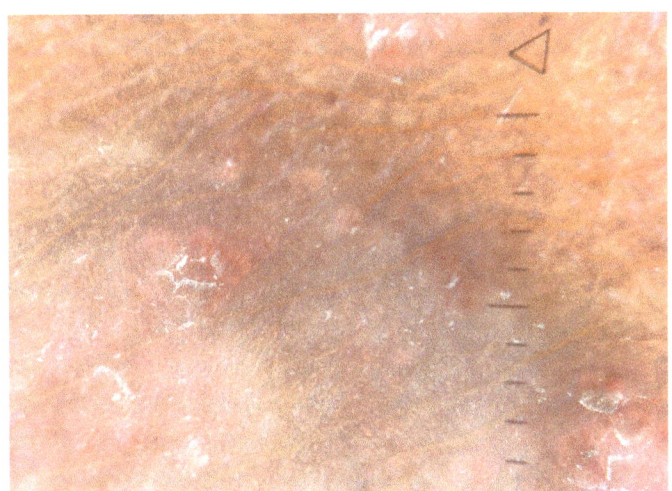

Fig. 75: Image shows eccrine opening white structureless areas absent pink background dotted vessels (same patient as **Fig. 74**).

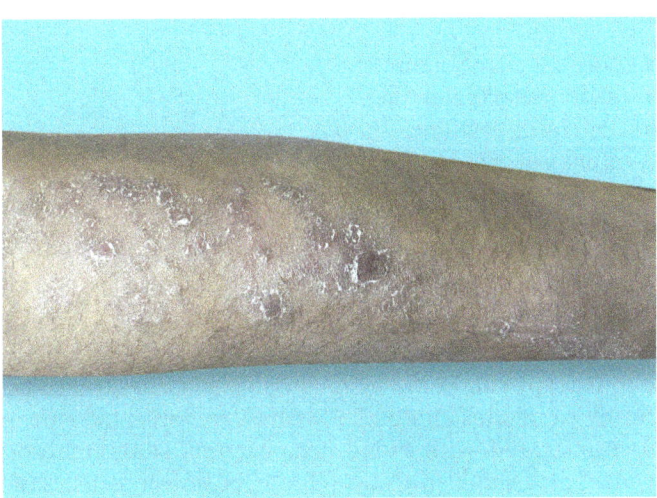

Fig. 78: Acute onset of papules following trauma.

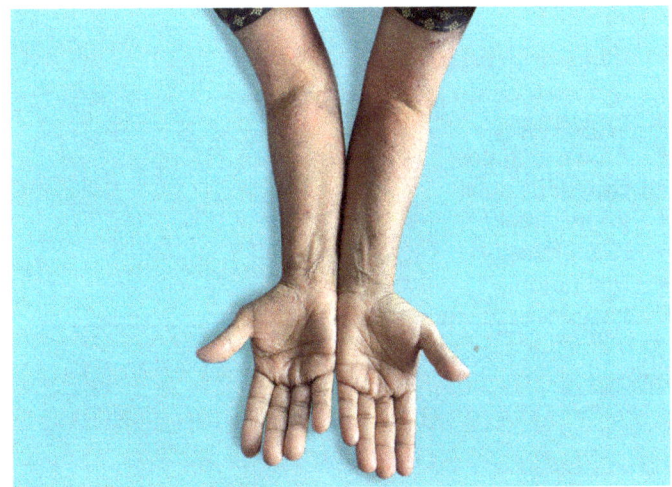

Fig. 76: Psoriasis etanercept after 10 injections.

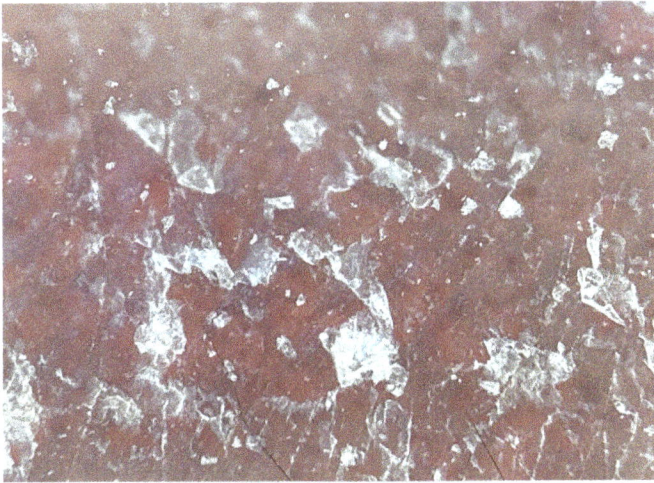

Fig. 79: Image showing uniform pink background diffuse white scale (same patient as **Fig. 78**).

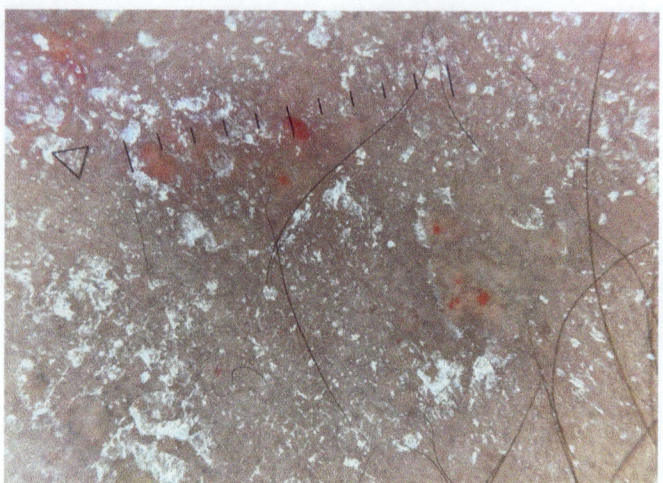

Fig. 80: Image showing dotted vessels hemorrhagic dots (same patient as **Figs. 78 and 79**).

- Regular distribution
- Scattered distribution
- Patchy distribution
- Ring-like distribution
- Distribution in clusters
- Minimal distribution
- Central distribution
- Peripheral distribution

Apart from regular red dots bushy glomerular vessels can be seen in patients with psoriatic erythroderma. Video-dermoscopy can better delineate the vascular structures. Bushy capillaries and basket weave capillaries have been demonstrated with video-dermoscopy. Diameter and density of the capillaries give a clue to the severity of psoriasis that correlates with psoriasis area severity index (PASI).

Bushy capillaries are frequently observed toward the center of the plaques. Homogenous bushy vessels were also demonstrated in psoriatic lesions of glans penis.

Hairpin bend vessels and twisted loops were demonstrated in the periphery of the plaques using video-dermoscopy.

Following are the dermoscopic features of vascular changes in psoriatic plaques:
- Red dots
- Red lines
- Bushy capillaries
- Radial capillaries
- Globules
- Globular rings
- Coma vessels
- Hairpin vessels
- Lacunar vessels
- Atypical vessels

Purpuric dots in patients with plaques psoriasis are considered dermoscopic signs suggestive of good therapeutic response to biological agents such as etanercept, infliximab, ustekinumab, and adalimumab while treating plaque psoriasis. However, the authors are of the view that persistence of these hemorrhagic spots beyond six injections of etanercept should warrant clinical reassessment of patient.

When the papules and or plaques are covered with scales the vascular details cannot be delineated. It is therefore, important to remove the scales and then examine the plaque using "dermoscopy".

Hemorrhagic spots indicate positive "Auspitz" sign. Using dermoscopy, subclinical Auspitz sign can easily demonstrated because of magnification. This is a useful indicator to assess the activity of the disease and plan management accordingly. Presence of red lines indicating linear vascular structure indicates atrophy due to overuse of topical corticosteroids or rarely topical tacrolimus.

Scales

Scales are the most easily observables dermoscopic findings. The color and distribution of scales give a clue to the diagnosis.

Following are the different colors of scale observed over a psoriatic plaque:
- White
- Whitish
- Silvery white
- Yellow
- Yellowish

Following are the different distributions of scale observed over a psoriatic plaque:
- Diffuse
- Patchy
- Clustered
- Peripheral
- Central

Other Dermoscopic Findings Seen in Psoriasis

- White structureless areas
- Orangish yellow structureless areas
- Brown dots
- Brown globules
- Gray-blue dots
- White streaks
- Hemorrhage
- Ulceration
- Pustules in pustular psoriasis

Dermoscopic Findings of Palmoplantar Psoriasis

Pink background is not frequently seen in colored race and in patients with barefoot walking. Diffuse distribution of white scale was more common than patchy distribution.

Rarely, annular pattern was demonstrated. The pinpoint vessels were found to be arranged along the furrows of dermatoglyphics.

TRICHOSCOPIC FINDINGS OF SCALP PSORIASIS[9,10] (FIGS. 81 TO 88)

Vascular patterns observed in the interfollicular spaces in scalp psoriasis include:
- Twisted red loops
- Simple red loops
- Arborizing red lines
- Red dots
- Red globules
- Glomerular vessels
- Signet ring vessels
- Red rings
- Hairpin vessels
- Radial capillaries
- Red lines
- Atypical vessels

Other features observed in scalp psoriasis include:
- Blotchy erythema
- Featureless red areas
- Honeycomb pigmented pattern
- Multi-hair follicular unit
- Yellow dots
- Hidden hairs
- White dots
- Perifollicular scales
- Perifollicular pigmentation
- Psoriatic hair cast was observed in erythrodermic patients.
- Absence of hair follicle may be attributed to chronicity or therapy

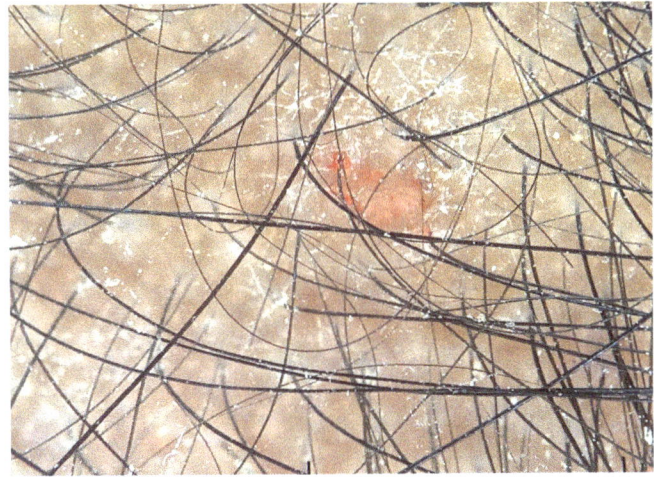

Fig. 82: Scaling and blotchy erythema with dotted vessel.

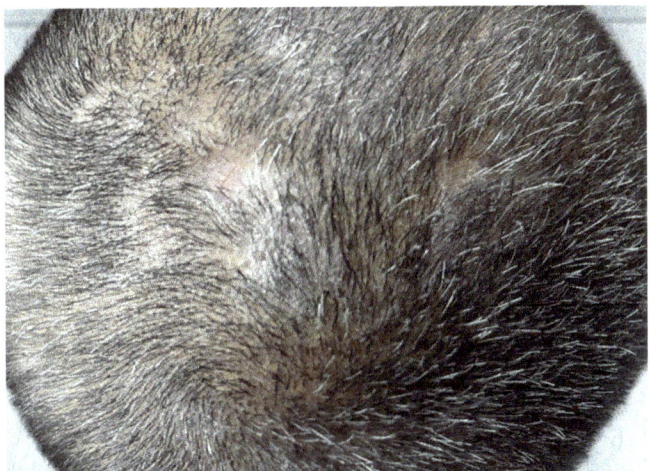

Fig. 83: Suspected case of scalp psoriasis.

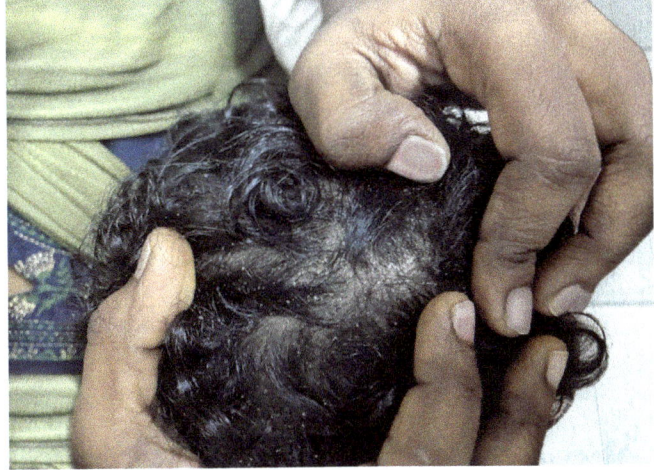

Fig. 81: Scalp psoriasis child.

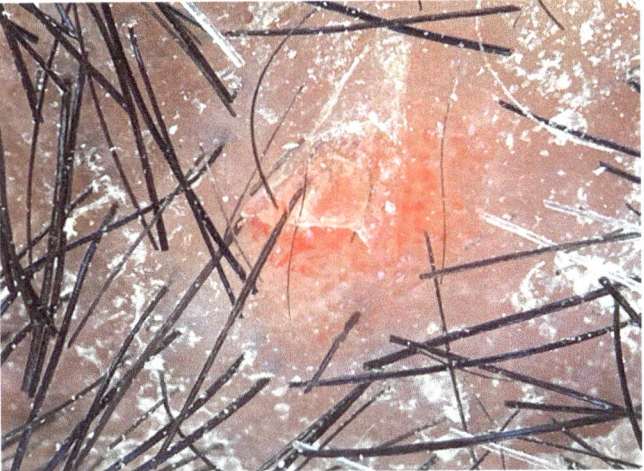

Fig. 84: Reddish background scaling dotted and hemorrhagic vessels.

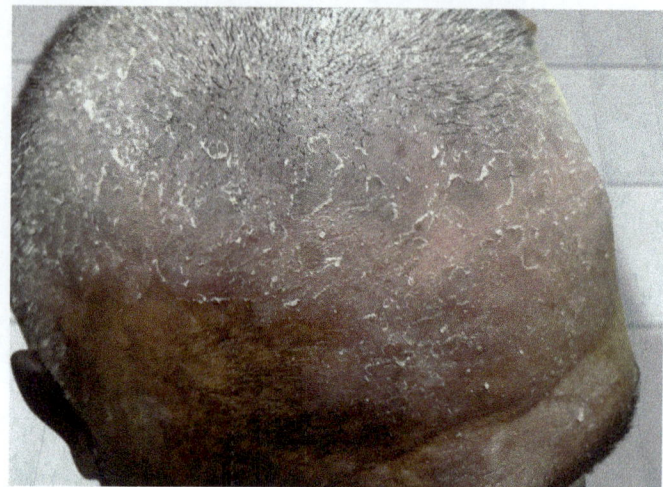

Fig. 85: Psoriasis scalp.

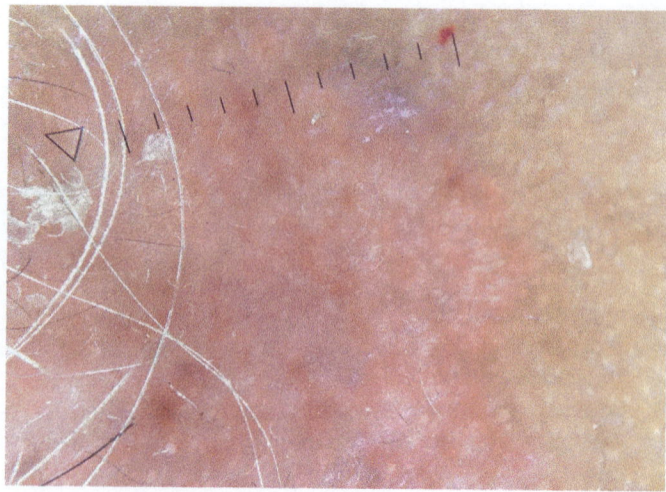

Fig. 88: Pink background, distinct margin, and silvery-white scale dotted vessel brown structureless area.

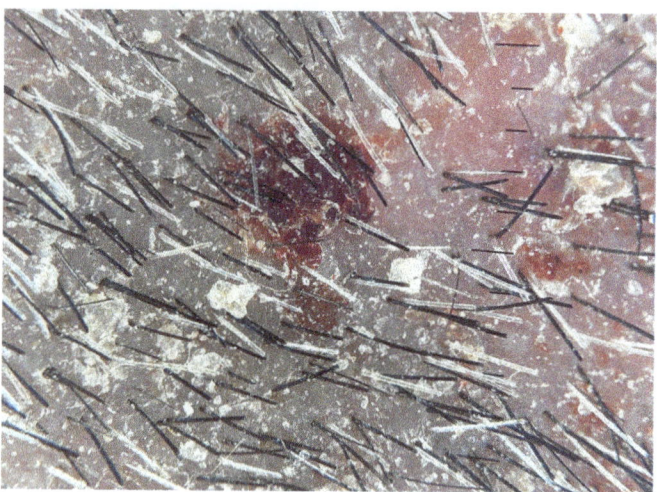

Fig. 86: Pinkish and grayish background hemorrhagic spots whitish scales.

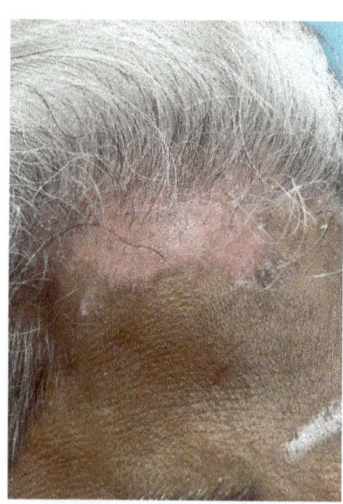

Fig. 87: Psoriasis scalp beyond the hair margin.

ONYCHOSCOPIC FINDINGS OF NAIL PSORIASIS[11-13] (FIGS. 89 TO 100)

It is important to examine and assess nail unit as a whole before deciding on the treatment. So is dermoscopic examination of all the components of nail unit namely the nail plate, nail bed, nailfolds, hyponychium, and free edge of the nail. In order to assess the patient better, pitting and splinter hemorrhage are common findings indicating involvement of nail matrix and nail bed, respectively.

Onychoscopic findings of nail psoriasis include:
- Nail plate pitting
- Nail plate thickening
- Nail plate crumbling
- Trachyonychia
- Beau's lines
- Leukonychia
- Lunular red spots
- Red spots
- Capillary dots
- Hemorrhagic dots
- Subungual hyperkeratosis
- Salmon spot

Globose and spindle-shaped vessels with white halo indicate capillary dilatation and acanthosis. Assessment of capillary density gives a clue to the severity of psoriasis as it correlates with PASI score. Red dots in the skin close to the proximal nailfold give a clue to differentiate nail changes of psoriasis from fungal infection and eczema, the two common mimickers. These proximal nailfold dotted vessels are significantly associated with polyarticular psoriatic arthritis.

CHAPTER 13 Dermoscopy in Psoriasis **137**

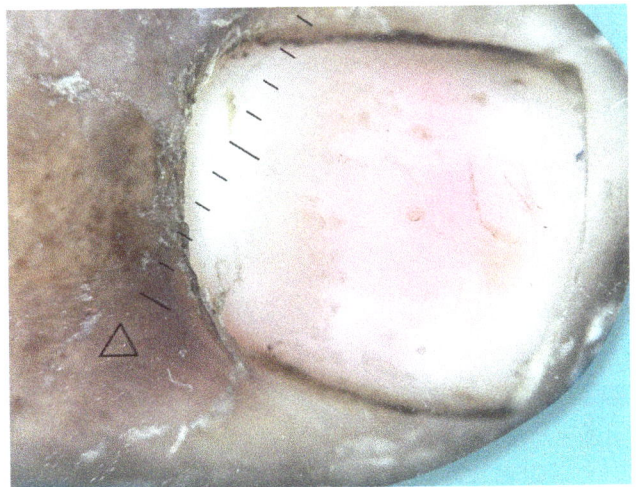

Fig. 89: Course pits and scaling of the proximal nailfold.

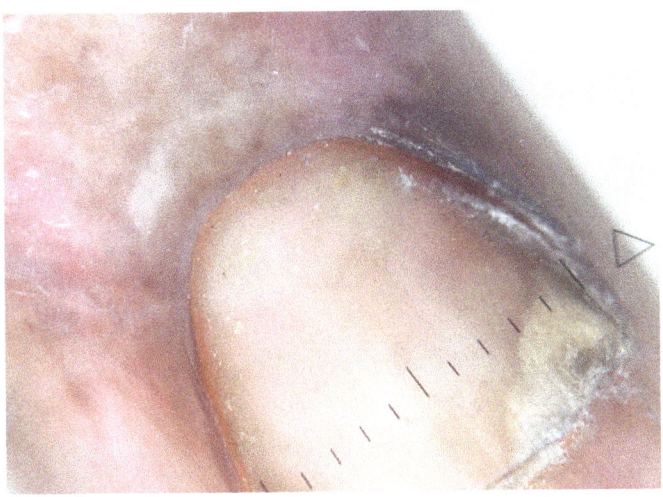

Fig. 92: Onycholysis along with salmon patches.

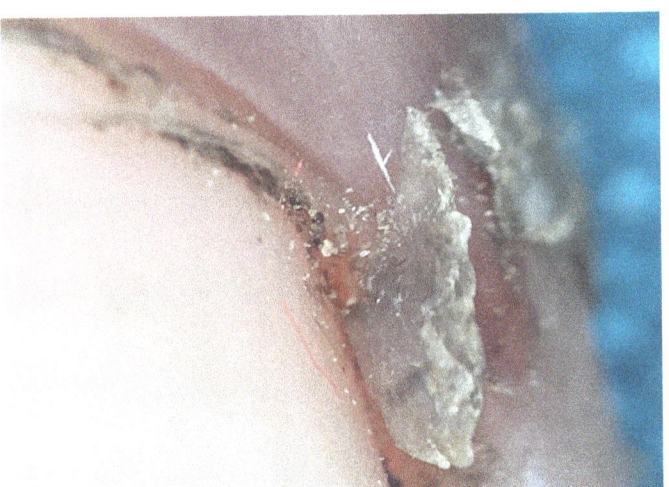

Fig. 90: Scaling and fissuring of the lateral nailfold.

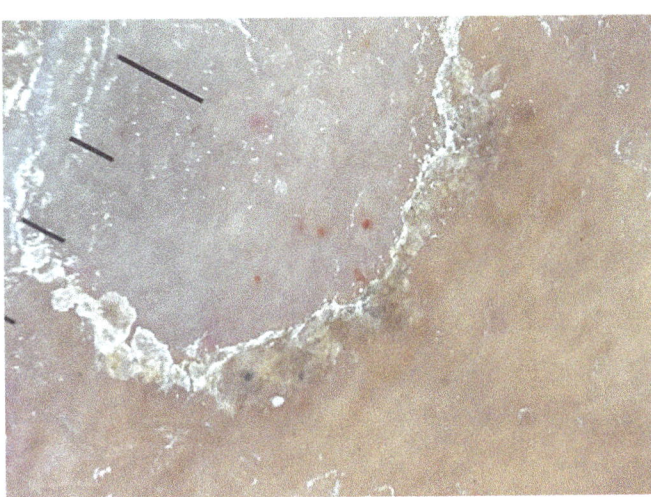

Fig. 93: Dotted vessels in proximal nailfold indicator of joint involvement.

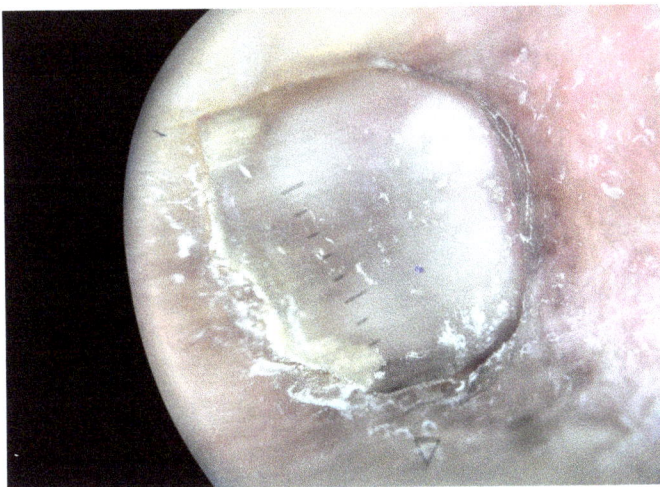

Fig. 91: Subungual hyperkeratosis.

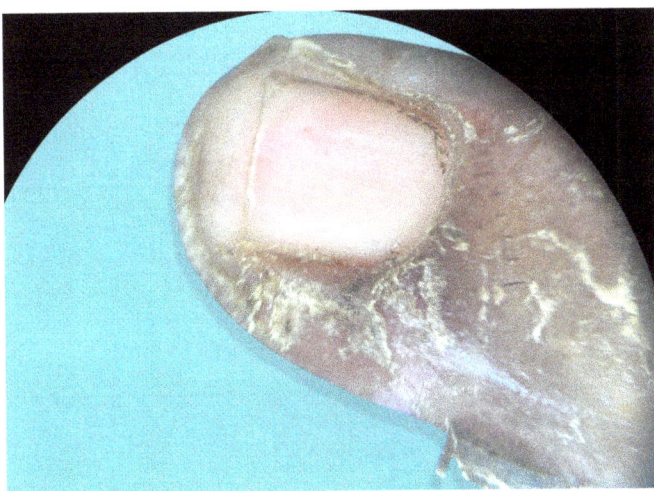

Fig. 94: Loss of cuticle and scaling of nailfolds.

CHAPTER 13 Dermoscopy in Psoriasis

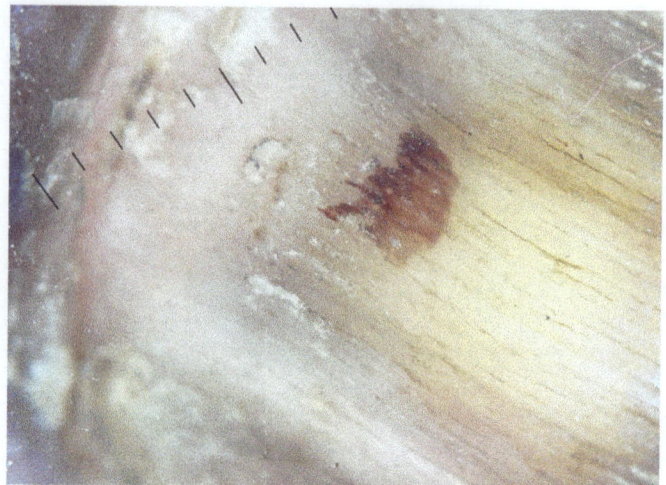

Fig. 95: Splinter hemorrhage.

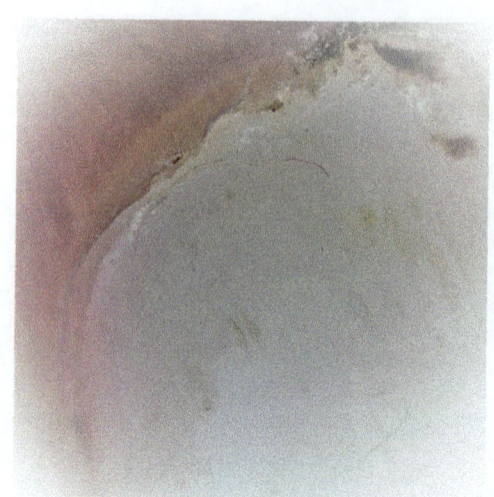

Fig. 98: Arcuate vessel.

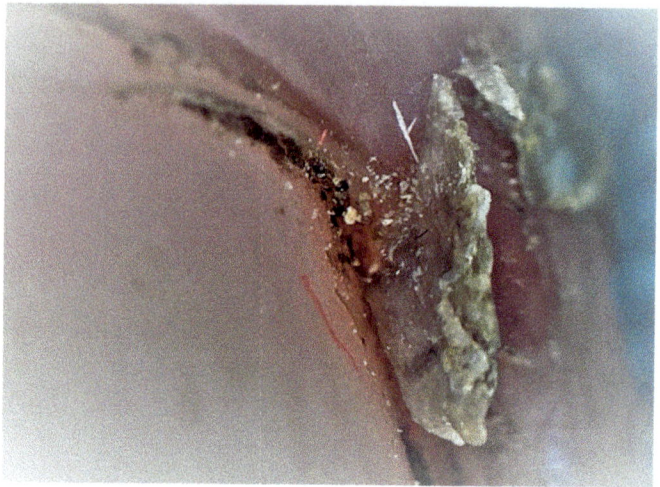

Fig. 96: Linear vessel.

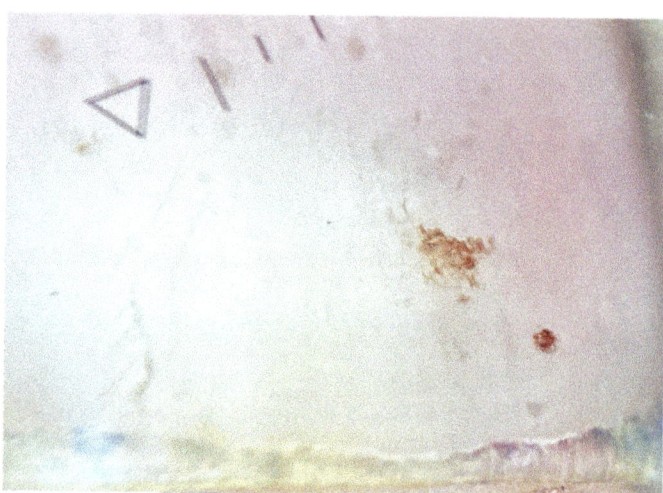

Fig. 99: Corkscrew vessel and splinter hemorrhage.

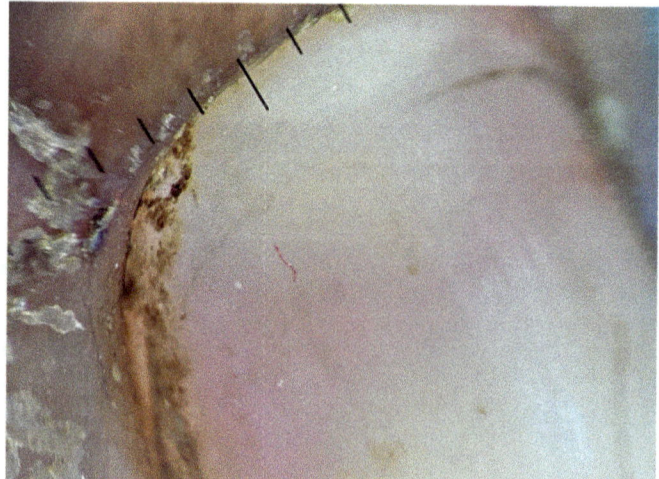

Fig. 97: Curvilinear vessel.

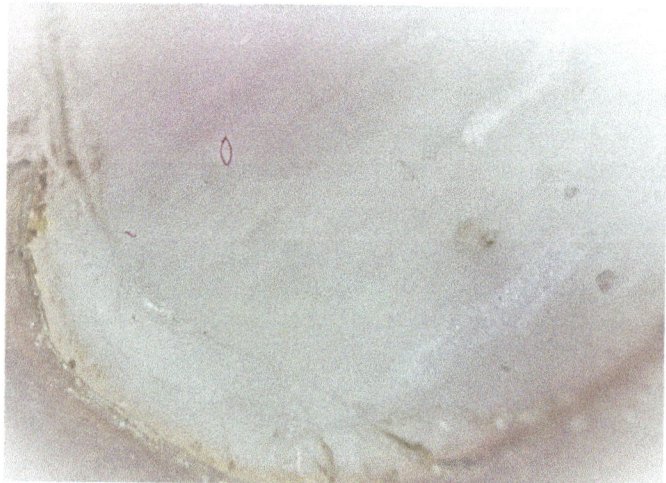

Fig. 100: Loop vessel comma vessel.

SUMMARY

- Demonstration of dotted vessels as a single finding is not pathognomonic to psoriasis as they can also be observed in conditions such as lichen planus, pityriasis, lichenoides chronica, etc.
- Presence of all the three important findings namely regularly distributed dotted vessels, diffuse whitish scales in a pink background has significant diagnostic sensitivity and specificity.
- Dermoscopy helps in assessment of therapeutic response and early diagnosis of complications.
- Digital dermoscopy gives detailed view of vascular changes.
- Scales are conspicuously absent in inverse psoriasis and psoriatic balanitis.
- Palmoplantar psoriasis reveals a thick hyperkeratotic surface making it difficult to visualize the pink background and vessel spots.

REFERENCES

1. Golińska J, Sar-Pomian M, Rudnicka L. Dermoscopy of plaque psoriasis differs with plaque location, its duration, and patient's sex. Skin Res Technol. 2021;27(2):217-26.
2. Vázquez-López F, Manjón-Haces JA, Maldonado-Seral C, Raya-Aguado C, Pérez-Oliva N, Marghoob AA. Dermoscopic features of plaque psoriasis and lichen planus: new observations. Dermatology. 2003;207:151-6.
3. Golińska J, Sar-Pomian M, Rudnicka L. Dermoscopic features of psoriasis of the skin, scalp and nails—a systematic review. J Eur Acad Dermatol Venereol. 2019;33(4):648-60.
4. Lallas A, Apalla Z, Argenziano G, Sotiriou E, Di Lernia V, Moscarella E, et al. Dermoscopic pattern of psoriatic lesions on specific body sites. Dermatology. 2014;228:250-4.
5. Stinco G, Buligan C, Maione V, Valent F, Patrone P. Videocapillaroscopic findings in the microcirculation of the psoriatic plaque during etanercept therapy. Clin Exp Dermatol. 2013;38:633-7.
6. Lallas A, Argenziano G, Zalaudek I, Apalla Z, Ardigo M, Chellini P, et al. Dermoscopic hemorrhagic dots: an early predictor of response of psoriasis to biologic agents. Dermatol Pract Concept, 2016;6:7-12.
7. Errichetti E, Stinco G. Dermoscopy in differential diagnosis of palmar psoriasis and chronic hand eczema. J Dermatol. 2016;43:423-5.
8. Abdel-Azim NE, Ismail SA, Fathy E. Differentiation of pityriasis rubra pilaris from plaque psoriasis by dermoscopy. Arch Dermatol Res. 2017;309:311-4.
9. Ross EK, Vincenzi C, Tosti A. Videodermoscopy in the evaluation of hair and scalp disorders. J Am Acad Dermatol. 2006;55:799-806.
10. Kim GW, Jung HJ, Ko HC, Kim MB, Lee WJ, Lee SJ, et al. Dermoscopy can be useful in differentiating scalp psoriasis from seborrhoeic dermatitis. Br J Dermatol. 2011;164:652-6.
11. Yadav TA, Khopkar US. Dermoscopy to detect signs of subclinical nail involvement in chronic plaque psoriasis: A study of 68 patients. Indian J Dermatol. 2015;60:272-5.
12. Errichetti E, Zabotti A, Stinco G, Quartuccio L, Sacco S, De Marchi G, et al. Dermoscopy of nail fold and elbow in the differential diagnosis of early psoriatic arthritis sine psoriasis and early rheumatoid arthritis. J Dermatol. 2016;43:1217-20.
13. Zabotti A, Errichetti E, Zuliani F, Quartuccio L, Sacco S, Stinco G, et al. Early psoriatic arthritis versus early seronegative rheumatoid arthritis: role of dermoscopy combined with ultrasonography for differential diagnosis. J Rheumatol. 2018;45:648-54.

Index

Page numbers followed by *b* refer to box, *f* refer to figure, *fc* refer to flowchart, and *t* refer to table.

A

Acanthosis 8*f*
Acitretin 66, 93, 110
　half-life of 93
　pretreatment evaluation for 93*fc*
Acne 38, 60
Acrodermatitis continua, early stage of 19*f*
Addison's disease 80
Alcohol 5, 6
　consumption 3
Alcoholic liver disease 79*f*
Alefacept 100, 101
　dosage of 101
　structure of 100*f*
Alopecia areata 80
Amfebutamone 21
Amoxicillin 104
Amyloidosis, secondary 113
Anemia, severe 59
Annular plaques 36*f*
Annular psoriasis 35, 36*f*
Annular pustular psoriasis 21
Anthralin 65, 89, 114
Antiestrogen therapy 103, 104
Antigliadin antibodies 113
Antihistamines 104
Antileukoproteinase, skin-derived 10
Antimicrobial therapy 104
Apical pulmonary fibrosis 113
Apremilast 97, 98, 98*f*
　dosage of 97
　mechanism of action of 97, 98*b*
Arcuate vessel 138*f*
Arthritis 73, 74
　high frequency of 70
　mutilans 33
Arthropathy 74, 113
　complications 114
　psoriasis 31, 54, 60, 108
　symmetrical 32*f*
Asymmetrical oligoarticular arthritis 33
Atherothrombotic diseases 75
Atopic dermatitis 37*f*, 41
Auranofin 103
　oral 102
Auspitz sign 16*f*, 17, 25*f*
Autoimmune diseases 78
Avitaminosis 55*f*
Azathioprine 103
　dosage of 103

B

Beau's lines 29
Beta blocker 3, 6, 13*f*
　exacerbation with 13*f*
　long-term 75*f*
Biological agents 85
Biological therapy, adverse effects of 102
Biomarkers 10
Blaschko's lines, psoriasis along 49*f*
Blood
　dyscrasias 59
　investigations 67
Body surface area 99
Bowen's disease 17
Bright red plaques 51*f*
Brodalumab 100
Bupropion 6

C

Calcineurin inhibitors 56, 89
Calcipotriene, use of 88
Calcipotriol 65
Calcium-channel blockers 6
Candida intertrigo 24
Candidal infection 26*f*
Captopril 6
Cardiac disease, perpetuation of 76*f*
Cardiovascular disease 11, 74-76
Caucasian population 3
Cautious during winter 118
Celiac disease 74, 80
Cellular immune system 9
Cellular markers 10
Central erythema 127*f*
Chronic kidney disease 80*f*
Chronic obstructive pulmonary disease 74, 78*f*
　treatment for 78*f*
Chylomicron 116
Circinate 21
Cirrhosis 59
　primary biliary 80
Classical erythematous plaque 43*f*, 52*f*
Coal tar 88
Colchicine 102
Cold laser 92
Combination therapy 92, 94, 104
Common skin manifestations 13
Corkscrew vessel 138*f*
Corticosteroids 65, 102
　administration 102*fc*
　safe usage of topical 87*b*
C-reactive protein 115
Crohn's disease 80
Curvilinear vessel 138*f*
Cushing's syndrome 87
Cutaneous complications 113
Cutaneous psoriasis, biomarkers of 10
Cuticle, loss of 137*f*
Cyclosporine 57*f*, 58*f*, 59, 66, 94, 106, 110, 114
　dosage of 95
　structural 94*fc*
　treatment, indication to 95
　withdrawal of 21

D

Dandruff, severe 14*f*
Day-to-day stress, management of 118
Dendritic cells, influence of 9
Dermatology life quality index 99
Dermoscopy 121*f*
Diabetes 74, 77, 113
　mellitus 80*f*
Dietary supplement 59, 106
Dilated papillary capillary 8*f*
Disease
　association 35
　mild-to-moderate 72
　type of 16
Distal interphalangeal joints, arthropathy of 54*f*
Dithranol 56, 65, 89

Dizygotic twin 2
Drug 6, 13
   antipsoriatic 59
   antithyroid 103
   interactions 94, 95
   lipid-lowering 6
   systemic 102
   therapy, evaluation of 84
Dyslipidemia 78f-80f, 113
   statin for 77f

E

Eczema 9f
   overlap 126f
   psoriasis resembling 29f
Eczematous patch 14f
Efalizumab 101, 102fc
   pharmacodynamics of 101
Elbows 16
Emollients 55, 86
Endogenous antioxidant, markers of 83
Enzyme transglutaminase 3
Epidermal thickening 8f
Epidermis, suprapapillary thinning of 8f
Epilepsy, case of 95
Erythema 16
   generalized 16
   marginated 26f
   pustule with surrounding 130f
   red 24f
Erythematous plaques, multiple 43f
Erythematous scaly papules 18
Erythroderma 22f, 50f, 71, 128f
   adult 8
   child with 9f
   congenital 50
   impending 128f
   infant with 52f
Erythrodermic psoriasis 8, 22, 22f-24f, 42, 44f, 49, 53f, 93, 108
   congenital 1, 24, 40, 52f, 60
   erythema of 22f
   recalcitrant 23f
Etanercept, psoriasis on 132f
Etretinate 93
Exanthematous pustulosis, acute generalized 66
Excimer laser 92
Eye involvement 29

F

Facial expression 60f
Fingertip pustular lesion 53f
Fish oil 104
Flexural psoriasis 24, 26f, 47, 48f
   female 26f
   male 26f
   sign of 15f

Fluoxetine 6
Fluticasone 65
Focal peripheral scaling 126f
Folate deficiency 113
Follicular papules, classical grouped 71f
Follicular psoriasis 36f
   with phrynoderma 55f
Folliculitis, follicular localization indicating 130f
Fumaric acid ester 103, 104f

G

Gastrointestinal system 78f
Genes, series of 5
Genetic diseases, multifactorial 2
Genetic factors 5
Genetic markers 10
Giant cell arteritis 80
Glomerulonephritis, chronic 80
Glyburide 6
Granulocyte colony-stimulating factor 6
Graves' disease 80
Guselkumab 98
   adverse effects of 99fc
Guttate lesions 18f
Guttate psoriasis 18, 18f, 44, 59, 106, 107
   child with 45f
   drop-like 45f
   episodes of 5
   over back 121f

H

Hair
   follicles, inflammation of 90
   loss 24, 78f
   margin 136f
Hairy skin 121f
Halobetasol propionate
   foam 90
   tazarotene lotion 90
Hashimoto's disease 80
Hemolytic anemia 80
Hemorrhagic spots 130f
   pinkish background 128f
Hepatic failure 113
Hepatitis 59, 110
   C virus infection 79f
Heritable disease 2
Home phototherapy 91
Honeycomb pattern 122f
Human immunodeficiency virus 5, 40, 42, 69, 69f, 70b, 70f, 71f, 111
Human leukocyte antigen 2, 3, 5, 73
Hydroxyurea 66, 96, 105, 110
   dosage of 96
   mechanism of action of 96f
Hyperkeratosis 7f, 8f
   massive 8f

Hyperkeratotic plaques 37f
Hyperostosis 38
Hypertension 74, 80f, 113
   patient with 75f
Hypothyroid 79f, 80f

I

Immune thrombocytopenia 80
Immunogenetic spin 9
Immunology 5
Immunopathogenesis 9
Impetigo herpetiformis 6, 66, 67, 67f, 68, 110
Infection 5, 13
   acute form of 95
   local 56
   secondary 87
Infertility, treatment for primary 68f
Inflamed skin lesions 3
inflammation, markers of 83
Inflammatory skin 5
Inflammatory trauma 13
Injurious local stimuli 5
Insulin resistance 77
Interferons 6
Interleukin inhibitor 99fc
   agents 99, 99fc
Iodide 21
Isomorphic skin lesion, development of 17
Itching 24
Ixekizumab 100
   dosage of 100, 100fc

J

Joint
   involvement of 2
   manifestations 5

K

Keratinocytes 91
Keratoderma 70f
Keratolysis punctata 14f
Keratolytics 55, 86
Ketoconazole 104
Kidney evaluation 96
Knees 16
Koebner's phenomenon 5, 13
Koebner's response 17
Kogoj's micropustules 6, 41

L

Laser 59, 92
Leukocyte, types of 9
Leukopenia 59
Lexette 90
Liarozole 104
Lichen planus 30f

Linear and dotted vessels 123*f*
Linear vessel 138*f*
Lithium 3, 6, 21
Liver
   disease 113
   enzymes, derangement of 67
   function tests 96
Loop vessel comma vessel 138*f*
Lymphoepithelial kazal-type inhibitor 41
Lymphoma, man developed 81*f*

M

Malignancy 81
Metabolic causes 5
Metabolic complication 113
Metabolic factors 6
Metabolic syndrome 1, 11, 74, 76
Methimazole 103, 103*f*
Methotrexate 58, 58*f*, 66, 84, 96, 106, 109, 110
   contraindications of 58, 97*f*
   cyclosporine to 106
   indications of 96*fc*
Methylprednisolone 65
Mimicking seborrheic dermatitis 55*f*
Mometasone 65
Monocyte chemoattractant protein 115
Monozygotic twin 2
Multifocal osteomyelitis, chronic recurrent 113
Multimodality therapeutic strategies 104
Multiple genes, involvement of 2
Multiple hemorrhagic
   dots 133*f*
   vessels 132*f*
Munro's microabscess, formation of 7*f*
Mycobacterium tuberculosis 110
Mycophenolate mofetil 66, 96, 110
Mycophenolic acid 96
Myocardial infarction 73, 75*f*, 76, 76*f*, 78*f*

N

Nail
   changes 31*f*
   dystrophy, severe 70
   pitting 15*f*, 50*f*
   psoriasis 29, 49, 59, 90, 101, 107, 108, 136
Nailfolds, scaling of 137*f*
Napkin psoriasis 47, 48*f*, 60
   infant with 48*f*
National Psoriasis Foundation 65
Nephritis 113
Neutrophil
   activation, markers of 83
   squirting 7*f*
Neutrophilic pustules 67
Nonhairy skin 121*f*

Nonsteroidal anti-inflammatory drugs 3, 75, 109
Normal skin lacks scaling 126*f*

O

Obesity 3, 5, 6, 76, 78*f*, 113
Ocular complications 114
Ocular psoriasis 29
Ocular symptoms 29
Oligoarthritis 32*f*
Omeprazole 104
Onycholysis 30, 30*f*, 137*f*
Ophthalmic complications 114
Oral antibiotics 59
Oral colchicine 103
Oral mucosal involvement 50*f*
Oral tacrolimus 102, 103
Ostraceous psoriasis 35
Oxyphenbutazone 21

P

Palm
   and soles, psoriasis of 28*f*
   psoriasis of 8*f*, 28*f*, 125*f*
   severe involvement of 70*f*
Palmoplantar keratoderma 70, 71*f*
Palmoplantar psoriasis 26, 27*f*, 28*f*, 107
   adult 126*f*
   dermoscopic findings of 134
   early
      lesions of 45*f*
      stage of 27*f*
   mimicking tinea pedes 27*f*
   pustular 6, 101
   severe form 27*f*
   sparing 28*f*
Palmoplantar pustulosis 19
Papules following trauma, acute onset of 133*f*
Parakeratosis 7*f*, 8*f*
   pustulosa 21
Penicillin 6, 104
Periumbilical erythema 15*f*
Phenylbutazone 21, 95
Photochemotherapy 91
Phototherapy, cyclosporine to 106
Pityriasis rubra pilaris 71, 71*f*
Plantar psoriasis 5, 16*f*, 22*f*, 42, 44*f*, 45*f*, 50*f*, 53*f*, 98, 44, 134
   single plaque of 45*f*
Plaque
   dermoscopy of 121*f*
   disease, chronic 18
   lesions, infant with 43*f*
   over back, exacerbation of 124*f*
Plaque psoriasis 52*f*
   chronic 123*f*
   girl with 43*f*

   persistence of 17*f*
   severe type of 44*f*
   treatment of chromic 88
Polyarthritis, symmetrical 33
Pregnancy 6
   systemic drugs in 66*b*, 110*b*
Progesterone 21
Proinflammatory cytokines 9
Propylthiouracil 103, 103*f*
Protein tyrosine phosphatase 3
Psoralen ultraviolet light A therapy, contraindications to 91*b*
Psoriasis 1, 2, 5, 8*f*, 9, 9*f*, 10, 14*f*, 15*f*, 16, 29*f*, 37*f*, 38, 40, 41, 46*f*, 48*f*, 54, 55*f*, 60, 69, 70*b*, 73, 73*f*, 75, 75*f*, 76-78, 86, 102, 110, 111, 114, 118, 122*f*, 126*f*, 127*f*, 131*f*
   adolescent girl with 54*f*
   adolescent with 117*f*
   adulthood 15, 42
   adult-onset 12
   affecting genitals 48*f*
   and hypothyroidism 79*f*
   and malignancy 111
   and pregnancy 64
   antimicrobial therapy of 103
   area 99
   autoimmune disease in 80*b*
   before treatment 131*f*
   biological therapy of 98
   blood of 115
   boy with 50*f*
      erythrodermic 60*f*
   case of 53*f*
   cause of 83
   child with 51*f*
   childhood 24, 61
   children with 97*b*
   classical flexural 47*f*
   classical palmoplantar 45*f*
   classical plaque type 44*f*
   classification of 33*b*
   clinical spectrum of 16*b*
   comorbidity in childhood 81
   complex 2
   concordance of 5
   congenital 13, 42, 50
   course of 13, 118
   current 33
   dermoscopic findings in 134, 120*f*
   dermoscopy in 120
   developing 3
   diagnosis of 83
   diagnostic clues of 41
   drugs exacerbating 6
   early papule 122*f*
   early pustular 20*f*
   early sign of 14*f*
   early-onset 3
   elbow 122*f*

erythrodermic 37f, 51f
etanercept 133f
expression of 115
follicularis 35
frequency of 2
gene for 40
generalized 93
gyrata 35
histological confirmation of 8, 41
history of 67
immunologic evolution of 9
immunosuppressive drugs for 81f
in special populations, treatment of 109
incidence of 2
indicator of 14f
infant, loose scales signaling 48f
infantile 50
inflammation, consequence of 76
inflammatory mediators of 74f
inverse 24, 47, 59, 106, 107
lady with severe 79f
large plaque type 36f
latent 33, 34
linear 18, 18f, 47
living with 117
localized pustular 19f, 21
man with 78f
march of 115
mild 33, 34, 34f, 64f
mimicking secondary syphilis 29f
moderate 33, 34, 34f
moderate-to-severe 33, 34, 34f, 35f, 79
mucosal 26, 49, 60, 107, 108
multiorgan failure due to 80
nail 30f
    dystrophy in 30f
    involvement in 30b, 30f
    with onychomycosis 31f
of skin, features of 120
onset of 76f
pathogenesis of 5, 76
pediatric 40
plaque type 13, 16, 17f, 19f, 59, 106, 107
prognosis of 118
psychological aspects of 117
renal disease and 79
scalp 136f
scaly plaque of 121f
severe 33, 34, 35f, 36f, 80f
    form of 36f, 69f
    plaque type 51f
severity grading for 16, 42
sign of 15f
signals of 12, 13, 14f, 15b
silvery scales of 47f
skin lesions of 32f
starting 23f
sudden onset of 69f
suspicion of 14f

systemic disease 74f
    associated with 74b
treatment of 72
    childhood 111
trigger of 13
twenty nail dystrophy in 31f
type and site of 106
type I 12f
type II 13f
type of 22, 24, 42, psoriasis 59
unstable 24, 24f, 29f, 51f
    form of 23f
with guarded prognosis 33, 35
with lichen planus 37f
with vitiligo 37f
woman with 64, 68f
Psoriasis in pregnancy
    systemic therapies for 110
    treatment of 65
Psoriasis in pregnancy and lactation
    phototherapy for 66, 109
    systemic therapies for 66, 110
    treatment of 109
Psoriasis vulgaris 17f, 18f, 26f, 43f, 93
    developed 46f
    plaque type 40
    treating 59
Psoriatic arthritis 10, 42, 83, 84t, 101, 106
    treatment of 108
Psoriatic arthropathy 31f, 58, 73
Psoriatic corona 25, 46f
Psoriatic erythroderma 23f, 129f
    back 129f
    congenital 15, 42
    erythema of 22f
Psoriatic lesions 13
Psoriatic march 115, 115f
    complications and 113
Psoriatic papule 122f
Psoriatic plaque 128f, 134
    background of 120
Psoriatic skin lesions 10
Psoriatic spondylitis 31
Psychosocial disability 117
Pulmonary disease 78
    significant 59
Pulmonary fibrosis 80
Pus, lake of 20f
Pustular lesions 70f
Pustular psoriasis 19, 19f, 21, 33f, 38, 50, 54f, 60, 80f, 93, 106, 107, 130f
    generalized 20f, 21, 21b
        acute 20f, 21
    gestational 66
    indicator of 53f
    nail dystrophy in 31f
    types of 21b
Pustules coalescing, superficial 53f
Pustulosis palmaris 38

R

Razoxane 96
Recalcitrant otitis externa 14f
Regular acanthosis 7f, 8f
Rehabilitation 117
    therapy goals of 118
Reiter's disease 70
    diagnosis of 70
Reiter's syndrome 36f, 71f
    scalp in 71f
Renal disease 74, 95
Renal endothelial cell proliferation 116
Renal failure 113
Resistant plaque psoriasis 124f
Retinoids 56, 58, 93, 94
    adverse effects of 94
    caution with use of 94
    mechanism of action of 94
Rheumatoid arthritis 78, 84t
Rifampicin 95, 104
Risankizumab 99
    dosage of 99
Rotational therapy 105, 106t
Rupioid lesions 36f
Rupioid psoriasis 35

S

Sacroiliitis 32f
Salicylates 21
Salicylic acid 89, 114
Salmon patches 137f
Saltwater baths 92
Scale 134
    types of 124f
Scaling and pink fissure 125f
Scalp
    mimicking seborrheic dermatitis, psoriasis of 25f
    scales 46f
    severe involvement of 47f
Scalp psoriasis 13, 24, 25, 25f, 44, 46f, 59, 106, 107
    child 135f
    mimicking lichen simplex chronicus 25f
    suspected case of 135f
    trichoscopic findings of 135
Sclerosis, multiple 80
Seborrheic dermatitis 25f
    greasy scales of 46f
    severe 14f, 54f
Secukinumab 99
    dosage of 100
Sequential therapy 105, 106, 106fc
    steps of 106fc
Serum and inflammatory biomarkers 10
Sex hormone binding globulin 115
Sharply marginated erythema 14f, 15f

Silvery white
   peripheral scales 126f
   psoriatic plaques 43f
Six-thioguanine 103
   dosage of 103
Sjögren's syndrome 80
Skin
   atrophy 56
   condition, severity of 64
   deep 1
   folds 70
   involvement, type of 71
   lesions 71f
Smoking 3, 5, 6
Splinter hemorrhage 138f
Spondylitis 33
Spongiform pustule 8f
Streaky lines, scales white 128f
Streptococcal infection 3, 5
Streptococcus 47
Stress 5, 6, 13
Striae distensae 56
Subfertility 113
Subungual hyperkeratosis 15f, 30f, 137f
Subungual keratosis 30f
Sulfasalazine 103, 104
   dosage of 104
   side effects of 104f
Sun exposed skin 23f
Sunlight 6
Symptomatic treatment 86
Systemic agents 105t, 114
Systemic complication 113
Systemic corticosteroid limitations 102fc

Systemic disease 1, 73
Systemic hypertension 75f
Systemic lupus erythematosus 80
Systemic steroids
   sudden withdrawal of 53f
   withdrawal of 20f
Systemic therapies 57, 93

T

TAPINAROF cream 90
Tar 56, 114
Target molecules 98fc
Tazarotene 56, 90, 114
T-cell 1
   abnormal regulation of 9
   agents targetting 100
Telangiectasia 56
Terbinafine 6, 21
Tetracycline antibiotics 3
Thrombocytopenia 59
Tildrakizumab 99
   dosage of 99
Tobacco smoking, habitual 76
Tofacitinib 98
Tongue, geographic 29f
Topical agents 105t
Topical corticosteroid 87, 131f, 132f
   reduction 131f
Topical immunomodulators 89
Topical retinoids 90
Topical steroids 56, 108
Topical therapy 86
Trauma 5
Trimethoprim-sulfamethoxazole 95

Tuberculosis, annual screening for 85
Tumor necrosis factor 73, 115

U

Ulcerative colitis 55, 80
Ultraviolet B 91
   efficacy of 56
Umbilical region 16
Upper respiratory infection 18
Urticaria 60, 118
   chronic 80

V

Vascular endothelial growth factor 115
Very low density lipoprotein 116
Vitamin D 88
   analog 88, 114
   topical 56
Vitiligo 80

W

White streak 123f
Whitish patchy scales 123f

Y

Ynovitis 38

Z

Zidovudine 69f-71f, 102, 103
   therapy 72
   dosage of 103

EU GSPR Authorised Reprsentative
Logos Europe, 9 rue Nicolas Poussin
1700, La Rochelle, France
Phone: +33 (0) 6 67 93 73 78
E-mail: contact@logoseurope.eu

www.ingramcontent.com/pod-product-compliance
Ingram Content Group UK Ltd.
Pitfield, Milton Keynes, MK11 3LW, UK
UKHW050431150426
5217IPUK00019B/1337